Explainable Artificial Intelligence in Stroke from the Clinical, Rehabilitation and Nursing Perspectives

Explainable Artificial Intelligence in Stroke from the Clinical, Rehabilitation and Nursing Perspectives

Editors

Jie Jia
Yan Hu
Dingguo Zhang

MDPI • Basel • Beijing • Wuhan • Barcelona • Belgrade • Manchester • Tokyo • Cluj • Tianjin

MDPI

Editors

Jie Jia
Department of Rehabilitation Medicine
Fudan University
Shanghai
China

Yan Hu
School of Nursing
Fudan University
Shanghai
China

Dingguo Zhang
Department of Electronic and Electrical Engineering
University of Bath
Bath
United Kingdom

Editorial Office
MDPI
St. Alban-Anlage 66
4052 Basel, Switzerland

This is a reprint of articles from the Special Issue published online in the open access journal *Brain Sciences* (ISSN 2076-3425) (available at: www.mdpi.com/journal/brainsci/special_issues/ai_stroke).

For citation purposes, cite each article independently as indicated on the article page online and as indicated below:

LastName, A.A.; LastName, B.B.; LastName, C.C. Article Title. *Journal Name* **Year**, *Volume Number*, Page Range.

ISBN 978-3-0365-6839-3 (Hbk)
ISBN 978-3-0365-6838-6 (PDF)

Contents

brain sciences

MDPI

Article

Application of Immersive Virtual-Reality-Based Puzzle Games in Elderly Patients with Post-Stroke Cognitive Impairment: A Pilot Study

Zhilan Liu [1,2,†], Zhijie He [1,†], Jing Yuan [2], Hua Lin [2], Conghui Fu [3], Yan Zhang [4], Nian Wang [2], Guo Li [2], Jing Bu [2], Mei Chen [3,*] and Jie Jia [1,4,5,6,*]

1 Department of Rehabilitation Medicine, Huashan Hospital, Fudan University, Shanghai 200040, China
2 Department of Geriatric Rehabilitation Medicine, Shanghai Fourth Rehabilitation Hospital, Shanghai 200040, China
3 Shanghai Jinshan Zhongren Aged Care Hospital, Shanghai 201501, China
4 National Clinical Research Center for Aging and Medicine, Huashan Hospital, Fudan University, Shanghai 200040, China
5 Department of Rehabilitation Medicine, Shanghai Jing'an District Central Hospital, Shanghai 200040, China
6 National Center for Neurological Disorders, Shanghai 200040, China
* Correspondence: chenmei_19850812@126.com (M.C.); shannonjj@126.com (J.J.); Tel.: +86-15821176620 (M.C.); +86-13617722357 (J.J.)
† These authors contributed equally to this work.

Abstract: Background: The society is aging in China, and the cognitive level of elderly post-stroke patients gradually declines. Face-to-face cognitive functional training is no longer sufficient. Immersive virtual reality (IVR) is a promising rehabilitation training device. In this study, we developed an IVR-based puzzle game to explore its effectiveness, feasibility, and safety in elderly stroke patients with cognitive dysfunction. Methods: A total of 30 patients with mild post-stroke cognitive impairment after stroke were randomly assigned to a control or IVR group. Patients in both groups received routine rehabilitation therapy. Patients in the control group received traditional cognitive training, and those in the IVR group received IVR-based puzzle game therapy. Before and after treatment, Montreal cognitive assessment (MOCA), trail-making test-A (TMT-A), digit symbol substitution test (DSST), digital span test (DST), verbal fluency test (VFT), and modified Barthel index (MBI) were evaluated in both groups. In addition, the IVR group was administered a self-report questionnaire to obtain feedback on user experience. Results: There was no significant difference in the baseline data between the two groups. After six weeks of treatment, the cognitive assessment scores were improved in both groups. Moreover, the IVR group showed more improvements than the control group in the DSST ($Z = 2.203$, $p = 0.028 < 0.05$, $\eta^2 = 0.16$); MOCA ($T = 1.186$, $p = 0.246 > 0.05$, $d = 0.44$), TMT-A ($T = 1.791$, $p = 0.084 > 0.05$, $d = 0.65$), MBI ($T = 0.783$, $p = 0.44 > 0.05$, $d = 0.28$), FDST ($Z = 0.78$, $p = 0.435 > 0.05$, $\eta^2 = 0.02$), BDST ($Z = 0.347$, $p = 0.728 > 0.05$, $\eta^2 = 0.004$), and VFT($Z = 1.087$, $p = 0.277 > 0.05$, $\eta^2 = 0.039$) did not significantly improve. The significant difference in DSST represents an improvement in executive function and visual–spatial cognitive characteristics. The other assessment scores did not show such features. Therefore, we did not observe significant differences through this measure. According to the results of the self-report questionnaire, most of the patients were satisfied with the equipment stability and training content. Several individuals reported mild adverse reactions. Conclusions: This pilot study suggests that IVR-based puzzle games are a promising approach to improve post-stroke cognitive function, especially executive cognitive function, and visual–spatial attention in older adults.

Keywords: immersive virtual reality; stroke; post-stroke cognitive impairment; aging

Citation: Liu, Z.; He, Z.; Yuan, J.; Lin, H.; Fu, C.; Zhang, Y.; Wang, N.; Li, G.; Bu, J.; Chen, M.; et al. Application of Immersive Virtual-Reality-Based Puzzle Games in Elderly Patients with Post-Stroke Cognitive Impairment: A Pilot Study. *Brain Sci.* **2023**, *13*, 79. https://doi.org/10.3390/brainsci13010079

Academic Editors: Konstantin Slavin and Andrew Clarkson

Received: 16 November 2022
Revised: 23 December 2022
Accepted: 28 December 2022
Published: 31 December 2022

1. Introduction

The population aging is proceeding at an accelerating rate in China. In 2020, the number of people over 65 years old was 1906.4 million, accounting for 13.5% of the total population [1]. The number of elderly people who are unable to live independently and need help due to cognitive decline and dementia has also relatively increased. Stroke is the leading cause of long-term physical and cognitive impairment and death in China. Cognitive degeneration is significantly faster in elderly patients after stroke than in healthy elderly people [2]. More and more studies are showing that the cognitive function of patients with stroke sequelae will continue to decline [3,4], including global cognition, attention, processing speed, memory, language, perceptual motor skills, and executive function [2,5]. The prevalence of dementia ranges from 7% to 49.8% 1 to 10 years after stroke [3,6,7]. Cognitive impairment not only affects the lives of individuals, caregivers, and families, but also places a heavy economic burden on medical resources. It has become one of the main causes of dysfunction, institutionalization, and death of the elderly in China.

Cognitive training has been proven to improve mild cognitive impairment after stroke [8,9]. The traditional cognitive training pattern usually uses paper and tools, requiring the therapist to interact face-to-face with the patient, and is limited by therapeutic tools that cannot meet the treatment needs. After long-term training, patients feel bored and lose their enthusiasm for training, so their compliance with treatment reduces. With the development of science and technology, cognitive training is no longer limited to the therapist's manual interventions. The elderly are increasingly aware and accepting of computer technology due to the pervasiveness the Internet, computers, mobile phones, and other electronic devices in daily life.

Compared with traditional cognitive training methods, immersive virtual reality (IVR) is an intelligent technology that uses a head-mounted device (HMD) or cave automatic virtual environment (CAVE) equipped with motion sensors to artificially create a virtual environment similar to the real world. Because it can present three-dimensional objects and create complex visual, auditory, and tactile multisensory virtual environments, it brings people an immersive feeling of daily activities, so is more and more popular in the medical and rehabilitation fields [10]. This nonintrusive multisource stimulation can more effectively improve the level of nerve remodeling in damaged brain regions, which is conducive to rehabilitation therapy [11].

Some studies have applied IVR to improve mood [12,13], balance gait [14–16], or limb function [17] in the elderly population; however, there is limited academic evidence on how the elderly after a stroke with cognitive impairment experience IVR [18]. Most studies have focused on cognitive dysfunction in the acute phase [17–19], but ignore cognitive decline in the chronic phase. On the other hand, the training content and scene design of IVR are relatively unitary. For example, Huang et al. [20] designed IVR recall scenarios to improve and maintain cognitive function in elderly patients with dementia. Researchers from South Korea improved attention and executive function in patients with MCI by designing a 3D VR program for shopping at a supermarket [21]. Manera et al. [22] tried to develop a kitchen and cooking game to assess and rehabilitate elderly people with MCI and Alzheimer's. Currently, there are still no systematic and comprehensive cognitive training programs for IVR applications on the market.

To solve these problems, we combined IVR with puzzle games. Puzzle games are patterns with different forms and content and a variety of training programs. Recent studies have indicated that puzzle games are enjoyable; repeatable; easy to operate by the elderly; and can improve attention, visuospatial, and executive functions [23–25]. Compared with the literature, the advantages of our method are: the IVR puzzle game system contains plentiful training content, which contains 3 major categories and 16 intelligible puzzle game items from which therapists and patients can choose. Our IVR uses a light HMD, stress-free smart sensor. It is easy for the elderly to understand and operate. Completion of the task is not dependent on motor function, and the proposed IVR is suitable for patients with varying degrees of limb impairment. It can also be combined with rehabilitation equipment during training, which is practical. The game interface is clear and real, producing a strong feeling of "faking the real". The system has an automatic feedback system and does not rely on human supervision. We selected elderly patients in the chronic phase after stroke and aimed to explore the initial effectiveness, feasibility and safety of this intelligent training system in elderly patients with post-stroke cognitive impairment.

2. Materials and Methods

2.1. Participants

This study was performed from January 2022 to October 2022. A total of 30 elderly patients with post-stroke cognitive impairment were recruited from the Department of Geriatric Rehabilitation, Shanghai Fourth Rehabilitation Hospital. The inclusion criteria were as follows: (1) stroke was diagnosed according to the criteria of Chinese Guidelines for the Prevention and Treatment of Cerebrovascular Diseases; (2) $60 \leq$ age < 90 years old, with stroke onset ≥ 6 months; (3) met the diagnostic criteria of PSCI [26]; (4) Montreal cognitive assessment scale (MoCA): $18 \leq$ MoCA < 26; (5) Fugl–Meyer motor scale > 85 for at least one upper and lower limb; (6) educational attainment ≥ 9 years. The exclusion criteria were as follows: (1) those who were difficult to evaluate or examine or could not cooperate with instructions; (2) patients with severe hearing impairment, visual impairment, mental disorders, or a history of epilepsy; (3) patients with previous vertigo; (4) those who were participating in other clinical studies of cognitive function at the same time. The discontinuation indicators were as follows: (1) patients who were unwilling to continue the trial; (2) intolerable or serious adverse events occurred, such as severe dizziness, vertigo, or other discomforts, and the investigator judged that the risk to the patients was greater than that to the beneficiaries; (3) during the study period, the patient's condition deteriorated or had a recurrent stroke; (4) unplanned discharge of the patient.

All individuals signed an informed consent form before the start of the study. The study was approved by the Ethics Committee of Huashan Hospital (KY2022-549) and registered with the Chinese Clinical Trial Registry (ChiCTR2200061932)

2.2. Study Design

In our study, PASS15 software (NCSS LLC., Kaysville, UT, USA) was used to calculate the sample size based on the assumption of equal variance of two samples. We set the power to 0.80 and α to 0.05. The Montreal cognitive assessment (MoCA) was used as the outcome index according to previous similar studies [27]. We considered the cognitive improvement effect of the IVR group was 3.2 higher than that of the non-IVR group as effective, the standard deviation of the individual MoCA was 2.2, and the loss rate was 20%. Finally, 15 cases in the experimental group and 15 cases in the control group were enrolled, for a total of 30 cases.

The 30 individuals were randomly divided into a control group (CG) or immersive virtual reality group (IVRG); each group has 15 individuals. All individuals received routine secondary medicine stroke prevention and 90 min of daily rehabilitation physiotherapy and occupational therapy. After that, individuals in the CG received traditional cognitive training and, those in the IVRG received IVR training. Traditional cognitive training included (1) processing speed and attention training: Schulte table training; (2) memory training: retelling content after seeing pictures such as cards and calendars; (3) computational ability training: performing addition and subtraction operations within 100; (4) executive and problem-solving ability training: such as using building block shapes, picture information classification, and reasoning simulation training. The training content of the IVRG system includes 3 categories: life skills training, exergames and entertaining games; a total of 16 game items are included (Figure 1). The difficulty level of each game is divided into five stars, where one star is the simplest and five stars is the most difficult. Investigators selected one item in each category in turn according to the patient's interest. Individuals in the IVRG wore head-mounted displays for training and started at the difficulty level of one star. The difficulty of the training was gradually adjusted from simple to complex, and each item lasted 5 min, with 2 min rest between the items. During the treatment, if individuals experienced any intolerable discomfort, the treatment was immediately stopped. The extra intervention time was the same in both groups: 15 min per day, 6 sessions per week, for a total of 6 weeks. Cognitive function was assessed for all subjects before and after 6 weeks of treatment, and self-report questionnaires were administered only for the IVR group after 6 weeks of training. Assessors were therapists who were specifically trained but not involved in the intervention study. The assessment was conducted in a quiet room in the Department of Rehabilitation Assessment. The evaluator was responsible for the evaluation, collecting the evaluation and questionnaire results of all subjects, and making the final statistical analysis.

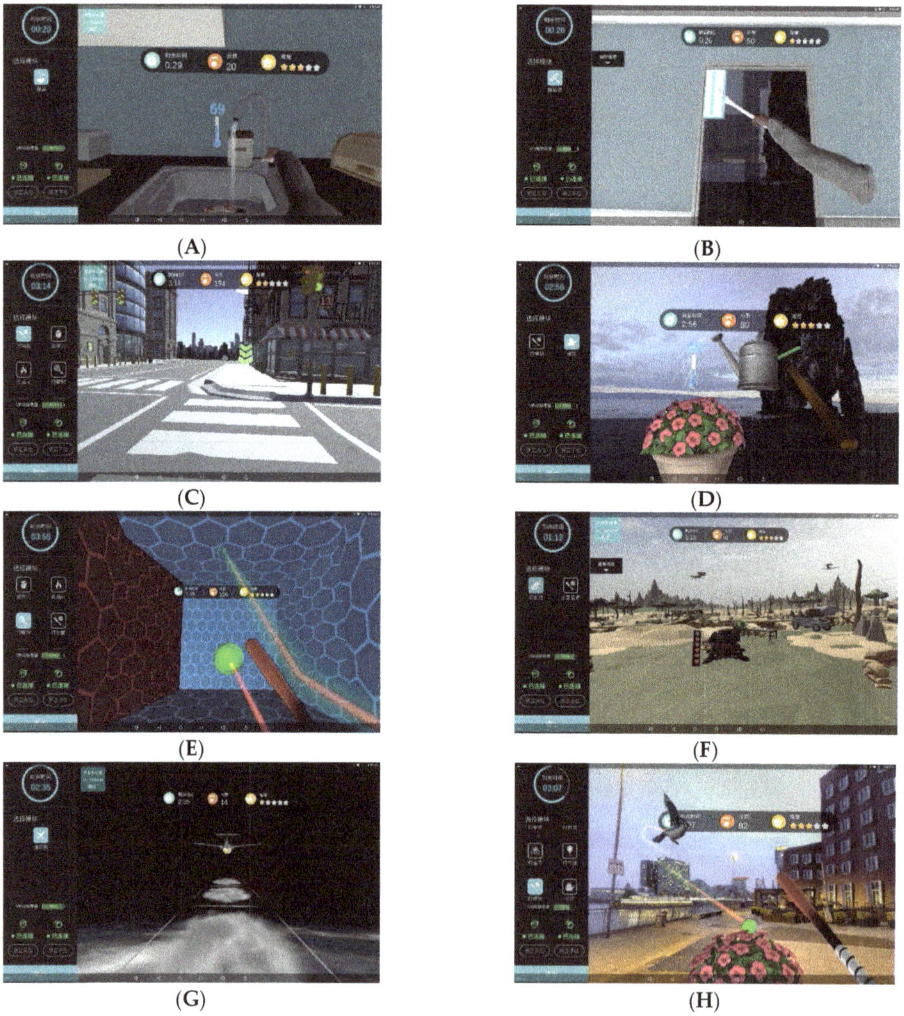

Figure 1. *Cont.*

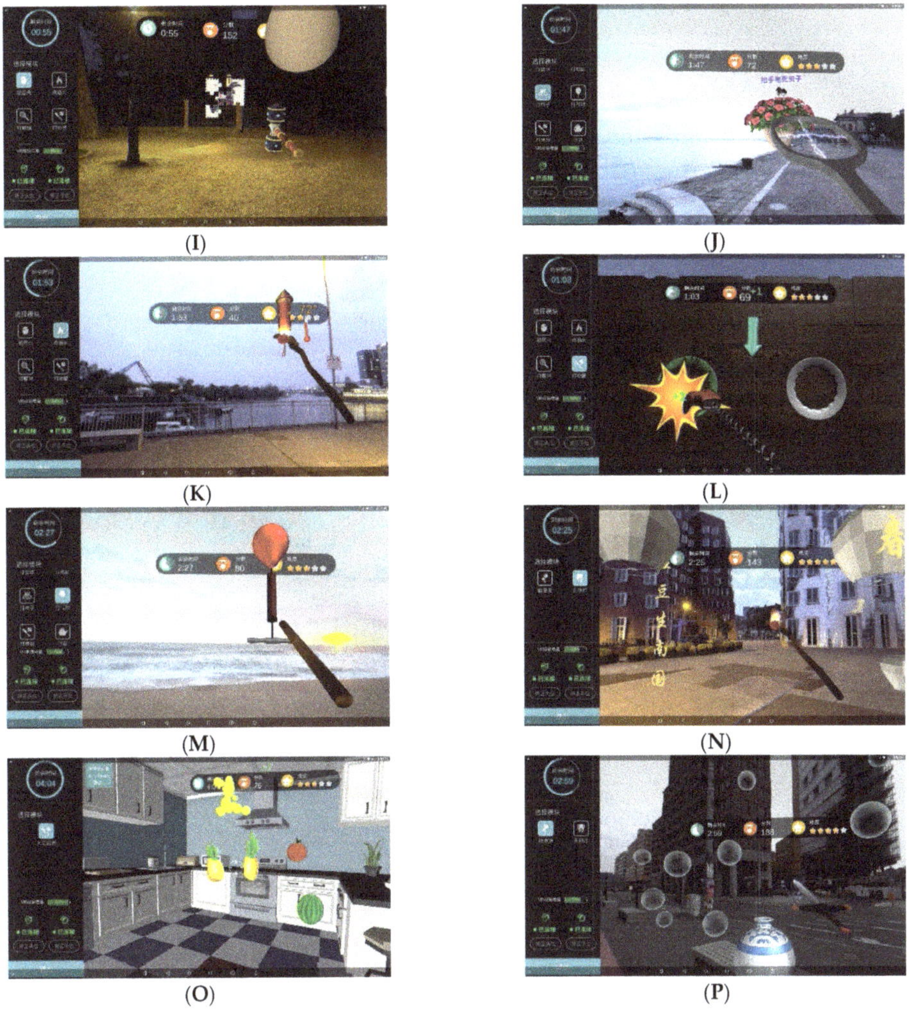

Figure 1. A total of 16 training items were available for researchers and individuals. (**A–D**) Life skills: cooking (**A**), cleaning a window (**B**), crossing a road (**C**), and watering flowers (**D**); (**E–H**) exergames: playing squash (**E**), shooting antiaircraft guns (**F**), flying gliders (**G**), and playing baseball (**H**); (**I–P**) entertaining games: breaking eggshells (**I**), swatting insects (**J**), lighting fireworks (**K**), whack-a-mole (**L**), pumping up a balloon (**M**), flying a Kongming lantern (**N**), Fruit Ninja (**O**), and Bubble Jab (**P**).

2.3. Assessments and Questionnaire

The global cognitive function was used as the primary outcome, and the MOCA-Beijing version was used for evaluation [28]. Each score was added to the final score if the patient's education years was $\leq$ 12 years plus 1 point, and the highest score was 30 points [29].

Secondary indicators include the trail-making test-A (TMT-A) [30], which assesses attention and information processing speed; the digit symbol substitution test (DSST) [31], which is used to measure executive function and visuospatial attention; the digital span test (DST) from the Wechsler adult intelligence scale IV in China [32], which is used to evaluate performance and memory; verbal fluency test (VFT), animal category [33], which used to assess language ability; and modified Barthel index (MBI) [34], which is used to assess activities of daily living.

TMT has good objectivity and is recommended by the National Institutes of Neurological Disorders and Stroke–Canadian Stroke Network (NINDS-CSN) as one of the three scales to evaluate executive function [35]. DSST is relatively independent of intelligence, education, and age, and is suitable for the elderly [31]. DST includes the forward digit span test (FDST) and backward digit span test (BDST). There are 10-digit strings in the FDST and 9-digit strings in the BDST. They measure immediate memory or short-term memory, attention, and working memory [32]. VFT is a simple measure of semantic fluency that requires individuals to name as many animals as possible in one minute and is widely used for cognitive assessment in older adults [36]. MBI is one of the most recommended methods for measuring activities of daily living, having good internal consistency, and is suitable for stroke patients [37].

The self-report questionnaire mainly consisted of 3 parts and 14 items to investigate the IVR group (Supplementary Materials Table S1). Part I inquired how often individuals used smart devices before the intervention. Part II was the satisfaction survey regarding IVR equipment and training content after 6 weeks of IVR intervention using a five-point Likert scale (ranging from "strongly disagree", designated as 1, to "strongly agree", designated as 5). In Part III, the visual analogue scale (VAS) was used to record the occurrence and degree of adverse reactions during the intervention.

2.4. *VR Equipment*

2.4.1. VR Integrity System Construction

Our study used a virtual reality post-stroke intelligent motor training system that was divided into 4 modules, including observation, doctor, patient, and server terminals. The observation and doctor terminals were installed on the same Android tablet. The doctor terminal, as a signal source for IVR all-in-one networking, was responsible for managing the patient's personal information and hardware equipment information and controlling the start and stop of the patient's rehabilitation. For the patient terminal, patients wore the HMD. The direction of motion in the HMD screen could be changed by turning the head. The sensor used 3DOF inertial motion technology and a built-in acceleration gyroscope. Wearing the smart sensor on the patient's limb or motion device, the angle and acceleration could be fed back to the patient to complete the training. The observation terminal was connected via Bluetooth, a sensor, and VR all-in-one, allowing the doctor to watch the scene of patient training in real time on the Android tablet, and to perform hand position, head position correction, and horizontal switching while guiding patient training. The architecture used by the server terminal was a Spring MVC, which was a module for web development based on the Spring framework, and the database was MYSQL5.6 established by MySQL AB. The system could save the patient's training data at any time, which were fed back to the doctor after processing (Figure 2).

2.4.2. Scene Modeling

The aim of scene modeling is to be as close to reality as possible based on interest. Therefore, as the most critical and directly touched limb in the scene, 1:1 modeling was used to restore the human arm function to the greatest extent possible. In addition, considering the acceptance of the virtual environment by the elderly, we created a comfortable environment to relax the individuals. For the game background, we selected quiet and relaxed venues such as beaches, street scenes, and parks. Background music was melodious, soothing, and calm. For the construction of the visual environment, we used 8K high-definition 360 degree panoramic shooting to create the most realistic scene.

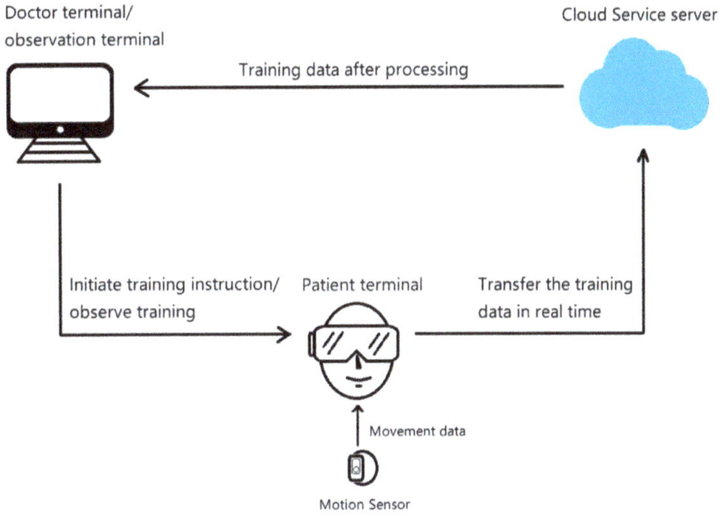

Figure 2. Product structure diagram for immersive virtual reality (IVR).

2.5. Statistical Analysis

SPSS version 20.0 (IBM Inc., Chicago, IL, USA) was used for statistical analysis. Measurement data were tested for normal distribution and homogeneity variance. Enumeration data were analyzed by Fisher's precision probability test. Normally distributed data are expressed as mean ± standard deviation, a paired-sample t-test was used for intragroup comparison, and the independent-sample t-test was used for intergroup comparison. Skewed distributions are expressed as the median (interquartile range), the Wilcoxon W test was used for intragroup comparison, and the Mann–Whitney U test was used for intergroup comparison. We considered differences with a two-sided $p < 0.05$ to be statistically significant. Self-report questionnaires were analyzed as percentages.

3. Results

3.1. Baseline Clinical Data

A total of 30 patients were included in our study, with an average age of 74.16 ± 7.08 years old, with 15 cases in the IVRG, and 15 cases in the CG. All patients completed the training, including 17 men and 13 women, 21 cases of cerebral infarction, and 9 cases of cerebral hemorrhage. There was no significant difference in the baseline data between the two groups ($p > 0.05$) (Table 1).

Table 1. Baseline clinical data of elderly stroke patients between the IVRG and CG.

	IVRG n = 15	CG n = 15	T	p Value
Age (Years)	74.93 ± 6.81	73.40 ± 7.5	0.586	0.562
Male/Female	9/6	8/7		1 [a]
Time since onset (months)	42.93 ± 34.54	29.27 ± 36.51	1.053	0.301
Type, n (%)				0.427 [a]
Cerebral infarction	12(80)	9(60)		
Cerebral hemorrhage	3(20)	6(40)		

IVRG, immersive virtual reality group; CG, control group; [a] Fisher's precision probability test.

3.2. Results of the Cognitive Evaluation

There were no significant differences in MOCA, TMT-A, MBI, DSST, FDST, BDST, or VFT scores between the IVR and control groups before treatment ($p > 0.05$) (Table 2). After 6 weeks of treatment, the scores for the MOCA (IVRG: T = 8.981, $p < 0.001$; CG: T = 13.229, $p < 0.001$), TMT-A (IVRG: T = 5.644, $p < 0.001$; CG: T = 4.112, $p = 0.001$), MBI (IVRG: T = −2.779, $p = 0.015$; CG: T = −6.089, $p = 0.000$) (Figure 3), DSST (IVGR: Z = 3.422, $p = 0.001$; CG: Z = 3.482, $p < 0.001$), FDST (IVGR: Z = 2.887, $p = 0.004$; CG: Z = 2.121, $p = 0.034$), BDST (IVGR: Z = 3.317, $p = 0.001$; CG: Z = 2.111, $p = 0.035$), and VFT (IVGR: Z = 3.332, $p = 0.001$; CG: Z = 3.429, $p = 0.001$) (Figure 4) in both groups significantly improved compared with those before treatment ($p < 0.05$). The comparison of scores after treatment between the two groups showed that the DSST scores of the IVR group (21,6) were higher than those of control group (14,11), and the difference was statistically significant (Z = 2.203, $p = 0.028 < 0.05$, $\eta^2 = 0.16$); MOCA (T = 1.186, $p = 0.246 > 0.05$, d = 0.44), TMT-A (T = 1.791, $p = 0.084 > 0.05$, d = 0.65), MBI (T = 0.783, $p = 0.44 > 0.05$, d = 0.28) (Figure 3), FDST (Z = 0.78, $p = 0.435 > 0.05$, $\eta^2 = 0.02$), BDST (Z = 0.347, $p = 0.728 > 0.05$, $\eta^2 = 0.004$), and VFT (Z = 1.087, $p = 0.277 > 0.05$, $\eta^2 = 0.039$) were not significantly improved. The size effect of the differences between groups in DSST was $\eta^2 = 0.16 > 0.14$ ($p = 0.028 < 0.05$), which means the significant difference in DSST was reliable.

Table 2. Comparisons of baseline cognitive evaluation between the IVR and control groups before treatment.

	IVRG (n = 15)	CG (n = 15)	T/Z	p-Value
MOCA	21.47 ± 2.67	21.27 ± 2.76	0.202	0.842 [a]
TMT A(s)	155 ± 67.48	159.4 ± 97.33	0.144	0.887 [a]
MBI	64.67 ± 11.41	59.33 ± 10.83	1.313	0.200 [a]
DSST	14,6	12,12	0.956	0.339 [b]
FDST	7,1	7,2	0.441	0.659 [b]
BDST	4,1	4,1	0.334	0.738 [b]
VFT	14,5	11,6	1.494	0.135 [b]

IVRG, immersive virtual reality group; CG, control group; MOCA, Montreal cognitive assessment; TMT-A, trail-making test-A; MBI, modified Barthel index; DSST, digit symbol substitution test; FDST: forward digit span test; BDST: backward digit span test; VFT, verbal fluency test; a, independent-sample t-test; b, Mann–Whitney U test.

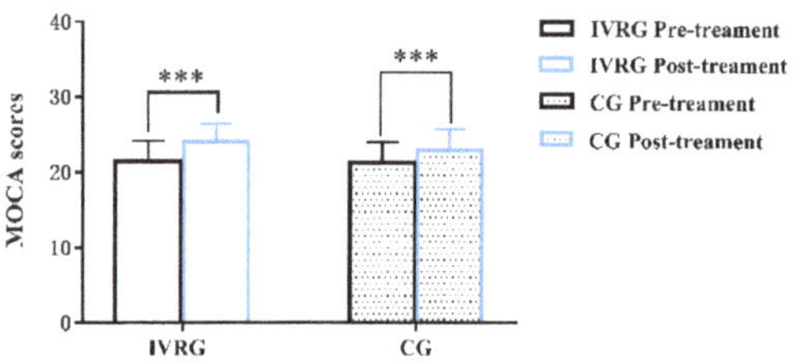

(A)

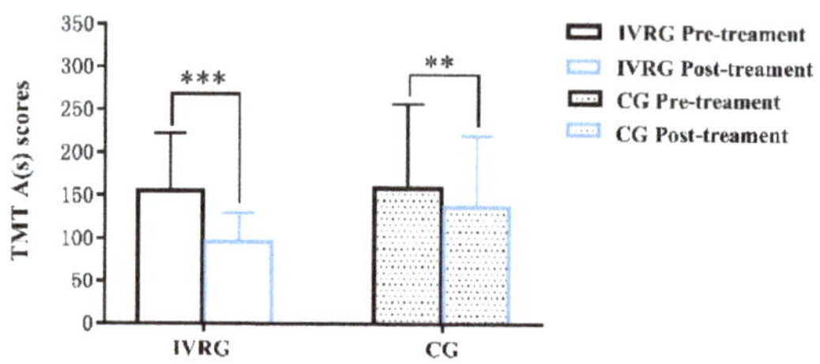

(B)

Figure 3. *Cont.*

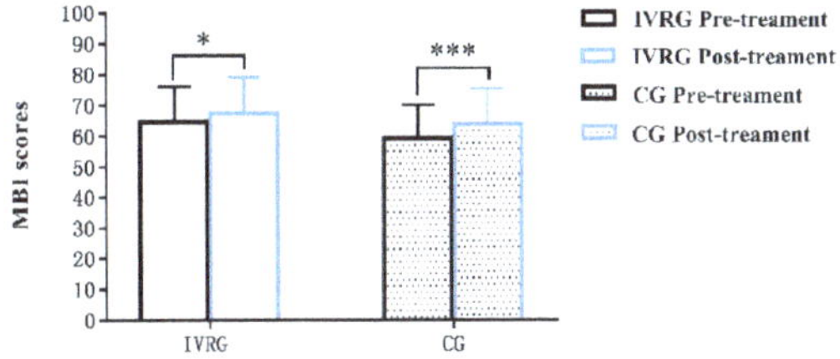

(**C**)

Figure 3. Bar plots for comparison of MOCA (**A**), TMT-A (**B**), and MBI (**C**) between the IVRG and CG before and after treatment. Significant differences were observed in intragroup. *, $p < 0.05$; **, $p < 0.01$; ***, $p < 0.001$. Abbreviation: MOCA, Montreal cognitive assessment; TMT-A, trail-making test-A; MBI, modified Barthel index; IVRG, immersive virtual reality group; CG, control group.

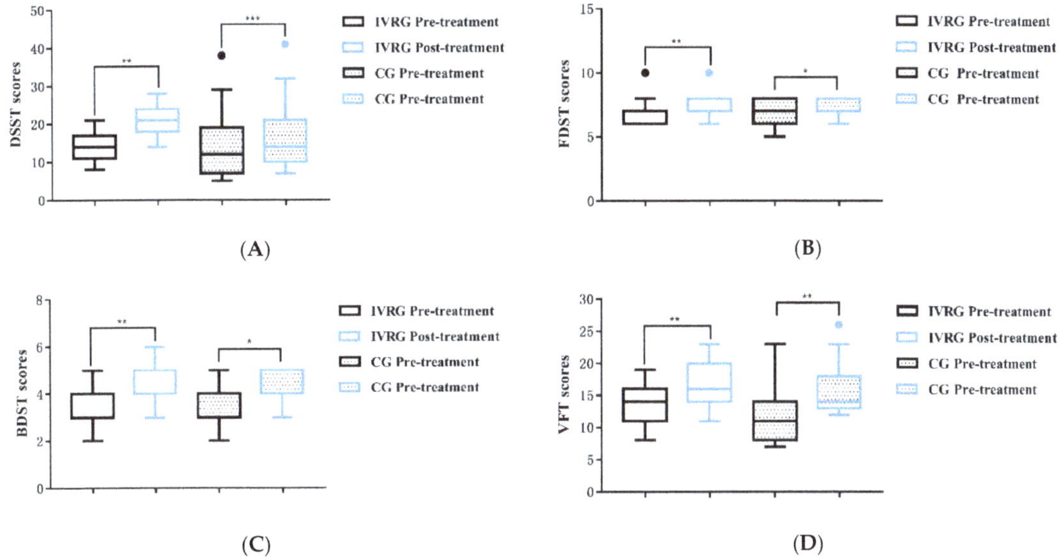

Figure 4. Boxplots comparing DSST (**A**), FDST (**B**), BDST (**C**), and VFT (**D**) between the IVRG and CG before and after treatment. Significant differences were observed in intragroup. *, $p < 0.05$; **, $p < 0.01$; ***, $p < 0.001$. Abbreviation: DSST: digit symbol substitution test; FDST: forward digit span test; BDST: backward digit span test; VFT: verbal fluency test; IVRG, immersive virtual reality group; CG, control group.

3.3. Self-Report Questionnaire

In the IVRG, 73.33% of the elderly stroke patients had never used smartphones. They used geriatric cellular phones with buttons or had no phones. A total of 60% of individuals had never used portable Android devices (PADs), and 20–13.33% of individuals seldom or sometimes used PADs to watch TV shows or play games. Of the individuals, 60% were still willing to use smart devices and 66.67% could completely understand the training directive. None of the individuals were dissatisfied with the training content, and 53.34% of them derived enjoyment from the IVR training process. More than 73.33% of individuals approved of the stability and maneuverability of our IVR device. A total of 73.34% of individuals were willing to promote the IVR device (Figure 5).

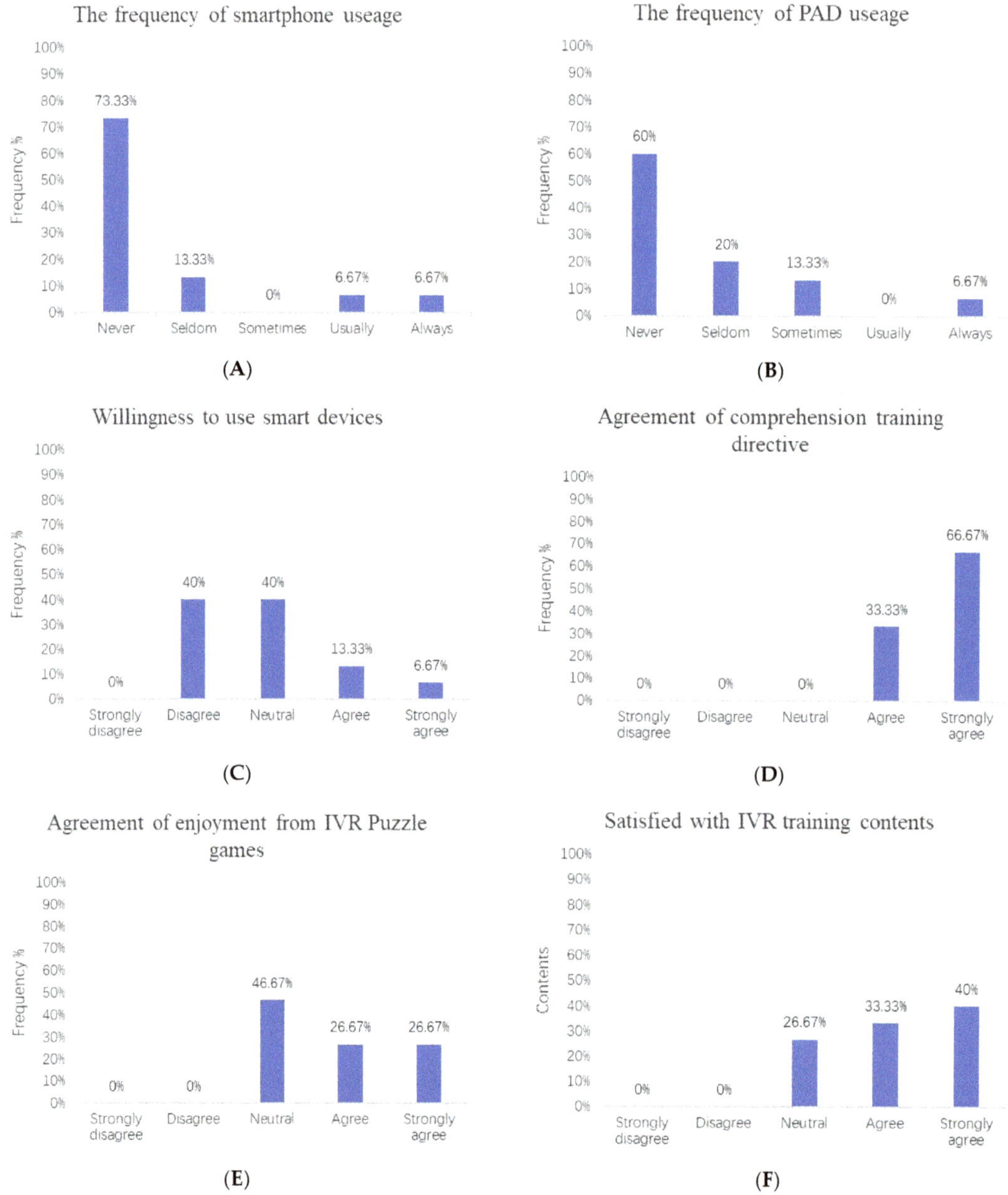

Figure 5. *Cont.*

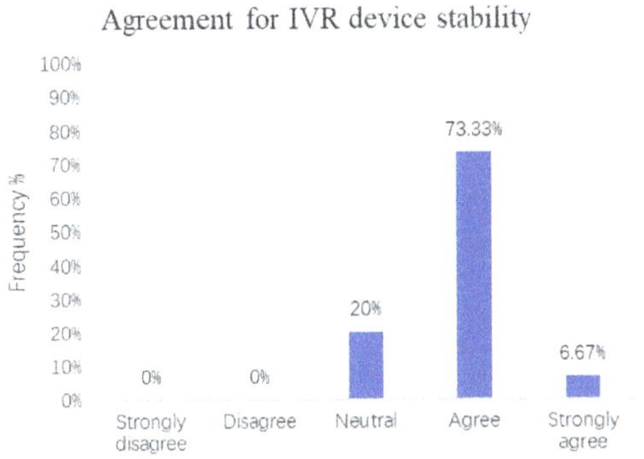

(G)

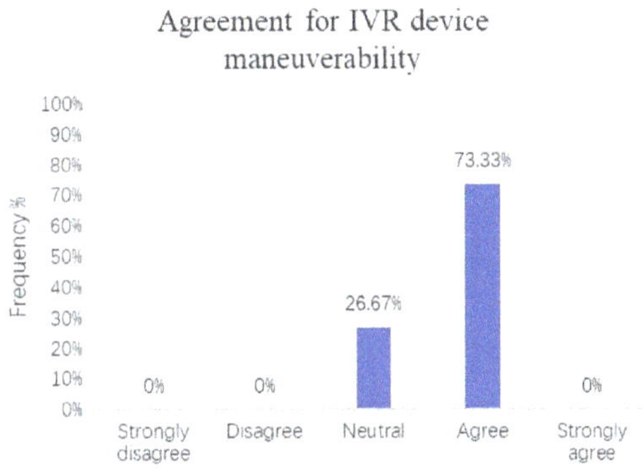

(H)

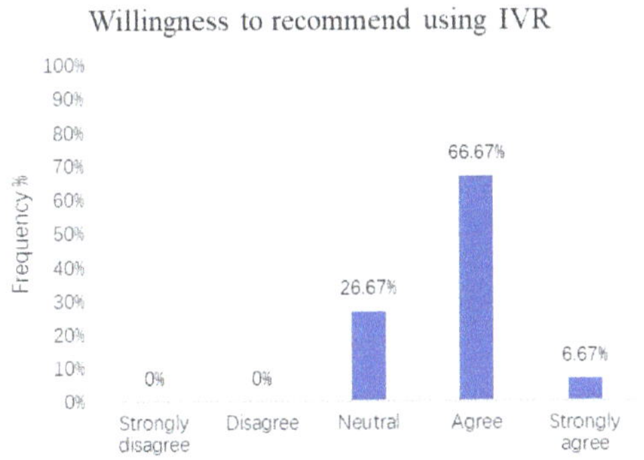

(I)

Figure 5. Histograms (**A–C**) depict the frequency of smart device usage experienced and the willingness to accept smart devices by the IVR group. Histograms (**D–I**) depict satisfaction with IVR equipment and training contents experience. PAD, portable android device; IVR, immersive virtual reality.

3.4. *Side Effects*

During IVR intervention, there were two individuals who reported dizziness without nausea and vomiting, and their VAS score was one. Two individuals reported dry eyes, and three individuals reported eye fatigue, of which two individuals had a VAS score of one and one individual had a VAS score of two (Figure 6). The other individuals did not report any adverse reactions that occurred.

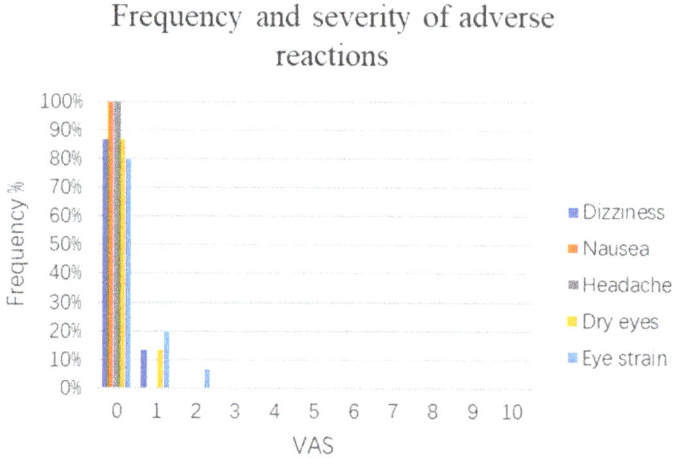

Figure 6. The bar diagram depicts the self-reported incidence and extent of adverse reactions associated with the IVR experience. The horizontal axis represents the percentage of adverse symptoms that occurred, including dizziness, nausea, headache, dry eyes, and eye strain. The vertical axis represents the severity of adverse symptoms experienced by individuals using a VAS, where 0 means no occurrence, and the higher the number, the more severe the adverse symptoms. Five colored lines are used to represent five adverse symptoms. VAS, visual analog scale.

4. Discussion

The purpose of this study was to investigate the initial effect and feasibility of IVR-based puzzle games in elderly patients with cognitive impairments after stroke. We initially found that IVR could improve their cognitive function, especially the executive functioning and visuospatial attention of elderly stroke patients. It is feasible to provide them with 15 min of IVR training 6 times a week.

4.1. Effectiveness of IVR-Based Puzzle Games

After six weeks of treatment, the global cognitive function (MoCA), attention and information processing speed (TMT-A), executive function and visuospatial attention (DSST), performance and memory (FDST and BDST), language ability (VFT), and activities of daily living (MBI) in both groups significantly improved. Moreover, the IVRG showed more improvements than the CG in the DSST ($Z = 2.203$, $p = 0.028 < 0.05$). This result is similar to those of a previous meta-analysis [38] of 894 patients from 23 randomized controlled trials, which showed significant improvements in executive and visuospatial function after VR interventions compared with conventional rehabilitation. However, there were no significant differences observed in global cognitive function, attention, verbal fluency, depression, or quality of life.

The significant difference in DSST represents an improvement in executive function and visual–spatial cognitive characteristics. The other assessment scores such as DST and MBI, did not show such improvements. Therefore, we did not observe significant differences in this measure. The DSST test required subjects to fill in the corresponding symbols of numbers on a blank form as fastest as possible within 90 s. In this process, the subjects needed to match nine digits corresponding to symbols and fill them in within the time limit. Executive functions include task setting, behavioral initiation, monitoring, and self-regulation [39]. In older adults, these domains all play an important role in cognitive tasks. For example, in our preset training, when completing the task of cooking, subjects needed to understand the whole cooking process, from washing vegetables under the tap, cutting dishes, to cooking. In this process, the system broadcasted the steps that needed to be completed by voice prompts, and only when the content of one stage was complete could the subject proceed to the next step, which required the subject to make appropriate choices and respond to the task.

The underlying mechanism through which IVR training improves cognitive function is unclear. The current possible hypothesis is that the virtual environment stimulates and activates brain metabolism, increases cerebral blood flow and neurotransmitter release [40,41], and reactivates and improves various cortical functions [41,42]. A study also found that the input of sensory function activates the brain regions associated with executive function [43]. Virtual reality technology is characterized by immersion, interactivity, and imagination [44]. Participants are isolated from the real world by different sensory capture devices [45]. IVR allows individuals to interact with virtual environments and three-dimensional entities to promptly obtain natural feedback information. The multiple sensory function declines experienced in elderly patients are associated with cognitive decline [46,47]. Especially for elderly patients, multisensory intervention learning is more beneficial than single-sensory intervention for those with cognitive decline [48,49]. Our IVR-based puzzle game system integrates interactive screens, immersive vision, voice prompts, and physical vibrations to stimulate the various senses of the participants in the virtual environment.

Exergames are thought to improve both motor function and cognition in older adults [43], which are defined as physical exercise that combines interaction with cognitive stimulation in a game environment. In our study design, the post-stroke elderly patients in the IVRG could choose a suitable or interesting game from options including playing squash or baseball, using an antiaircraft gun, and gliding. The subjects who chose to play squash or baseball were given a stick or, which they could swing as if they were hitting the ball in a game. The antiaircraft gun and gliding required the subject to use a pedal or limb linkage. A HMD was used as the aiming direction, and the head needed to be moved to aim in the shooting direction. The patient also needed to shake their arm or pedal the bicycle. The faster the speed, the more bullets could be emitted. Our results support previous findings. Htut et al. [50] found that virtual-reality-based game exercise not only improved the balance and muscle endurance of the elderly but also increased the patient's enthusiasm and improved the global cognitive level on the MOCA more than traditional physical activity. Huang [11] suggested that the combination of immersive VR and exergames enhanced the sense of presence during exercise and had the potential to further improve executive function in older adults after 4 weeks of exergame training. Executive function plays an important role in improving the ability to perform activities daily living. However, unfortunately, the IVRG did not show significant advantages over the non-IVRG in our results. This may be related to the standard of the MBI scale. Although the MBI is reliable and effective, it lacks detailed assessment of the cognitive field and the participation in some social activities [51]. Moreover, our puzzle games are extensive but goal-oriented, so need further improvement. The complexity of future life skills training projects and steps need to be further upgraded.

IVR may improve the visual–spatial function of elderly patients through the characteristics of ecological validity [52]. IVR may mistakenly make subjects believe that they are in the real world through immersive stimulation. The interference from the outside world can be eliminated, and the participants can be immersed in the virtual world through increased attention and reduced distraction [19]. In addition, in our study, for the VR background, we selected diversified and comfortable natural environments, and the kitchen, road, and room were all three-dimensional simulated spaces that accurately mimicked real environments, which could improve the patient's visual spatial ability through visual stimulation. Kim et al. [53] mentioned in their discussion that for their virtual background, they selected natural landscapes such as mountains, fields, ski resorts, and football fields. Visual attention and short-term visuospatial memory in the VR group were significantly improved in acute stroke patients with cognitive impairment, which was similar to our finding.

IVR can not only be used to train executive ability, spatial disorientation, but also to improve episodic and verbal memory, attention [52], and living ability [18,54]. However, because different training items have varying training effects, the results of our study are different from those of previous studies. Gamito et al. [55] used several activities of daily living as VR cognitive function training content, such as purchasing items, finding routes, finding characters, recognizing signs, and calculating. After 4–6 weeks of two to three sessions per week, stroke patients had improved memory and attention but not visual function. Previous studies have been conducted to help patients improve episodic memory by showing them familiar environments, including streets, residences, and childhood scenes [56,57]. The task of listing supermarket shopping items has also been used to help elderly patients improve age-related memory decline [21,58]. Combined with our research, most of our training was aimed at the patient completing a task but did not involve memorizing or recalling. However, the performance and memory of the IVRG group were improved compared with those before treatment. The reason may be that VR can improve the memory function of the elderly by enhancing concentration [56–58].

Our IVR-based puzzle game training program provided variety and enjoyment. It integrates diversified and plentiful life skills, exergames, and entertainment modules. It could improve cognitive function in terms of episodic memory, verbal memory, attention and daily living ability, and had a significant effect on executive ability and spatial orientation. However, previous studies have also pointed out that [55,59] there is insufficient evidence that the cognitive function of the IVR group improved more than that of the non-IVR group. Therefore, we hope that IVR may maintain and, if possible, improve cognitive function in elderly patients with chronic stroke. There are a large number of elderly patients with stroke sequelae in China. At present, the rehabilitation of patients after stroke is carried out in rehabilitation hospitals. The disadvantages are short hospitalization time, shortage of ward beds, and lack of therapists, so are not suitable for long-term rehabilitation of elderly patients. In the long run, community-based rehabilitation can meet the needs of some patients, but only if there are enough therapists. According to the results, the therapeutic effect of IVR with a smart device is consistent with that of therapists and is acceptable to elderly stroke patients, which makes it possible for IVR to replace manual therapy and have the opportunity to be widely used [60,61].

4.2. Feasibility and Safety of IVR in Elderly Stroke Patients

The results of self-report Part I (Figure 5A–C) showed that most elderly patients had no experience with using smart devices, and nearly half of them were unwilling to use smart devices. However, the results of the final survey of IVR are encouraging. Almost all the elderly patients gave positive answers to our training content and the manipulability of the IVR equipment, and they were willing to try this new training method. Morganti [62] also reported that elderly participants were initially unfamiliar with the VR device, but after continuous training, they showed enthusiasm for the rehabilitation exercise. In Part II (Figure 5D–F), more than half of the older participants approved of the content of the puzzle games, indicating that they were receptive to such games. The IVR-based puzzle games attracted these older patients for several reasons. On the one hand, a comfortable visual backdrop and gentle auditory experience attracted the participants and enabled them to quickly immerse in the training environment during the training process. The built-in automatic voice broadcast system of the HMD interactive system encouraged participants when they completed one stage of the task to enhance their self-confidence and desire to make further efforts, which could have increase participants' motivation to persist in completing the training. On the other hand, the three categories of puzzle games were easily understood by the elderly, and the instructions of the game were acceptable and operable. Participants could have fun while training.

It should be noted that one-quarter of the participants had a neutral attitude toward the game contents, which means that the puzzle games need to be further improved to be more suitable for the interests of the elderly. We will adjust the game contents to include activities such as tai chi, painting, cross-stitch, square dancing, chess, cards, and other puzzle activities in the future.

HMD and smart sensors are linked to VR through a network and Bluetooth. If the network is unstable or the Bluetooth disconnects during patient training, it will affect the stability and control performance of the device, including the inability of the doctor, on the observation side, to keep abreast of the patient's training. About three-quarters of the participants were satisfied with the device, and the rest were neutral (Figure 5G–H). This may be related to network instability during training as well as the interruption of smart sensor transmission.

Considering that all the elder stroke patients were wearing a HMD and using IVR equipment for the first time, we were not sure how well the patients would accept them, so each training session was no longer than 15 min. Similar to other studies [56–58], the incidence of dizziness in elderly stroke patients was very low, which automatically resolved after the end of the intervention. In the beginning, we were concerned about the vision problems of the elderly: whether they could see the pictures on the screen after wearing the HMD or whether those who wore glasses would feel uncomfortable wearing the HMD. The participants were tested and asked whether they could see clearly on the screen before training, and no patients complained about related problems after adjusting the position of the HMD. It is feasible for the elderly who wear glasses to wear a HMD at the same time. One patient reported mild dry eyes and eye strain before the intervention, but the IVR did not significantly worsen his symptoms; in addition, he successfully completed the entire study task. A small number of patients will experience eye fatigue, which can be relieved after rest. Dizziness, nausea, headache, dry eyes, eye strain, and other adverse reactions were not reported in the remaining patients. This means that the vast majority of elderly patients with mild cognitive decline after stroke well-tolerated IVR and were receptive to it.

Reliable, sensitive, and safe training environments are provided by precise control and manipulation in a virtual environment. IVR-based puzzle games have great potential to be used for cognitive intervention in elderly patients with mild cognitive decline after stroke. Moreover, if this interactive technology can be used for social contact, interest activities, and other long-term rehabilitation training goals [63], it may become possible to reduce therapist workload by increasing training initiative [48].

4.3. Limitations and Prospects

There are some limitations to this study. The sample size in this study was relatively small, so future studies with larger sample sizes are needed. Moreover, six weeks is too short for patients who need rehabilitation for a long time, and the long-term effects of IVR on cognition are unclear. Cognitive assessment scales were used to evaluate the outcomes in our study, but there was a lack of objective measurement tools. Participants could not be blinded to the trial design, but, fortunately, no participants withdrew from the study. Further studies may address these shortcomings in the future by increasing the sample size; using a longer-duration intervention and follow-up; applying task-related electroencephalograph (EEG), functional near-infrared spectroscopy (fNIRS), and functional magnetic resonance imaging (fMRI) for objective evaluation. Considering that improvements in the cognitive domain are related to training content, it is suggested that systematic training content should also be added to improve memory and performance on command tasks.

5. Conclusions

Overall, our research preliminarily demonstrated that IVR-based puzzle games may improve global cognitive, episodic memory, verbal memory, attention, and daily living ability, especially executive ability and spatial orientation, in elderly patients with post-stroke cognitive impairments. This intelligent interactive experience has better applicability in the elderly. The IVR-based puzzle game was well accepted and tolerated in elderly stroke patients and can be recommended for use. Our study changes the traditional two-dimensional training mode to increase the authenticity of the training scene, and brought enjoyment to the elderly patients. Virtual reality technology may have the same efficacy as conventional cognitive rehabilitation; as a noninvasive intervention, it may have the advantages of interest and rich content. It may have application value and development prospects in improving the cognitive function of the elderly with chronic stroke.

Supplementary Materials: Details of self-report questionnaire and the example of VR training video can be found in the supplemental file (Supplementary Materials); https://www.mdpi.com/article/10.3390/brainsci13010079/s1.

Author Contributions: Conceptualization, Z.L., Z.H., M.C. and J.J.; methodology, Z.L., Z.H., J.Y. and H.L.; validation, J.Y., H.L., M.C. and J.J.; formal analysis, Z.L., Z.H. and J.Y.; investigation, Z.L., Z.H., C.F., N.W., G.L. and J.B.; resources, J.Y., Y.Z. and J.J.; data curation, H.L. and M.C.; writing—original draft preparation, Z.L. and Z.H.; writing—review and editing, Z.L., Z.H., J.Y., H.L., C.F., Y.Z., M.C. and J.J.; visualization, Z.L., Z.H. and J.Y.; supervision, Y.Z., M.C. and J.J.; project administration, M.C. and J.J.; funding acquisition, J.J. All authors have read and agreed to the published version of the manuscript.

Funding: This research was funded by the National Key Research and Development Program Project of China (2018YFC2002300 and 2018YFC2002301), National Natural Integration Project (91948302), the National Natural Science Foundation of China (82021002), Shanghai Science and Technology Innovation Action Plan (22YF1404200), Shanghai Jing'an District Health System Key Discipline Construction (2021ZB02), Medical Research Program of Shanghai Jing'an District Science (2021QN06), Shanghai Jing'an District Science and Technology Commission, and Shanghai Jin'an District Health Commission (2022MS15).

Institutional Review Board Statement: The study was conducted in accordance with the Declaration of Helsinki, and approved by the Ethics Committee of Huashan Hospital (KY2022-549).

Informed Consent Statement: Informed consent was obtained from all subjects involved in the study. Written informed consent was obtained from the patients to publish this paper.

Data Availability Statement: Not applicable.

Acknowledgments: We thank all patients for their participation in the study.

Conflicts of Interest: The authors declare no conflict of interest.

References

1. Zheng, Z. From the past to the future: What we learn from China's 2020 Census. *China Popul. Dev. Stud.* **2021**, *5*, 101–106. [CrossRef]
2. Lo, J.W.; Crawford, J.D.; Desmond, D.W.; Bae, H.J.; Lim, J.S.; Godefroy, O.; Roussel, M.; Kang, Y.; Jahng, S.; Kohler, S.; et al. Long-Term Cognitive Decline After Stroke: An Individual Participant Data Meta-Analysis. *Stroke* **2022**, *53*, 1318–1327. [CrossRef] [PubMed]
3. Pendlebury, S.T.; Rothwell, P.M. Incidence and prevalence of dementia associated with transient ischaemic attack and stroke: Analysis of the population-based Oxford Vascular Study. *Lancet Neurol.* **2019**, *18*, 248–258. [CrossRef] [PubMed]
4. Altieri, M.; Di Piero, V.; Pasquini, M.; Gasparini, M.; Vanacore, N.; Vicenzini, E.; Lenzi, G.L. Delayed poststroke dementia: A 4-year follow-up study. *Neurology* **2004**, *62*, 2193–2197. [CrossRef]
5. Hurford, R.; Charidimou, A.; Fox, Z.; Cipolotti, L.; Werring, D.J. Domain-specific trends in cognitive impairment after acute ischaemic stroke. *J. Neurol.* **2013**, *260*, 237–241. [CrossRef]
6. Hénon, H.; Pasquier, F.; Leys, D. Poststroke Dementia. *Cerebrovasc. Dis.* **2006**, *22*, 61–70. [CrossRef]
7. Morley, J.E. An Overview of Cognitive Impairment. *Clin. Geriatr. Med.* **2018**, *34*, 505–513. [CrossRef]
8. Miotto, E.C.; Bazan, P.R.; Batista, A.X.; Conforto, A.B.; Figueiredo, E.G.; Martin, M.; Avolio, I.B.; Amaro, E.J.; Teixeira, M.J. Corrigendum: Behavioral and Neural Correlates of Cognitive Training and Transfer Effects in Stroke Patients. *Front. Neurol.* **2021**, *12*, 785008. [CrossRef]
9. Unverzagt, F.W.; Guey, L.T.; Jones, R.N.; Marsiske, M.; King, J.W.; Wadley, V.G.; Crowe, M.; Rebok, G.W.; Tennstedt, S.L. ACTIVE cognitive training and rates of incident dementia. *J. Int. Neuropsychol. Soc.* **2012**, *18*, 669–677. [CrossRef]
10. Parsons, T.D. Virtual Reality for Enhanced Ecological Validity and Experimental Control in the Clinical, Affective and Social Neurosciences. *Front. Hum. Neurosci.* **2015**, *9*, 660. [CrossRef]
11. Huang, K. Exergaming Executive Functions: An Immersive Virtual Reality-Based Cognitive Training for Adults Aged 50 and Older. *Cyberpsychol. Behav. Soc. Netw.* **2020**, *23*, 143–149. [CrossRef] [PubMed]
12. Liu, Q.; Wang, Y.; Yao, M.Z.; Tang, Q.; Yang, Y. The Effects of Viewing an Uplifting 360-Degree Video on Emotional Well-Being Among Elderly Adults and College Students Under Immersive Virtual Reality and Smartphone Conditions. *Cyberpsychol. Behav. Soc. Netw* **2020**, *23*, 157–164. [CrossRef] [PubMed]

13. Niki, K.; Yahara, M.; Inagaki, M.; Takahashi, N.; Watanabe, A.; Okuda, T.; Ueda, M.; Iwai, D.; Sato, K.; Ito, T. Immersive Virtual Reality Reminiscence Reduces Anxiety in the Oldest-Old Without Causing Serious Side Effects: A Single-Center, Pilot, and Randomized Crossover Study. *Front. Hum. Neurosci.* **2020**, *14*, 598161. [CrossRef] [PubMed]
14. Yang, W.C.; Wang, H.K.; Wu, R.M.; Lo, C.S.; Lin, K.H. Home-based virtual reality balance training and conventional balance training in Parkinson's disease: A randomized controlled trial. *J. Med. Assoc.* **2016**, *115*, 734–743. [CrossRef] [PubMed]
15. Muhla, F.; Clanche, F.; Duclos, K.; Meyer, P.; Maiaux, S.; Colnat-Coulbois, S.; Gauchard, G.C. Impact of using immersive virtual reality over time and steps in the Timed Up and Go test in elderly people. *PLoS ONE* **2020**, *15*, e0229594. [CrossRef]
16. Muhla, F.; Duclos, K.; Clanche, F.; Meyer, P.; Maiaux, S.; Colnat-Coulbois, S.; Gauchard, G.C. Does the Management of Visual and Audible Motion Information during an Immersive Virtual Reality Timed Up and Go Test Impact Locomotor Performance in the Elderly? *Gerontology* **2022**, *68*, 456–464. [CrossRef]
17. Kiper, P.; Szczudlik, A.; Agostini, M.; Opara, J.; Nowobilski, R.; Ventura, L.; Tonin, P.; Turolla, A. Virtual Reality for Upper Limb Rehabilitation in Subacute and Chronic Stroke: A Randomized Controlled Trial. *Arch. Phys. Med. Rehabil.* **2018**, *99*, 834–842. [CrossRef]
18. Laver, K.E.; George, S.; Thomas, S.; Deutsch, J.E.; Crotty, M. Virtual reality for stroke rehabilitation. *Cochrane Database Syst. Rev.* **2017**, *11*, CD008349. [CrossRef]
19. Olk, B.; Dinu, A.; Zielinski, D.J.; Kopper, R. Measuring visual search and distraction in immersive virtual reality. *R. Soc. Open. Sci.* **2018**, *5*, 172331. [CrossRef]
20. Huang, L.C.; Yang, Y.H. The Long-term Effects of Immersive Virtual Reality Reminiscence in People With Dementia: Longitudinal Observational Study. *JMIR Serious Games* **2022**, *10*, e36720. [CrossRef]
21. Maeng, S.; Hong, J.P.; Kim, W.; Kim, H.; Cho, S.; Kang, J.M.; Na, K.; Oh, S.; Park, J.W.; Bae, J.N.; et al. Effects of Virtual Reality-Based Cognitive Training in the Elderly with and without Mild Cognitive Impairment. *Psychiatry Investig.* **2021**, *18*, 619–627. [CrossRef] [PubMed]
22. Manera, V.; Petit, P.; Derreumaux, A.; Orvieto, I.; Romagnoli, M.; Lyttle, G.; David, R.; Robert, P.H. 'Kitchen and cooking,'a serious game for mild cognitive impairment and Alzheimer's disease: A pilot study. *Front. Aging Neurosci.* **2015**, *7*, 00024. [CrossRef] [PubMed]
23. Chesham, A.; Gerber, S.M.; Schütz, N.; Saner, H.; Gutbrod, K.; Müri, R.M.; Nef, T.; Urwyler, P. Search and Match Task: Development of a Taskified Match-3 Puzzle Game to Assess and Practice Visual Search. *JMIR Serious Games* **2019**, *7*, e13620. [CrossRef] [PubMed]
24. Krebs, C.; Falkner, M.; Niklaus, J.; Persello, L.; Kloppel, S.; Nef, T.; Urwyler, P. Application of Eye Tracking in Puzzle Games for Adjunct Cognitive Markers: Pilot Observational Study in Older Adults. *JMIR Serious Games* **2021**, *9*, e24151. [CrossRef]
25. Nef, T.; Chesham, A.; Schutz, N.; Botros, A.A.; Vanbellingen, T.; Burgunder, J.M.; Mullner, J.; Martin, M.R.; Urwyler, P. Development and Evaluation of Maze-Like Puzzle Games to Assess Cognitive and Motor Function in Aging and Neurodegenerative Diseases. *Front. Aging Neurosci.* **2020**, *12*, 87. [CrossRef]
26. Dong, Q.; Guo, Q.; Luo, B.; Xu, Y. Expert consensus on the management of cognitive impairment after stroke. *Chin. J. Stroke* **2017**, *12*, 519–531.
27. Rogers, J.M.; Duckworth, J.; Middleton, S.; Steenbergen, B.; Wilson, P.H. Elements virtual rehabilitation improves motor, cognitive, and functional outcomes in adult stroke: Evidence from a randomized controlled pilot study. *J. Neuroeng. Rehabil.* **2019**, *16*, 56. [CrossRef]
28. Huang, L.; Chen, K.L.; Lin, B.Y.; Tang, L.; Zhao, Q.H.; Lv, Y.R.; Guo, Q.H. Chinese version of Montreal Cognitive Assessment Basic for discrimination among different severities of Alzheimer's disease. *Neuropsychiatr. Dis. Treat.* **2018**, *14*, 2133–2140. [CrossRef]
29. Ziad, S.; Nasreddine, M.; Natalie, A.; Phillips, P.; Dirian, B.V.R.B. The Montreal Cognitive Assessment, MoCA: A Brief Screening Tool For Mild Cognitive Impairment. *J. Am. Geriatr. Soc.* **2005**, *53*, 695–699.
30. Mateen, B.A.; Bussas, M.; Doogan, C.; Waller, D.; Saverino, A.; Kiraly, F.J.; Playford, E.D. The Trail Making test: A study of its ability to predict falls in the acute neurological in-patient population. *Clin. Rehabil.* **2018**, *32*, 1396–1405. [CrossRef]
31. Rosano, C.; Newman, A.B.; Katz, R.; Hirsch, C.H.; Kuller, L.H. Association between lower digit symbol substitution test score and slower gait and greater risk of mortality and of developing incident disability in well-functioning older adults. *J. Am. Geriatr. Soc.* **2008**, *56*, 1618–1625. [CrossRef] [PubMed]
32. Cui, J.; Wang, J.; Fan, H.; Yao, J.; Chen, N.; Duan, J.; Zou, Y. Norm development of the Chinese edition of Wechsler Adult Intelligence Scale-Fourth Edition. *Chin. Ment. Health J.* **2017**, *31*, 635–641.
33. Manly, J.J.; Jacobs, D.M.; Sano, M.; Bell, K.; Merchant, C.A.; Small, S.A.; Stern, Y. Effect of literacy on neuropsychological test performance in nondemented, education-matched elders. *J. Int. Neuropsychol. Soc.* **1999**, *5*, 191–202. [CrossRef] [PubMed]
34. Collin, C.; Wade, D.T.; Davies, S.; Horne, V. The Barthel ADL Index: A reliability study. *Int. Disabil. Stud.* **1988**, *10*, 61–63. [CrossRef]
35. Hachinski, V.; Iadecola, C.; Petersen, R.C.; Breteler, M.M.; Nyenhuis, D.L.; Black, S.E.; Powers, W.J.; Decarli, C.; Merino, J.G.; Kalaria, R.N.; et al. National Institute of Neurological Disorders and Stroke-Canadian Stroke Network vascular cognitive impairment harmonization standards. *Stroke* **2006**, *37*, 2220–2241. [CrossRef]
36. Zhao, Q.; Guo, Q.; Hong, Z. Clustering and switching during a semantic verbal fluency test contribute to differential diagnosis of cognitive impairment. *Neurosci. Bull.* **2013**, *29*, 75–82. [CrossRef]

37. Shah, S.; Vanclay, F.; Cooper, B. Improving the sensitivity of the Barthel Index for stroke rehabilitation. *J. Clin. Epidemiol.* **1989**, *42*, 703–709. [CrossRef]
38. Zhang, Q.; Fu, Y.; Lu, Y.; Zhang, Y.; Huang, Q.; Yang, Y.; Zhang, K.; Li, M. Impact of Virtual Reality-Based Therapies on Cognition and Mental Health of Stroke Patients: Systematic Review and Meta-analysis. *J. Med. Internet. Res.* **2021**, *23*, e31007. [CrossRef]
39. Alvarez, J.A.; Emory, E. Executive function and the frontal lobes: A meta-analytic review. *Neuropsychol. Rev.* **2006**, *16*, 17–42. [CrossRef]
40. You, S.H.; Jang, S.H.; Kim, Y.H.; Hallett, M.; Ahn, S.H.; Kwon, Y.H.; Kim, J.H.; Lee, M.Y. Virtual reality-induced cortical reorganization and associated locomotor recovery in chronic stroke: An experimenter-blind randomized study. *Stroke* **2005**, *36*, 1166–1171. [CrossRef]
41. Carrieri, M.; Petracca, A.; Lancia, S.; Basso, M.S.; Brigadoi, S.; Spezialetti, M.; Ferrari, M.; Placidi, G.; Quaresima, V. Prefrontal Cortex Activation Upon a Demanding Virtual Hand-Controlled Task: A New Frontier for Neuroergonomics. *Front. Hum. Neurosci.* **2016**, *10*, 53. [CrossRef]
42. García-Betances, R.I.; Arredondo Waldmeyer, M.T.; Fico, G.; Cabrera-Umpiérrez, M.F. A Succinct Overview of Virtual Reality Technology Use in Alzheimer's Disease. *Front. Aging Neurosci.* **2015**, *7*, 00080.
43. Monteiro-Junior, R.S.; Vaghetti, C.A.; Nascimento, O.J.; Laks, J.; Deslandes, A.C. Exergames: Neuroplastic hypothesis about cognitive improvement and biological effects on physical function of institutionalized older persons. *Neural. Regen. Res.* **2016**, *11*, 201–204. [CrossRef] [PubMed]
44. Flannery, R.J. Treating learned helplessness in the elderly dementia patient: Preliminary inquiry. *Am. J. Alzheimer's Dis. Other Demen* **2002**, *17*, 345–349. [CrossRef]
45. Park, M.J.; Kim, D.J.; Lee, U.; Na, E.J.; Jeon, H.J. A Literature Overview of Virtual Reality (VR) in Treatment of Psychiatric Disorders: Recent Advances and Limitations. *Front. Psychiatry* **2019**, *10*, 505. [CrossRef] [PubMed]
46. Li, N.; Chen, G.; Xie, Y.; Chen, Z. Aging Effect on Visuomotor Adaptation: Mediated by Cognitive Decline. *Front. Aging Neurosci.* **2021**, *13*, 742928. [CrossRef] [PubMed]
47. Campos, J.L.; Marusic, U.; Mahoney, J.R. Editorial: The intersection of cognitive, motor, and sensory processing in aging: Links to functional outcomes, Volume I. *Front. Aging Neurosci.* **2022**, *14*, 1009532. [CrossRef]
48. Bauer, A.C.; M.Andringa, G. The Potential of Immersive Virtual Reality for Cognitive Training in Elderly. *Gerontology* **2020**, *66*, 614–623. [CrossRef] [PubMed]
49. Freiherr, J.; Lundstrom, J.N.; Habel, U.; Reetz, K. Multisensory integration mechanisms during aging. *Front. Hum. Neurosci.* **2013**, *7*, 863. [CrossRef]
50. Htut, T.Z.; Hiengkaew, V.; Jalayondeja, C.; Vongsirinavarat, M. Effects of physical, virtual reality-based, and brain exercise on physical, cognition, and preference in older persons: A randomized controlled trial. *Eur. Rev. Aging Phys. Act.* **2018**, *15*, 10. [CrossRef]
51. Ohura, T.; Hase, K.; Nakajima, Y.; Nakayama, T. Validity and reliability of a performance evaluation tool based on the modified Barthel Index for stroke patients. *BMC Med. Res. Methodol.* **2017**, *17*, 131. [CrossRef] [PubMed]
52. Kober, S.E.; Wood, G.; Hofer, D.; Kreuzig, W.; Kiefer, M.; Neuper, C. Virtual reality in neurologic rehabilitation of spatial disorientation. *J. Neuroeng. Rehabil.* **2013**, *10*, 17. [CrossRef]
53. Kim, B.R.; Chun, M.H.; Kim, L.S.; Park, J.Y. Effect of Virtual Reality on Cognition in Stroke Patients. *Ann. Rehabil. Med.* **2011**, *35*, 450. [CrossRef] [PubMed]
54. Cunha, N.M.D.; Nguyen, D.; Naumovski, N.; Mckune, A.J.; Kellett, J.; Georgousopoulou, E.N.; Frost, J.; Isbel, S. A Mini-Review of Virtual Reality-Based Interventions to Promote Well-Being for People Living with Dementia and Mild Cognitive Impairment. *Gerontology* **2019**, *65*, 430–440.
55. Gamito, P.; Oliveira, J.; Coelho, C.; Morais, D.; Lopes, P.; Pacheco, J.; Brito, R.; Soares, F.; Santos, N.; Barata, A.F. Cognitive training on stroke patients via virtual reality-based serious games. *Disabil. Rehabil.* **2017**, *39*, 385–388. [CrossRef] [PubMed]
56. Optale, G.; Urgesi, C.; Busato, V.; Marin, S.; Piron, L.; Priftis, K.; Gamberini, L.; Capodieci, S.; Bordin, A. Controlling Memory Impairment in Elderly Adults Using Virtual Reality Memory Training: A Randomized Controlled Pilot Study. *Neurorehabilit. Neural. Repair.* **2010**, *24*, 348–357. [CrossRef]
57. Huygelier, H.; Schraepen, B.; van Ee, R.; Vanden Abeele, V.; Gillebert, C.R. Acceptance of immersive head-mounted virtual reality in older adults. *Sci. Rep.* **2019**, *9*, 4519. [CrossRef]
58. Plechatá, A.; Sahula, V.; Fayette, D.; Fajnerová, I. Age-Related Differences With Immersive and Non-immersive Virtual Reality in Memory Assessment. *Front. Psychol.* **2019**, *10*, 1330. [CrossRef]
59. Wiley, E.; Khattab, S.; Tang, A. Examining the effect of virtual reality therapy on cognition post-stroke: A systematic review and meta-analysis. *Disabil. Rehabil. Assist. Technol.* **2022**, *17*, 50–60. [CrossRef]
60. Jonsdottir, J.; Baglio, F.; Gindri, P.; Isernia, S.; Castiglioni, C.; Gramigna, C.; Palumbo, G.; Pagliari, C.; Di Tella, S.; Perini, G.; et al. Virtual Reality for Motor and Cognitive Rehabilitation From Clinic to Home: A Pilot Feasibility and Efficacy Study for Persons With Chronic Stroke. *Front. Neurol.* **2021**, *12*, 601131. [CrossRef]
61. Broeren, J.; Claesson, L.; Goude, D.; Rydmark, M.; Sunnerhagen, K.S. Virtual Rehabilitation in an Activity Centre for Community-Dwelling Persons with Stroke. *Cerebrovasc. Dis.* **2008**, *26*, 289–296. [CrossRef] [PubMed]

62. Morganti, F. Virtual interaction in cognitive neuropsychology. *Stud. Health Technol. Inf.* **2004**, *99*, 55–70.
63. Baker, S.; Waycott, J.; Robertson, E.; Carrasco, R.; Neves, B.B.; Hampson, R.; Vetere, F. Evaluating the use of interactive virtual reality technology with older adults living in residential aged care. *Inf. Process. Manag.* **2020**, *57*, 102105. [CrossRef]

brain sciences

MDPI

Article

Repetitive Transcranial Magnetic Stimulation of the Brain Region Activated by Motor Imagery Involving a Paretic Wrist and Hand for Upper-Extremity Motor Improvement in Severe Stroke: A Preliminary Study

Tianhao Gao [1], Yiqian Hu [1], Jie Zhuang [2], Yulong Bai [1,3] and Rongrong Lu [1,3,*]

1 Department of Rehabilitation Medicine, Huashan Hospital, Fudan University, Shanghai 200040, China
2 School of Psychology, Shanghai University of Sport, Shanghai 200438, China
3 National Center for Neurological Disorders, Shanghai 200040, China
* Correspondence: 0356213@fudan.edu.cn; Tel.: +86-21-52887820

Abstract: Approximately two-thirds of stroke survivors experience chronic upper-limb paresis; however, treatment options are limited. Repetitive transcranial magnetic stimulation (rTMS) can enhance motor function recovery in stroke survivors, but its efficacy is controversial. We compared the efficacy of stimulating different targets in 10 chronic stroke patients with severe upper-limb motor impairment. Motor imagery-based brain–computer interface training augmented with virtual reality was used to induce neural activity in the brain region during an imagery task. Participants were then randomly assigned to two groups: an experimental group (received high-frequency rTMS delivered to the brain region activated earlier) and a comparison group (received low-frequency rTMS delivered to the contralesional primary motor cortex). Behavioural metrics and diffusion tensor imaging were compared pre- and post rTMS. After the intervention, participants in both groups improved somewhat. This preliminary study indicates that in chronic stroke patients with severe upper-limb motor impairment, inducing activation in specific brain regions during motor imagery tasks and selecting these regions as a target is feasible. Further studies are needed to explore the efficacy of this intervention.

Keywords: stroke; motor imagery; brain–computer interface; virtual reality; rTMS; DTI

Citation: Gao, T.; Hu, Y.; Zhuang, J.; Bai, Y.; Lu, R. Repetitive Transcranial Magnetic Stimulation of the Brain Region Activated by Motor Imagery Involving a Paretic Wrist and Hand for Upper-Extremity Motor Improvement in Severe Stroke: A Preliminary Study. *Brain Sci.* **2022**, *13*, 69. https://doi.org/10.3390/brainsci13010069

Academic Editors: Catherine Sweeney-Reed and Konstantin V. Slavin

Received: 5 November 2022
Revised: 14 December 2022
Accepted: 25 December 2022
Published: 29 December 2022

1. Introduction

Stroke is the second most common cause of death globally, and its prevalence is projected to increase in the coming years in parallel with an increase in life expectancy [1]. Notwithstanding considerable improvements in managing the acute phase of stroke, some residual disability persists in most patients, necessitating rehabilitation [2], which incurs a heavy economic burden on families and society [3]. Hemiplegia is the most common impairment following a stroke [4,5], and approximately 37–50% of stroke survivors live with chronic severe upper-limb paresis, characterised by limited active range of motion (AROM), limited strength, impaired coordination from the shoulder to the hand and fingers, and severely diminished ability to perform activities of daily living (ADL) [6]. Therefore, rehabilitation interventions that are both effective and applicable for recovery from severe upper-limb motor impairment are an urgent clinical need.

Transcranial magnetic stimulation (TMS) is a brain stimulation technique that modulates brain activity noninvasively. This is accomplished by inducing electrical currents via rapidly changing magnetic field pulses. When TMS is applied in repetitive trains of stimulation, i.e., repetitive TMS (rTMS), its effects on cortical excitability can outlast the period of stimulation [7]. Two general types of rTMS protocols are used in stroke rehabilitation. The first is excitatory high-frequency (HF) rTMS stimulation, which is applied over the ipsilesional primary motor cortex (M1) or adjacent brain areas. The mechanism behind these protocols may strengthen synaptic connections in descending motor pathways [8]. The second protocol involves applying low-frequency (LF) rTMS over a contralesional M1, which may reduce the interhemispheric inhibition exerted by the contralesional M1 on the ipsilesional M1, thus promoting cortical reorganisation in the ipsilesional hemisphere. Both protocols have been reported to improve motor recovery in post-stroke patients [8]. However, the inter-individual variability of the responses to rTMS intervention remains high. Several studies [9,10] have investigated the efficacy of rTMS in promoting the recovery of upper-limb motor function in stroke patients, but the results are contradictory.

The question of how to precisely select the stimulation target is presently one of the most concerning issues in this space. In previous studies, the stimulated target and the protocol were heterogeneous. Some studies [11] indicate that HF-rTMS may contribute more to the functional connectivity reorganisation of the ipsilesional motor network and realise greater benefit to motor recovery than LF-rTMS. Other studies [12] have indicated that LF-rTMS has a positive effect on grip strength and lower-limb function, as assessed using the Fugl–Meyer Assessment (FMA) scale. Presently, however, applying LF-rTMS to the contralesional M1 for hand motor recovery in the post-acute stage of stroke is recommended based on level A evidence ("definitely effective or ineffective"), and HF-rTMS of the ipsilesional M1 is recommended based on level B evidence ("probably effective or ineffective") [13]. However, in some stroke patients with severe brain injury, motor-evoked potentials (MEPs) cannot be recorded on the affected side of the brain; consequently, the stimulus target cannot be precisely determined. Furthermore, the residual function of the injured cortex may not be sufficient to dominate the paretic extremity for the completion of simple activities [14]. In contrast, the results of other studies indicate that, among these stroke patients, HF-rTMS over the contralesional side may improve motor function to some degree [9,11]. Because the accuracy of this neural modulation technique is correlated with the outcome of this intervention, the choice of stimulation target is crucial. Therefore, it is worth researching whether such a functional area exists in stroke patients with severe motor impairment and, if it exists, whether HF-rTMS over this region can further improve the motor function of a paretic wrist and hand.

In chronic stroke patients, a recent model known as the "bimodal-balance recovery" hypothesis has attempted to define the role of contralesional and ipsilesional cortices [15]. This hypothesis highlights the role of contralesional motor cortices varied based on the amount of ipsilesional reserve and neural pathways available to contribute to recovery. In patients with mild motor impairment, contralesional influence is believed to be in inhibitory, whereas in patients with severe motor impairment, the contralesional influence is thought to be supportive for paretic limb motor function. More recently, Lin et al. [16] further investigated the relationship between interhemispheric balance and motor performance and confirmed the above hypothesis. Therefore, it is worth further investigating the role of different hemispheres in chronic stroke patients. Moreover, in chronic stroke patients with severe upper-limb motor impairment, it is difficult to locate the brain regions activated by a motor task focused on the affected wrist and hand because there is no actual movement of the paretic wrist and hand. However, motor imagery ability is retained even in patients with severe motor impairment [17]. Furthermore, several studies have revealed that motor imagery possesses many of the same properties—in terms of temporal regularities, programming rules, and biomechanical constraints—observed in the corresponding real action [18,19]. In our previous research [20,21], we also found that even stroke patients with severe upper-limb motor impairment could elicit activation of the associated brain regions during motor imagery involving their paretic wrist and hand using a motor imagery-based brain–computer interface (BCI) with different end effectors. After several sessions of BCI training, the motor imagery (MI)-related electroencephalogram (EEG) activity had more discriminable patterns. These changes gradually converged, appearing predominantly in the centro-parietal cortical region (e.g., C3 and C4). Considering the aforementioned theoretical basis, we further investigated whether HF-rTMS stimulation applied over the brain regions activated during MI would improve motor function of the paretic upper limb in stroke patients. In this study, we first had stroke patients with severe upper-limb motor impairment undergo MI-based BCI training augmented with virtual reality to induce neural activity in the brain region typically activated during MI tasks. Subsequently, HF-rTMS was delivered to this activated brain region. This preliminary study investigates the feasibility and efficacy of this stimulation protocol.

2. Materials and Methods

2.1. Participants

This study is a randomised, parallel, controlled, single-blinded clinical trial. Ten stroke patients who had suffered a stroke at least six months previously and continued to experience severe chronic upper-limb motor impairment were recruited for this preliminary study. A clinical assessment of the motor impairment of the participants was performed by a physiatrist who was unaware of the randomisation assignment of the participants. The inclusion criteria were as follows: (1) aged 18–90 years old at the time of randomisation; (2) more than 6 months since their first clinical cortical or subcortical, ischaemic, or haemorrhagic stroke, confirmed via computed tomography (CT) or magnetic resonance imaging (MRI); (3) no active extension of the paretic wrist and scores of grade 0–1 on the manual muscle test (MMT) for wrist extension; (4) no cognition impairment, with a Montreal Cognitive Assessment (MOCA) score of $\geq$26; and (5) no hearing or visual impairments. The exclusion criteria included the following: (1) patients with contraindications for MRI or rTMS, (2) participation in other clinical trials, and (3) pregnancy. The study was approved by the Ethics Committee of Huashan Hospital and was conducted in accordance with the tenets of the Declaration of Helsinki. All participants provided written informed consent before participating. This study was registered with the China Clinical Trial Registration Centre (registration number: ChiCTR2000036423).

2.2. Intervention

The intervention was divided into two phases. The first phase involved inducing the brain regions typically activated during MI involving the paretic wrist and hand using an MI-based BCI system augmented with virtual reality (VR). In the second phase, rTMS was used to stimulate the brain, with the participants randomly divided into two groups: an experimental group and a comparison group. The stimulation target of the experimental group was the aforementioned brain regions activated by MI-based BCI augmented with VR, while the comparison group received an LF-rTMS intervention applied over the contralateral M1. An overview of the study design showing the timeline, intervention, and measured outcomes is presented in Figure 1.

2.2.1. Inducing Neural Activity in Associated Brain Regions during Motor Imagery Involving a Paretic Wrist and Hand

An 11-channel, high-resolution EEG system, g.USBamp (g.tec Medical Engineering, Schiedlberg, Austria), was used for this study. The electrodes were attached to the scalp, per the 10–20 international electrode placement system, as follows: FC3, FC4, C5, C3, C1, CZ, C2, C4, C6, CP3, and CP4. The ground electrodes were placed on the medial frontal cortex. The reference electrodes were fixed at the left and right mastoids, and the average value from the bilateral electrodes was used as the reference. The EEG signals were collected at a sampling rate of 256 Hz.

This process is described in detail in our previous research [20]. Each session lasted 30 min (four cycles of six minutes each, with two-minute intervals) and was conducted five days a week for four weeks.

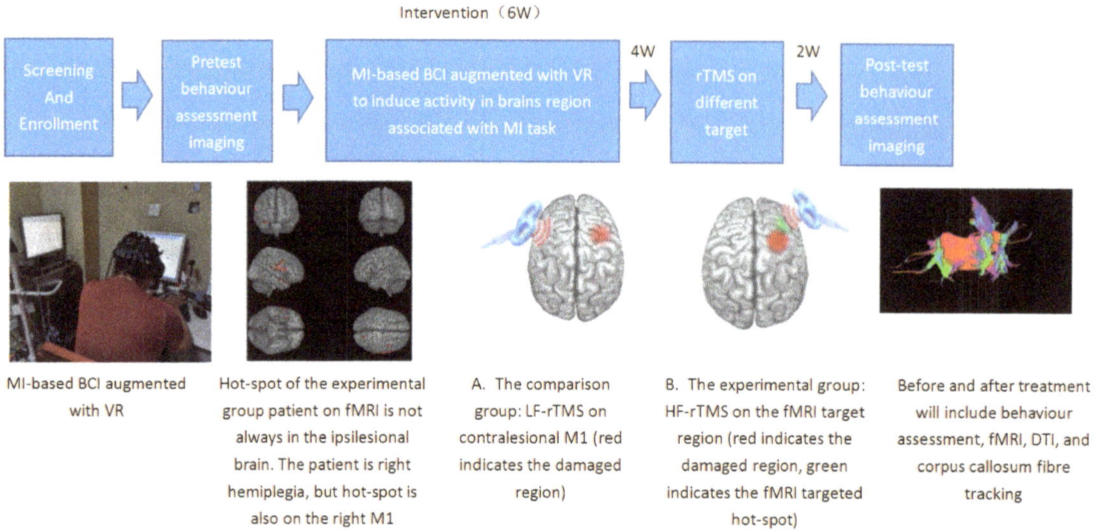

Figure 1. Overview of study design showing the timeline, intervention, and outcome measures. MI, motor imagery; BCI, brain–computer interface; VR, virtual reality; rTMS, repetitive transcranial magnetic stimulation; LF, low frequency; HF, high frequency; fMRI, functional magnetic resonance imaging; DTI, diffusion tensor imaging.

2.2.2. Activated Brain Regions during MI Tasks Determined Using fMRI

fMRI was performed to determine the brain regions activated during the MI task. We used a block design with three tasks: A is a prompt to imagine the grasping movement of the left hand, B is a prompt to imagine the grasping movement of the right hand, and C is a prompt to rest. Each task lasted for 20 s. During the MI task, short videos of the grasping movement of the left hand, the grasping movement of the right hand, and a blank screen were shown to the participants. The three tasks were performed in the order ABC, BCA, and CAB, and each sequence was repeated three times (Figure 2). The participants were instructed to do the following: (1) mentally imagine the action of grasping using their left/right hand following the video instruction and (2) just rest without any action or imagery when presented with blocks of blank screen.

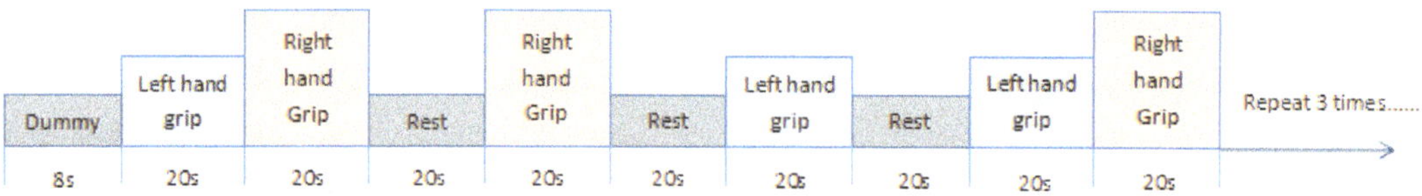

Figure 2. fMRI tasks.

The participants were scanned in a 3.0 Tesla Siemens MAGNETOM Prisma whole-body 60 cm bore human scanner equipped with 80 mT/m gradients and a 200 T/m/s slew rate (Siemens Healthineers, Erlangen, Germany) at Shanghai University of Sport. We used an eight-channel head coil for radio frequency (RF) transmission and reception. We collected sagittal T1-weighted images as the localiser and performed a semiautomated high-order shimming programme to ensure global field homogeneity. A three-dimensional fast spoiled gradient echo pulse sequence was chosen for acquiring high-resolution structural images with the following parameters: repetition time (TR) = 8.156 s, inversion time (TI) = 450 ms, echo time (TE) = 3.18 ms, voxel size = $1 \times 1 \times 1$ mm^3, 166 contiguous slices, field of view (FOV) = 25.6 cm^2, flip angle = 12°, sense factor = 2. A single session of functional images, which are sensitive to blood oxygen level-dependent (BOLD) contrast, were acquired using an echo planar imaging (EPI) sequence (TR = 2 s, TE = 30 ms, voxel size = $3 \times 3 \times 3$ mm^3, FOV = 19.2 cm^2, flip angle = 90°, SENSE factor = 1, 42 contiguous oblique axial slices parallel to the anterior commissure–posterior commissure line, interleaved acquisition) before and after BCI training. Three initial RF excitations were performed to achieve steady state equilibrium, and these were excluded from subsequent analyses.

Preprocessing was carried out using statistical parametric mapping (SPM) version 12 (SPM12; Wellcome Institute of Cognitive Neurology, London, UK) running under MATLAB (Mathworks Inc., Natick, MA, USA). In each functional session, all EPI images were realigned to the first EPI image to correct for head motion, followed by slice time correction, co-registration between functional images and structural images, and spatial normalisation to a standard Montreal Neurological Institute (MNI) EPI template. A cut-off of 25 mm was chosen for discrete cosine transform functions, and all normalised EPI images were smoothed with a 6 mm full-width half-maximal Gaussian smoothing kernel. Statistical modelling was performed using a general linear model implemented in SPM12. To minimise potential nuisance variables in comparisons across sessions, the two functional sessions were concatenated into a single session per the procedures in previous research.

For the fixed-effect analysis, the design matrix comprised the following independent events: MI of left hand, MI of right hand, rest (null event) before intervention, MI of left hand, MI of right hand, and rest after intervention together with a set of linear trend predictors, six head motion parameters, and a confound-mean predictor. To detect neural activation of the entire block, each 20 s block was modelled using a canonical hemodynamic response function (HRF), and the onset of each block was taken as the onset of the block in the SPM analysis model with a duration of 20 s.

Significant activations were thresholded at $p < 0.001$, voxel-level uncorrected and at $p < 0.05$, cluster-level corrected, and for multiple comparisons unless otherwise stated. The SPM coordinates are reported in the MNI space. Brain regions were identified using the automated anatomical labelling (AAL) atlas [22] and Brodmann templates, as implemented in MRIcron.

2.2.3. Transcranial Magnetic Stimulation

Measurement of Cortical Excitability

We used MEG-TD (Wuhan Yiruide Medical Equipment New Technology Co., Ltd., Wuhan, China) in this study. MEG-TD generates a bidirectional pulse waveform with a pulse width of 340 ± 20 μs and the pulse rise time of 60 ± 10 μs.

Electromyography (EMG) data were recorded from the first dorsal interosseous (FDI) using standard Ag/AgCl electrodes and a ground electrode positioned on the wrist. The EMG signals were amplified with a band pass filter of 10 Hz to 2 kHz. Because the participants in our study had no detectable MEP in the lesioned hemisphere, the motor threshold and MEP of the contralesional hemisphere were recorded. To determine the resting motor threshold (RMT), TMS was administered a commercially available figure-of-eight coil (YRD, maximum magnetic field intensity = 2 T, diameter = 9 cm; Wuhan Yiruide Medical Equipment New Technology Co., Ltd., Wuhan, China) using MEG-TD. The coil was placed in a tangent direction to the head, with the centre towards stimulating target. The RMT was assessed per the guidelines of the International Federation for Clinical Neurophysiology, and the minimum TMS intensity capable of producing at least five MEPs of 50 μV amplitude in 10 consecutive stimuli was estimated [23]. TMS intensity was adjusted to achieve an MEP of 1 mV peak-to-peak amplitude in the FDI muscle, and 10 consecutive MEPs were subsequently recorded.

Repetitive TMS

The 10 participants were randomly divided into two groups, with five participants in each group. rTMS was delivered according to the group assignment using MEG-TD with a figure-of-eight coil. For the comparison group, LF-rTMS was delivered to the contralesional M1 per the stimulation protocol recommended by the guideline (100 pulses of 1 Hz stimulation per session, with a 1 s interval between sessions and 12 sessions per treatment, totaling 1200 pulses at 80% rMT) [13]. In the experimental group, HF-rTMS was delivered to the brain regions activated during the MI task. We first determined the associated brain regions using fMRI and then converted the fMRI data, per the 10–20 international electrode placement system, to locate the stimulation target. The stimulation scheme was 10 Hz stimulation for 3 s per session, with an 8 s interval between sessions, 30 sessions per treatment, totalling 1200 pulses at 100% rMT. rTMS was conducted once a day, five times a week for 10 times in total.

2.3. *Assessments*

2.3.1. Primary Outcome

The change in upper-limb motor impairment at the end of the treatment was assessed using the motor status scale (MSS). MSS measures shoulder, elbow (maximum score = 40), wrist, hand, and finger movements (maximum score = 42), and it affords a reliable and valid assessment of upper limb impairment and disability following a stroke [24].

2.3.2. Secondary Outcomes

Secondary measures included the FMA scale (used for the upper extremities, range of motion, or wrist motor function) and the action research arm test (ARAT).

2.3.3. Commissural Fibres across the Corpus Callosum

Diffusion tensor imaging (DTI) was also performed to assess the white matter integrity of the fibres across the corpus callosum. Fractional anisotropy (FA) was measured at the corpus callosum because it is one of the most important white matter structures in the brain; the corpus callosum connects the two cerebral hemispheres and transmits information between them [25]. Previous research indicates that the anisotropy of the corpus callosum may be corelated with motor impairment and with functional gains following rehabilitation intervention [26,27].

DTI analysis was performed using the software library of the Oxford Centre for Functional Magnetic Resonance Imaging of the Brain. Skull-stripped DTI images were registered to b = 0 images to correct for eddy current distortions and simple head motion. Diffusion tensors were fitted to each voxel of the diffusion-weighted images, and Markov chain Monte Carlo sampling was used to build up distributions at these voxels. The resulting DTI images were then co-registered to the T1-weighted anatomical images. For fibre tracking, we adapted the two-step fibre-tracking method described by Wahl [28]. First, we placed a rectangular region of interest (ROI) in the primary motor regions of the precentral gyri (M1) of both hemispheres. Following the tracking step, a second ROI on the corpus callosum was added where the fibres from the first tracking emerged, and a second tracking was performed. After obtaining the DTI data, the FA value of the entire transcallosal motor tract was determined. The assessments were conducted before and after rTMS intervention.

2.4. *Statistical Analysis*

The Statistical Package for the Social Sciences (SPSS) version 20.0 (IBM, Chicago, IL, USA) was used to complete the statistical analysis. Considering the small sample size of this study, Wilcoxon signed-ranks test was used for within-group comparison before and after the intervention. Mann–Whitney U-test was used for between-group comparison. The level of significance was set at $p < 0.05$.

3. Results

3.1. *Participants*

We recruited ten participants: nine male and one female, and all ten participants were right-handed. Demographic information is presented in Table 1. All participants completed the two phases of the intervention and all the assessments. All the participants were assessed with the kinaesthetic and visual imagery questionnaire (KVIQ) [29], and all of their scores were above 25, which indicated they could actually perform motor imagery.

Table 1. Demographic characteristics of the participants (n = 10).

Participant	Group	Sex	Age (y)	Diagnosis	Affected UE	Post-Stroke Duration (mo)
1	Experimental	M	43	Haemorrhagic	Left	8
2	Experimental	M	68	Ischaemic	Left	16
3	Experimental	M	42	Haemorrhagic	Left	20
4	Experimental	M	75	Ischaemic	Left	6
5	Experimental	F	58	Haemorrhagic	Right	7
6	Comparison	M	65	Haemorrhagic	Left	11
7	Comparison	M	32	Haemorrhagic	Left	6
8	Comparison	M	56	Ischaemic	Right	8
9	Comparison	M	66	Ischaemic	Left	7
10	Comparison	M	41	Haemorrhagic	Left	20

M, male; UE, upper extremity; y. year; mo, month.

3.2. *Activated Brain Regions during Motor Imagery Tasks and the Stimulation Target*

fMRI was performed before and after MI-based BCI augmented with VR to determine the activated regions during MI tasks involving the paretic wrist and hand. The characters of each participant and the stimulating target of the experimental group are presented in Table 2.

3.3. *Behavioural Outcome Metrics*

There was no significant difference between the two groups for all measured behavioural outcomes before the intervention (Table 3). Compared with the pre-rTMS scores, the MSS scores of both groups (experimental group: pre 14.72 $\pm$ 6.01; post 16.72 $\pm$ 7.14; comparison group: pre 14.04 $\pm$ 6.07; post 14.88 $\pm$ 6.42) improved, but there was no significant improvement ($p = 0.066$ and $p = 0.109$). There was also no significant difference when comparing the two groups.

After the intervention, the FMA scores of both groups improved to a certain extent; however, there was no significant difference within and between the groups. All the participants could not flex or extend their wrists at baseline, but they regained some AROM after the rTMS intervention. For the experimental group, the AROM for wrist flexion was 16.00 $\pm$ 26.08 after the rTMS intervention, while it was 6.00 $\pm$ 8.94 for the comparison group. There was also no change in the ARAT scores, which indicate the practical functional capacity of the hand. The changes in the measured behavioural outcomes are presented in Figure 3.

3.4. *Commissural Fibres across the Corpus Callosum*

FA was measured at the corpus callosum before and after the rTMS intervention, and there was no significant difference between the FA values of the two groups. After the rTMS intervention, FA in the experimental group showed a trend of increase, while the FA values of the comparison group did not change significantly (Table 4).

Table 2. Characteristics of each participant and the stimulating target of the experimental group.

	Affected Hemisphere	Activated Brain Regions in fMRI	Activated Brain Regions Converted According to 10–20 International System	Activated Brain Regions
Participant 1	Right	Mainly in the right premotor cortex (BA 6) and precentral gyrus (M1, BA 4)	FC4	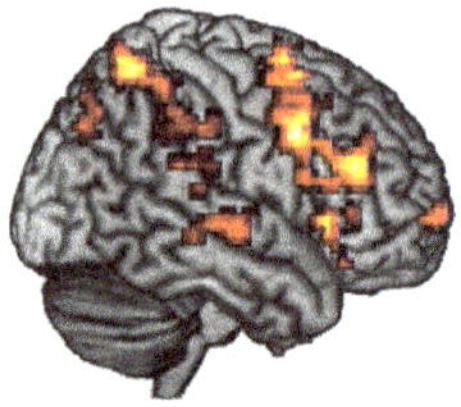
Participant 2	Left	Mainly in the right precentral gyrus (M1, BA 4), premotor cortex, and supplementary motor cortex (SMA, BA 6)	C2	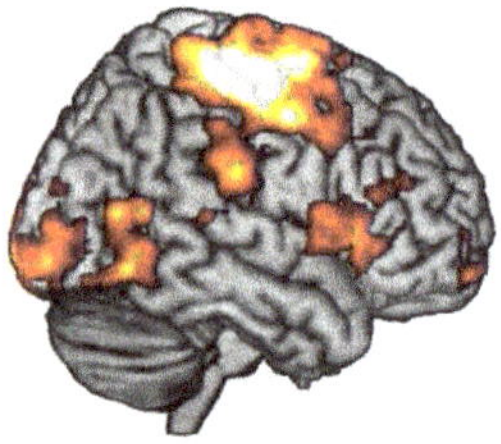
Participant 3	Right	Mainly in the left precentral gyrus (M1, BA 4) and premotor cortex (BA 6)	C3	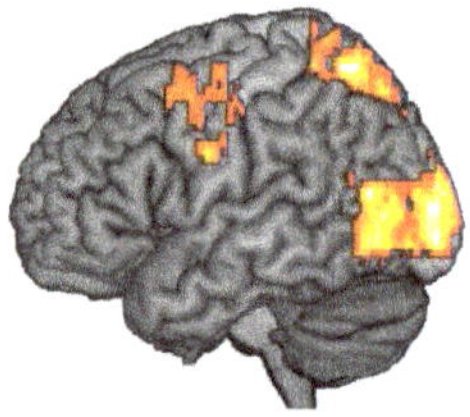
Participant 4	Right	Mainly in the left precentral gyrus (M1, BA 4) and premotor cortex (BA 6)	C1	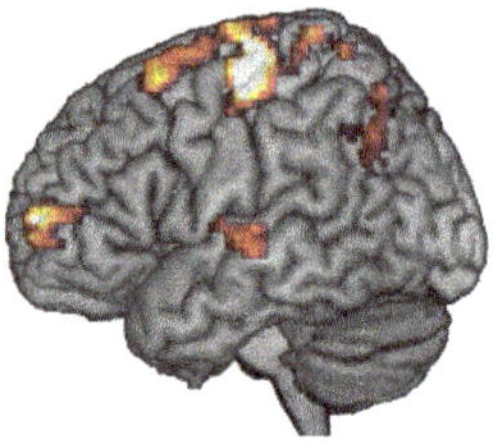
Participant 5	Right	Mainly in the right precentral gyrus (M1, BA 4) and premotor cortex (BA 6)	C1	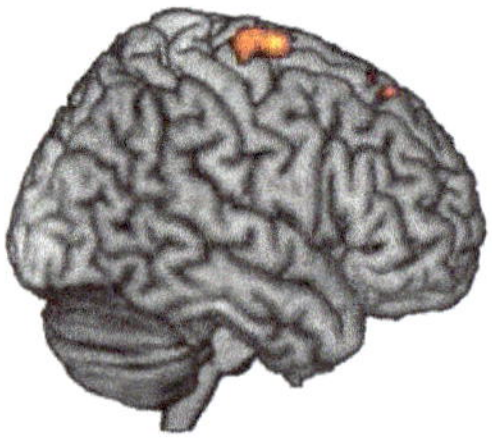

Table 3. Behavioural Outcome Metrics.

Participant	Group	Pre MSS	Post MSS	Pre FMA	Post FMA	Pre ARAT	Post ARAT	Pre AROM Flexion	Post AROM Flexion	Pre AROM Extension	Post AROM Extension
1	Experimental	18.80	21.80	12.00	15.00	4.00	18.00	0°	0°	0°	0°
2	Experimental	13.00	13.00	10.00	10.00	0.00	0.00	0°	0°	0°	0°
3	Experimental	15.00	18.20	11.00	13.00	0.00	2.00	0°	20°	0°	0°
4	Experimental	21.20	24.20	16.00	22.00	5.00	8.00	0°	60°	0°	25°

Table 3. *Cont.*

Participant	Group	Pre MSS	Post MSS	Pre FMA	Post FMA	Pre ARAT	Post ARAT	Pre AROM Flexion	Post AROM Flexion	Pre AROM Extension	Post AROM Extension
5	Experimental	5.60	6.40	5.00	6.00	0.00	0.00	0°	0°	0°	0°
6	Comparison	16.40	17.00	11.00	12.00	0.00	0.00	0°	20°	0°	0°
7	Comparison	22.80	24.20	22.00	24.00	8.00	8.00	0°	10°	0°	20°
8	Comparison	11.00	13.20	9.00	12.00	0.00	2.00	0°	0°	0°	0°
9	Comparison	6.60	6.60	6.00	6.00	0.00	0.00	0°	0°	0°	0°
10	Comparison	13.40	13.40	11.00	12.00	0.00	0.00	0°	0°	0°	0°

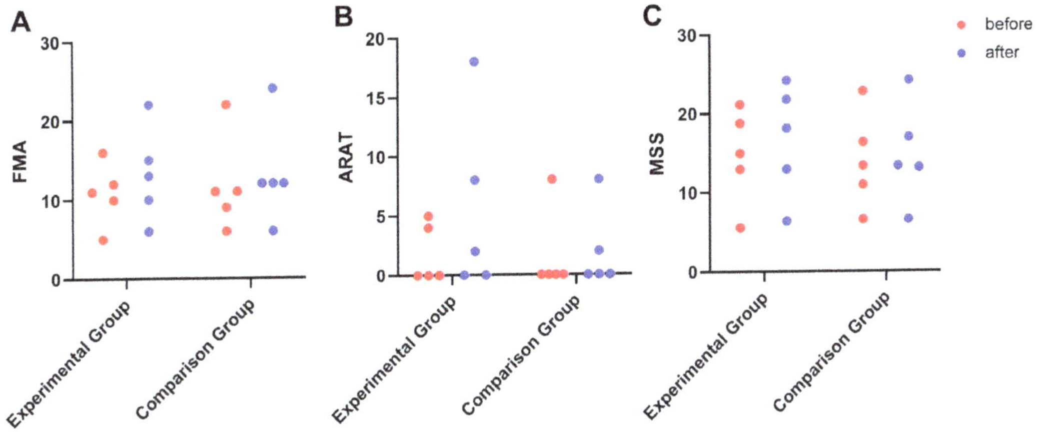

Figure 3. Behavioural Outcomes in Experimental group and Comparison group. (**A**) For FMA; (**B**) for ARAT; (**C**) for MSS.

Table 4. FA for fibres across corpus callosum.

	Experimental Group		Comparison Group				
	Baseline	Post rTMS	Baseline	Post rTMS	Sig. [a]	Sig. [b]	Sig. [c]
FA	0.53 ± 0.05	0.56 ± 0.06	0.55 ± 0.04	0.56 ± 0.06	0.059	0.828	0.909

[a,b] FA (pre–post), within-group comparisons in experimental group and comparison group, respectively. [c] FA between groups.

4. Discussion

Rehabilitation is critical for reducing stroke-related disability [30], and there is growing recognition that cortical neuroplasticity supporting adaptive recovery may extend for years after stroke [31]. However, up to 50% of stroke survivors still have persistent, severe upper-extremity paresis even after receiving rehabilitation treatment. TMS is a safe, non-invasive method of stimulating the cerebral cortex [32]. When used at low or high frequencies, rTMS may potentially enhance the ability of the brain to relearn task-specific functions as well as augment the effects of rehabilitation via modulating corticomotor excitability [33]. However, the reported efficacy of this intervention differs significantly. Furthermore, in light of the negative results from the NICHE trial [34], evidence for the efficacy of LF-rTMS to the contralesional M1 for motor recovery during the chronic stage of stroke is controversial. Meanwhile, the conventional approach of facilitating excitability of the ipsilesional primary motor cortex also fails to produce motor improvement in stroke survivors with severe loss of ipsilesional substrate [35]. Previous studies indicate that different stimulation targets may affect the efficacy of rTMS for the recovery of upper-limb motor function differently [36]. Therefore, it is worth considering how to select appropriate targets before rTMS intervention is applied. In this study, the brain regions activated by MI were selected as the intervention target, and we investigated the effect of stimulating this target on the recovery of upper-limb motor function in chronic stroke patients with severe upper-limb motor impairment.

Our results indicate that MI ability is retained even in stroke patients with severe motor impairment, and this ability can be further enhanced after specific feedback training, which is consistent with the findings of previous research [17], including our previous study [20]. Therefore, in stroke patients with severe motor impairment, selecting the brain regions activated during MI tasks as rTMS intervention targets is feasible and has certain potential value. Our preliminary results also confirm the feasibility of identifying intervention targets using this approach. In addition, we further compared this new target with the conventional target [13]. After the intervention, the MSS scores of both groups increased, but there was no significant difference between and within the two experimental groups. The results of other behavioural assessments also indicate some improvement, but the improvements were not statistically significant. For this study, we recruited stroke patients in the chronic stage. Brain plasticity in this stage might experience a more complicated reconstruction and follow other recovery patterns [37]. In a chronic stroke brain, there may be a new functional cerebral architecture, one that is not as effective as that in the intact brain but still attempts to generate some form of motor signal to the downstream neurons in the most effective way it can. Both the ipsilesional and contralesional motor sensory regions may be involved in this process [38]. Lin et al. [16] confirmed that balance and recovery have a bimodal dependence. They also identified a threshold of the clinical score useful to stratify stroke patients (UEFM = 43). Above this threshold, better motor performance is associated with low transcallosal inhibition from the contralesional hemisphere, while below this threshold, better performance is associated with higher transcallosal inhibition. In our study, we recruited patients whose UEFM were all below 43. As Lin et al. indicated in their study, the contralesional hemisphere might play a supportive role in the recovery of the aforementioned participants. However, in our results, we did have participants (2,3,4) that showed the recovery pattern that Lin et al. pointed out in their study. Still, participants (1,5) showed the activation of ipsilesional brain regions during motor imagery task, which was contrary to the results of Lin et al.'s study. This indicates that there are different types of brain remodelling in chronic stroke patients. Therefore, an individualised target selection may further increase the therapeutic effect of rTMs. Considering the preliminary nature and small sample size of our study, we could not make a concrete conclusion. Further studies should be performed to investigate the relationship between the two hemispheres in chronic stroke patients.

In this study, we converted the activated brain regions determined using fMRI per the 10–20 international electrode placement system. Although it would be more precise to locate the target using an rTMS navigator, considering the coverage of the navigator, it is more feasible to perform the conversion per the 10–20 international electrode placement system for rTMS stimulation.

We also traced the transcallosal fibres in our participants. In healthy individuals, interhemispheric neural activity between the homologous motor cortices is well-balanced through the opposing inhibitory influences exerted by the M1s of both hemispheres [39]. Previous research indicates that increased transcallosal fibre microstructure may be predictive of the interhemispheric inhibitory capacity in healthy individuals [40]. Investigating fibres via the corpus callosum can reflect brain plasticity from a structural perspective. In this study, we found that FA increased in the experimental group ($p = 0.059$) after rTMS intervention. Because our participants were stroke patients with severe upper-limb impairment, the FA of fibres across the corpus callosum may primarily reflect fibres from the contralesional M1 to the ipsilesional M1. With improvements in upper-limb motor function, the increased FA may indicate the specific role of the contralesional M1 in recovery from severe brain injury. These results are also in agreement with the findings of the study by Grefkes [41], in which they concluded that movement of a stroke-affected hand showed additional inhibitory influences from the contralesional to ipsilesional M1 that correlated with the degree of motor impairment. Further studies are needed to confirm the effect of rTMS delivered to different brain regions and how it affects the balance between the two hemispheres and the recovery from motor impairment.

There are some limitations to this study. First, this is a preliminary study, and only 10 participants were recruited, which certainly impacts its efficacy. Second, in this study, there were exactly 10 sessions of rTMS interventions. Whether increasing the number of intervention sessions will further increase the efficacy of rTMS treatment also needs to be verified in future studies. Third, although all participants underwent task-oriented training focused on the upper limbs, we did not further define the implementation time of the training. In future research, we will implement task-oriented training immediately after rTMS, which may yield the benefit of improving recovery. Therefore, we will increase the sample size and optimise the intervention plan based on the results of this study and continue to conduct randomised, controlled studies to investigate the effect of using task-activated brain regions as the intervention target for the improvement of upper-limb motor function in chronic stroke patients with severe upper-limb motor impairment.

5. Conclusions

In chronic stroke patients with severe upper-limb motor impairment, determining the brain regions activated during an MI task and selecting them as the target of an rTMS intervention is feasible. Due to the preliminary nature of this study, further studies are needed to explore the efficacy of this intervention.

Author Contributions: Conceptualization, T.G. and R.L.; data curation, T.G.; formal analysis, T.G., Y.H., J.Z. and R.L.; funding acquisition, R.L.; investigation, T.G. and Y.H.; methodology, T.G., J.Z. and R.L.; project administration, Y.B. and R.L.; supervision, T.G., Y.H., J.Z., Y.B. and R.L.; validation, Y.B. and R.L.; writing—original draft, T.G. and R.L.; writing—review and editing, Y.B. and R.L. All authors have read and agreed to the published version of the manuscript.

Funding: This research was funded by the Shanghai Municipal Health Commission (grant number 20194Y0103) and National Natural Science Foundation of China (grant numbers 81902280).

Institutional Review Board Statement: This study was conducted in accordance with the Declaration of Helsinki and approved by the ethics committee of Huashan Hospital, Fudan University (protocol code ChiCTR2000036423 and date of approval 23 August 2020).

Informed Consent Statement: Informed consent was obtained from all subjects involved in the study or their legal representatives. Written or electronic informed consent has been obtained from all the subjects or their legal representatives to publish this paper.

Data Availability Statement: The data presented in this study are available on request from the corresponding author.

Acknowledgments: We wish to express our gratitude to the participants and their families in this study, and we also want to thank Yi Wu for his support in the conduction of this study and Zhijie He for helping to revise this paper.

Conflicts of Interest: The authors declare no conflict of interest.

References

1. GBD 2019 Stroke Collaborators. Global, regional, and national burden of stroke and its risk factors, 1990–2019: A systematic analysis for the Global Burden of Disease Study 2019. *Lancet Neurol.* **2021**, *20*, 795–820. [CrossRef]
2. Virani, S.S.; Alonso, A.; Benjamin, E.J.; Bittencourt, M.S.; Callaway, C.W.; Carson, A.P.; Chamberlain, A.M.; Chang, A.R.; Cheng, S.; Delling, F.N.; et al. Heart Disease and Stroke Statistics-2020 Update: A Report from the American Heart Association. *Circulation* **2020**, *141*, e139–e596. [PubMed]
3. Chen, W.W.; Gao, R.L.; Liu, L.S.; Zhu, M.L.; Wang, W.; Wang, Y.J.; Wu, Z.S.; Li, H.J.; Gu, D.F.; Yang, Y.J. Summary of China Cardiovascular Disease Report 2016. *Chin. Circ. J.* **2017**, *32*, 521–530.
4. Pollock, A.; Farmer, S.E.; Brady, M.C.; Langhorne, P.; Mead, G.E.; Mehrholz, J.; van Wijck, F. Interventions for improving upper limb function after stroke. *Cochrane Db Syst Rev.* **2014**, *2014*, CD010820. [CrossRef] [PubMed]

5. Stinear, C.M.; Lang, C.E.; Zeiler, S.; Byblow, W.D. Advances and challenges in stroke rehabilitation. *Lancet Neurol.* **2020**, *19*, 348–360. [CrossRef] [PubMed]
6. Broeks, J.G.; Lankhorst, G.J.; Rumping, K.; Prevo, A.J. The long-term outcome of arm function after stroke: Results of a follow-up study. *Disabil. Rehabil.* **1999**, *21*, 357–364. [CrossRef]
7. Fitzgerald, P.B.; Fountain, S.; Daskalakis, Z.J. A comprehensive review of the effects of rTMS on motor cortical excitability and inhibition. *Clin. Neurophysiol.* **2006**, *117*, 2584–2596. [CrossRef]
8. Hildesheim, F.E.; Silver, A.N.; Dominguez-Vargas, A.U.; Andrushko, J.W.; Edwards, J.D.; Dancause, N.; Thiel, A. Predicting Individual Treatment Response to rTMS for Motor Recovery After Stroke: A Review and the CanStim Perspective. *Front. Rehabil. Sci.* **2022**, *3*, 795335. [CrossRef]
9. Wang, Q.; Zhang, D.; Zhao, Y.Y.; Hai, H.; Ma, Y.W. Effects of high-frequency repetitive transcranial magnetic stimulation over the contralesional motor cortex on motor recovery in severe hemiplegic stroke: A randomized clinical trial. *Brain Stimul.* **2020**, *13*, 979–986. [CrossRef]
10. Dionisio, A.; Duarte, I.C.; Patricio, M.; Castelo-Branco, M. The Use of Repetitive Transcranial Magnetic Stimulation for Stroke Rehabilitation: A Systematic Review. *J. Stroke Cerebrovasc.* **2018**, *27*, 1–31. [CrossRef]
11. Guo, Z.; Jin, Y.; Bai, X.; Jiang, B.; He, L.; Mcclure, M.A.; Mu, Q. Distinction of High- and Low-Frequency Repetitive Transcranial Magnetic Stimulation on the Functional Reorganization of the Motor Network in Stroke Patients. *Neural Plast.* **2021**, *2021*, 8873221. [CrossRef] [PubMed]
12. He, Y.; Li, K.; Chen, Q.; Yin, J.; Bai, D. Repetitive Transcranial Magnetic Stimulation on Motor Recovery for Patients with Stroke: A PRISMA Compliant Systematic Review and Meta-analysis. *Am. J. Phys. Med. Rehab.* **2020**, *99*, 99–108. [CrossRef]
13. Lefaucheur, J.P.; Aleman, A.; Baeken, C.; Benninger, D.H.; Brunelin, J.; Di Lazzaro, V.; Filipovic, S.R.; Grefkes, C.; Hasan, A.; Hummel, F.C.; et al. Evidence-based guidelines on the therapeutic use of repetitive transcranial magnetic stimulation (rTMS): An update (2014–2018). *Clin. Neurophysiol.* **2020**, *131*, 474–528. [CrossRef] [PubMed]
14. Salehi, D.N.; Kamali, F.; Shariat, A.; Jaberzadeh, S. Comparison of Transcallosal Inhibition Between Hemispheres and Its Relationship with Motor Behavior in Patients with Severe Upper Extremity Impairment After Subacute Stroke. *J. Stroke Cerebrovasc.* **2022**, *31*, 106469. [CrossRef] [PubMed]
15. Di Pino, G.; Pellegrino, G.; Assenza, G.; Capone, F.; Ferreri, F.; Formica, D.; Ranieri, F.; Tombini, M.; Ziemann, U.; Rothwell, J.C.; et al. Modulation of brain plasticity in stroke: A novel model for neurorehabilitation. *Nat. Rev. Neurol.* **2014**, *10*, 597–608. [CrossRef]
16. Lin, Y.L.; Potter-Baker, K.A.; Cunningham, D.A.; Li, M.; Sankarasubramanian, V.; Lee, J.; Jones, S.; Sakaie, K.; Wang, X.; Machado, A.G.; et al. Stratifying chronic stroke patients based on the influence of contralesional motor cortices: An inter-hemispheric inhibition study. *Clin. Neurophysiol.* **2020**, *131*, 2516–2525. [CrossRef] [PubMed]
17. Ietswaart, M.; Johnston, M.; Dijkerman, H.C.; Joice, S.; Scott, C.L.; Macwalter, R.S.; Hamilton, S.J. Mental practice with motor imagery in stroke recovery: Randomized controlled trial of efficacy. *Brain* **2011**, *134*, 1373–1386. [CrossRef]
18. Decety, J. Neural representations for action. *Rev. Neurosci.* **1996**, *7*, 285–297. [CrossRef] [PubMed]
19. Decety, J.; Jeannerod, M.; Prablanc, C. The timing of mentally represented actions. *Behav. Brain Res.* **1989**, *34*, 35–42. [CrossRef]
20. Hu, Y.Q.; Gao, T.H.; Li, J.; Tao, J.C.; Bai, Y.L.; Lu, R.R. Motor Imagery-Based Brain-Computer Interface Combined with Multimodal Feedback to Promote Upper Limb Motor Function after Stroke: A Preliminary Study. *Evid.-Based Compl. Alt.* **2021**, *2021*, 1116126. [CrossRef]
21. Lu, R.R.; Zheng, M.X.; Li, J.; Gao, T.H.; Hua, X.Y.; Liu, G.; Huang, S.H.; Xu, J.G.; Wu, Y. Motor imagery based brain-computer interface control of continuous passive motion for wrist extension recovery in chronic stroke patients. *Neurosci. Lett.* **2020**, *718*, 134727. [CrossRef]
22. Tzourio-Mazoyer, N.; Landeau, B.; Papathanassiou, D.; Crivello, F.; Etard, O.; Delcroix, N.; Mazoyer, B.; Joliot, M. Automated anatomical labeling of activations in SPM using a macroscopic anatomical parcellation of the MNI MRI single-subject brain. *Neuroimage* **2002**, *15*, 273–289. [CrossRef] [PubMed]
23. Groppa, S.; Oliviero, A.; Eisen, A.; Quartarone, A.; Cohen, L.G.; Mall, V.; Kaelin-Lang, A.; Mima, T.; Rossi, S.; Thickbroom, G.W.; et al. A practical guide to diagnostic transcranial magnetic stimulation: Report of an IFCN committee. *Clin. Neurophysiol.* **2012**, *123*, 858–882. [CrossRef]
24. Ferraro, M.; Demaio, J.H.; Krol, J.; Trudell, C.; Rannekleiv, K.; Edelstein, L.; Christos, P.; Aisen, M.; England, J.; Fasoli, S.; et al. Assessing the motor status score: A scale for the evaluation of upper limb motor outcomes in patients after stroke. *Neurorehab. Neural Repair* **2002**, *16*, 283–289. [CrossRef]
25. van der Knaap, L.J.; van der Ham, I.J. How does the corpus callosum mediate interhemispheric transfer? A review. *Behav. Brain Res.* **2011**, *223*, 211–221. [CrossRef] [PubMed]
26. Stewart, J.C.; Dewanjee, P.; Tran, G.; Quinlan, E.B.; Dodakian, L.; Mckenzie, A.; See, J.; Cramer, S.C. Role of corpus callosum integrity in arm function differs based on motor severity after stroke. *Neuroimage Clin.* **2017**, *14*, 641–647. [CrossRef] [PubMed]
27. Stewart, J.C.; O'Donnell, M.; Handlery, K.; Winstein, C.J. Skilled Reach Performance Correlates with Corpus Callosum Structural Integrity in Individuals with Mild Motor Impairment After Stroke: A Preliminary Investigation. *Neurorehab. Neural Repair* **2017**, *31*, 657–665. [CrossRef]

28. Wahl, M.; Lauterbach-Soon, B.; Hattingen, E.; Jung, P.; Singer, O.; Volz, S.; Klein, J.C.; Steinmetz, H.; Ziemann, U. Human motor corpus callosum: Topography, somatotopy, and link between microstructure and function. *J. Neurosci.* **2007**, *27*, 12132–12138. [CrossRef]
29. Malouin, F.; Richards, C.L.; Jackson, P.L.; Lafleur, M.F.; Durand, A.; Doyon, J. The Kinesthetic and Visual Imagery Questionnaire (KVIQ) for assessing motor imagery in persons with physical disabilities: A reliability and construct validity study. *J. Neurol. Phys. Ther.* **2007**, *31*, 20–29. [CrossRef]
30. Veerbeek, J.M.; van Wegen, E.; van Peppen, R.; van der Wees, P.J.; Hendriks, E.; Rietberg, M.; Kwakkel, G. What is the evidence for physical therapy poststroke? A systematic review and meta-analysis. *PLoS ONE* **2014**, *9*, e87987.
31. Dimyan, M.A.; Cohen, L.G. Neuroplasticity in the context of motor rehabilitation after stroke. *Nat. Rev. Neurol.* **2011**, *7*, 76–85. [CrossRef]
32. Rossi, S.; Hallett, M.; Rossini, P.M.; Pascual-Leone, A. Safety, ethical considerations, and application guidelines for the use of transcranial magnetic stimulation in clinical practice and research. *Clin. Neurophysiol.* **2009**, *120*, 2008–2039. [CrossRef]
33. Corti, M.; Patten, C.; Triggs, W. Repetitive transcranial magnetic stimulation of motor cortex after stroke: A focused review. *Am. J. Phys. Med. Rehab.* **2012**, *91*, 254–270. [CrossRef]
34. Harvey, R.L.; Edwards, D.; Dunning, K.; Fregni, F.; Stein, J.; Laine, J.; Rogers, L.M.; Vox, F.; Durand-Sanchez, A.; Bockbrader, M.; et al. Randomized Sham-Controlled Trial of Navigated Repetitive Transcranial Magnetic Stimulation for Motor Recovery in Stroke. *Stroke* **2018**, *49*, 2138–2146. [CrossRef]
35. Li, X.; Lin, Y.L.; Cunningham, D.A.; Wolf, S.L.; Sakaie, K.; Conforto, A.B.; Machado, A.G.; Mohan, A.; O'Laughlin, K.; Wang, X.; et al. Repetitive Transcranial Magnetic Stimulation of the Contralesional Dorsal Premotor Cortex for Upper Extremity Motor Improvement in Severe Stroke: Study Protocol for a Pilot Randomized Clinical Trial. *Cerebrovasc. Dis.* **2022**, *51*, 557–564. [CrossRef]
36. Chang, P.W.; Lu, C.F.; Chang, S.T.; Tsai, P.Y. Functional Near-Infrared Spectroscopy as a Target Navigator for rTMS Modulation in Patients with Hemiplegia: A Randomized Control Study. *Neurol. Ther.* **2022**, *11*, 103–121. [CrossRef]
37. Ward, N.S. Mechanisms underlying recovery of motor function after stroke. *Postgrad. Med. J.* **2005**, *81*, 510–514. [CrossRef]
38. Pundik, S.; Mccabe, J.P.; Hrovat, K.; Fredrickson, A.E.; Tatsuoka, C.; Feng, I.J.; Daly, J.J. Recovery of post stroke proximal arm function, driven by complex neuroplastic bilateral brain activation patterns and predicted by baseline motor dysfunction severity. *Front. Hum. Neurosci.* **2015**, *9*, 394. [CrossRef] [PubMed]
39. Ferbert, A.; Priori, A.; Rothwell, J.C.; Day, B.L.; Colebatch, J.G.; Marsden, C.D. Interhemispheric inhibition of the human motor cortex. *J. Physiol.* **1992**, *453*, 525–546. [CrossRef] [PubMed]
40. Fling, B.W.; Benson, B.L.; Seidler, R.D. Transcallosal sensorimotor fiber tract structure-function relationships. *Hum. Brain Mapp.* **2013**, *34*, 384–395. [CrossRef] [PubMed]
41. Grefkes, C.; Nowak, D.A.; Eickhoff, S.B.; Dafotakis, M.; Kust, J.; Karbe, H.; Fink, G.R. Cortical connectivity after subcortical stroke assessed with functional magnetic resonance imaging. *Ann. Neurol.* **2008**, *63*, 236–246. [CrossRef] [PubMed]

brain sciences

MDPI

Systematic Review

Sensorimotor Rhythm-Based Brain–Computer Interfaces for Motor Tasks Used in Hand Upper Extremity Rehabilitation after Stroke: A Systematic Review

Jianghong Fu [1], Shugeng Chen [1] and Jie Jia [1,2,3,*]

1 Department of Rehabilitation Medicine, Huashan Hospital, Fudan University, Shanghai 200040, China
2 National Clinical Research Center for Aging and Medicine, Huashan Hospital, Fudan University, Shanghai 200040, China
3 National Center for Neurological Disorders, Shanghai 200040, China
* Correspondence: shannonjj@126.com; Tel./Fax: +86-021-5288-7820

Abstract: Brain–computer interfaces (BCIs) are becoming more popular in the neurological rehabilitation field, and sensorimotor rhythm (SMR) is a type of brain oscillation rhythm that can be captured and analyzed in BCIs. Previous reviews have testified to the efficacy of the BCIs, but seldom have they discussed the motor task adopted in BCIs experiments in detail, as well as whether the feedback is suitable for them. We focused on the motor tasks adopted in SMR-based BCIs, as well as the corresponding feedback, and searched articles in PubMed, Embase, Cochrane library, Web of Science, and Scopus and found 442 articles. After a series of screenings, 15 randomized controlled studies were eligible for analysis. We found motor imagery (MI) or motor attempt (MA) are common experimental paradigms in EEG-based BCIs trials. Imagining/attempting to grasp and extend the fingers is the most common, and there were multi-joint movements, including wrist, elbow, and shoulder. There were various types of feedback in MI or MA tasks for hand grasping and extension. Proprioception was used more frequently in a variety of forms. Orthosis, robot, exoskeleton, and functional electrical stimulation can assist the paretic limb movement, and visual feedback can be used as primary feedback or combined forms. However, during the recovery process, there are many bottleneck problems for hand recovery, such as flaccid paralysis or opening the fingers. In practice, we should mainly focus on patients' difficulties, and design one or more motor tasks for patients, with the assistance of the robot, FES, or other combined feedback, to help them to complete a grasp, finger extension, thumb opposition, or other motion. Future research should focus on neurophysiological changes and functional improvements and further elaboration on the changes in neurophysiology during the recovery of motor function.

Keywords: brain–computer interfaces; motor task; sensorimotor rhythm; stroke; hand rehabilitation

Citation: Fu, J.; Chen, S.; Jia, J. Sensorimotor Rhythm-Based Brain–Computer Interfaces for Motor Tasks Used in Hand Upper Extremity Rehabilitation after Stroke: A Systematic Review. *Brain Sci.* **2023**, *13*, 56. https://doi.org/10.3390/brainsci13010056

Academic Editors: Simona Lattanzi and Konstantin V. Slavin

Received: 16 November 2022
Revised: 5 December 2022
Accepted: 25 December 2022
Published: 28 December 2022

1. Introduction

Stroke causes the highest morbidity associated with disability-adjusted life years lost in China, with two million new cases annually [1]. Up to 66% of stroke survivors experience upper limb and hand motor impairments, which results in functional limitations in activities of daily living and decreased life quality [2,3], and leads to a heavy burden for the family and society. Hand rehabilitation after a stroke is difficult during neurorehabilitation. Traditional rehabilitation methods cannot fully meet the need of patients and the expectations of doctors [4]. Various methods were being applied in hand function rehabilitation, including central interventions such as mirror therapy, transcranial magnetic stimulation, transcranial direct current stimulation, brain–computer interfaces (BCIs), motor imagery, etc., peripheral interventions such as a robot, physical therapy, functional electrical stimulation, etc., and medicine such as botulinum for spasticity [5]. BCIs have been proven to be effective for hand motor recovery after stroke [6–8]. According to its working mechanism, BCIs can be classified as assistive or rehabilitative devices based on their clinical applications. In some laboratories, assistive BCIs are used as communication tools for amyotrophic lateral sclerosis patients [9,10] or as daily activity assistance for tetraplegia, such as drinking assistance [11,12]. Meanwhile, rehabilitative BCIs are mainly used in promoting functional recovery for such as stroke patients.

There were various kinds of rehabilitative BCIs equipment. In practice, the workflow of BCI is acquiring brain signals, extracting features, transforming the signal into command via external devices, and activating the sensory feedback. In non-invasive systems, BCIs involve brain activities measured by different kinds of equipment, such as electroencephalograph (EEG), functional magnetic resonance imaging, and functional near-infrared imaging, and the user's movement intention such as motor imagery or motor attempt is decoded in real-time from the ongoing electrical activity of the brain by extracting relevant features [6]. Based on different features, such as common spatial pattern (CSP), and event-related desynchronization (ERD), different movement intentions can be classified by linear discriminant analysis (LDA) classifier, support vector machine. The algorithm converts the brain signals into information, then the external devices, such as the computer screen, robot, functional electrical stimulation (FES), or orthosis received the information and provide feedback to the subjects. The whole process forms a closed loop called neural feedback [13,14]. Auditory, visual, tactile, and proprioceptive feedback is commonly adopted in BCI, and their combination is used extensively in clinical experiments [15–17]. Motor imagery (MI), motor attempt (MA), or motor execution (ME) can activate several signal rhythm changes in the cerebral cortex [18,19], which can be captured and used to modulate the amplitude of sensorimotor rhythm (SMR) to control external devices. In addition, BCIs are a kind of active rehabilitation device. They achieved control of devices by catching the subject's initiative. In particular, the motor task is not only the start factor for BCIs, but also the repeated training of task can promote motor recovery. Well-designed motor tasks and befitting feedback for the patients can enhance the BCI training and lead to a successful rehabilitation process.

Motor tasks usually concern the movement intention or the actual movement of the paretic limb. As we all know, hand recovery is a long and rough process. Several stroke patients in the acute stage can hardly move their hands, neither completely nor incompletely grasp, and they encounter kinds of difficulties, such as opening the fingers or moving their thumb or other fingers independently. The recovery of the hand function conforms to some rules, such as the six Brunnstrom recovery stages [20], but many of the hand functions stagnate at some specific stages. According to Brunnstrom recovery stage for stroke, in stage I, there is no muscle contraction at all; in stage II, there is subtle flexion of the hand; in stage III, the hand can flex more actively but cannot be opened; in stage IV, patients can volitionally extend the thumb and other fingers partially; in the stage V, patients can hold a ball or a cylinder, and they can extend their fingers simultaneously; and in the stageVI, the paretic hand can almost accomplish every kind of functional grasping and extending, but the speed and coordination are a little bit worse than the contralateral limb. The recovery rules can also be applied to shoulders, elbows, forearms, and wrists. It is obvious that an improvement from no active movement to active movement is a hard step, and the separation movement, from finger grasping to finger opening, is also a difficult process. Therefore, facing a series of difficulties, the task specificity of hand motions is of great importance, and the correlation with feedback is the main link and is discussed in detail in the review.

Clinical efficacy in hand function rehabilitation of stroke patients has been revealed by several reviews. Remsik et al. [21] considered BCIs as a method of hand function rehabilitation after stroke with a review. Monge–Pereira et al. [22] suggested EEG-based BCIs interventions may be a promising rehabilitation approach in subjects with stroke by a systematic review. Carvalho et al. [23] suggested that neurofeedback training with EEG-based BCIs might promote both clinical and neurophysiologic changes in stroke patients. Bai et al. [24] investigated the effectiveness of BCIs in restoring upper extremity function after stroke. Even though they have testified to the effectiveness of the BCIs, hardly have they forced deeply on these questions: Why was a motor task chosen in each BCI trial, and is it suitable for a stroke patient? Some stroke patients received BCIs training but gained small improvements. Except for other reasons such as a lack of treatment times, short treatment duration, etc., can the motor tasks help promote better motor recovery? Thus, this review concentrates on the motor tasks and feedback of BCI clinical trials based on upper limb and hand interventions with BCIs systems in patients after stroke, which is truly suitable for them to solve their problems. We use the traditional method to search articles and draw clinical recommendations. This review aims: (1) to explore the motor tasks design in EEG-based BCIs clinical trials, (2) to analyze the association between motor tasks and the neurologic mechanism, and (3) to discuss the feedback combing the motor tasks that were suitable for stroke patients.

2. Methods

2.1. Search Strategy

We searched articles in PubMed, Embase, Cochrane library, and Web of Science. At the same time, we screened the reference of previous systematic reviews in PubMed in case of missed articles. For PubMed, JF and SC took advantage of subject terms and entry terms for each subject, extended each subject term with the virtue of mesh categories, and then searched the corresponding entry terms separately. These subject terms and entry terms can be the reference for other databases. However, due to different search strategies in each database, other databases went through the same process to retrieve articles. The specific search strategy for each database can be found in Supplement S1.

2.2. Study Selection

The inclusion criterion is following the PICO principle:

(1) Subjects were hemiplegic paralysis, and were diagnosed with ischemic or hemorrhagic stroke;
(2) Subjects received EEG-based BCIs training, which described the motor tasks in detail in the papers, and the control group received conventional therapy or sham BCI training;
(3) The Fugl–Meyer Assessment Upper Extremity Scale (FMA-UE), Action Research Arm Test (ARAT), the Jebsen Hand Function Test, etc. were used for functional recovery assessments;
(4) We concentrated on randomized controlled trials.

The PEDro scale was used to assess the methodological quality of the controlled studies (details are shown in Table 1).

Table 1. Methodological quality assessment of the enrolled studies.

Author/PEDro Item	1	2	3	4	5	6	7	8	9	10	11	Total
Ramos–Murguialday et al., 2013a [17]	1	1	1	1	1	1		1		1	1	8
Angand Guan et al., 2014a [25]	1	1		1			1	1		1	1	6
Li et al., 2014a [15]	1	1	1	1				1	1	1	1	7
Angand Chua et al., 2014a [26]	1	1	1	1			1	1		1		6
Rayegani et al., 2014a [27]	1	1		1			1			1	1	5
Ang et al., 2015a [16]	1	1		1	1			1	1	1	1	7
Pichiorri et al., 2015a [28]	1	1	1	1				1		1	1	6
Kim et al., 2016 [29]	1	1	1	1			1	1		1	1	7
Frolov et al., 2017a [30]	1	1		1			1			1	1	5
Biasiucci et al., 2018a [7]	1	1	1	1	1		1	1	1	1	1	9
Ramos–Murguialday et al., 2019a [31]	1	1	1	1	1	1	1			1	1	8
Chen et al., 2020 [32]	1	1		1				1	1	1	1	6
Miao et al., 2020 [33]		1		1				1	1	1	1	5

Table 1. *Cont.*

Author/PEDro Item	1	2	3	4	5	6	7	8	9	10	11	Total
Cheng et al., 2020 [34]	1	1		1			1	1	1	1	1	8
Chen et al., 2021 [35]	1	1		1				1	1	1	1	7

1. Eligibility criteria were specified; 2. subjects were randomly allocated to groups; 3. allocation was concealed; 4. the groups were similar at baseline regarding the most important prognostic indicators; 5. there was blinding of all subjects; 6. there was blinding of all therapists; 7. there was blinding of all assessors; 8. measures of at least one key outcome were obtained from more than 85% of the subjects initially allocated to groups; 9. all subjects for whom outcome measures were available received the treatment or control condition as allocated; 10. the results of between-group statistical comparisons are reported; 11. the study provides both point measures and measures of variability.

3. Results

We searched articles in PubMed, Embase, Cochrane library, Web of Science, and Scopus and obtained a total of 442 articles. After screening, 15 randomized controlled studies were eligible for analysis. We mainly concentrated on the motor task design and the corresponding BCI system feedback in their research (characteristics of the enrolled studies are shown in Table 2).

Table 2. Characteristics of the enrolled studies.

Study, Year	Country	n(E/C), Study Design	Experimental (E)/Control Group (C)	Feedback	Outcome Measures	Dosage	Main Results
Ramos–Murguialday et al., 2013a [17]	Germany	16/16, RCT	E: PT rehab + BCI-orthosis MA task: attempt to open and close the hand and arm extension C: PT rehab + sham BCI	The hand orthosis drives extending fingers, and arm orthosis assists the upper arm extension.	FMA-UE, GAS, MAL, MAS	40 min/d, 5 d/wk, 4 wk, 20 d	FMA-UE scores improved more in the experimental than in the control group, FMA-UE scores (3.41 ± 0.563, $p = 0.018$).
Angand Guan et al., 2014a [25]	Singapore	6/8, RCT	E: mobilization + BCI-robot MI task: imagine hand grasping C: mobilization + robot	The haptic knob robot for the hand grasping action.	FMA-UE	1.5 h/d, 3 d/wk, 6 wk, 18 d	FMA-UE score improved in all groups, but no intergroup differences were found at any time point.
Li et al., 2014a [15]	China	7/7, RCT	E: Con-rehab + BCI-FES, visual and auditory feedback MI task: imagine the upper extremity movements according to the direction of the arrow C: Con-rehab + FES	Once patients correctly imagined the movement five times in succession, FES was triggered, which stimulated the affected upper extremity's extensor carpus radialis muscles.	FMA-UE, ARAT, EEG	1–1.5 h/d, 3 d/wk, 24 d	A significant improvement in the motor function of the upper extremity for the BCI group was confirmed ($p < 0.05$ for ARAT), simultaneously with the activation of bilateral cerebral hemispheres.
Angand Chua et al., 2014a [26]	Singapore	11/14, RCT	E: BCI-Manus robot MI task: imagine moving the paretic arm and hand forward to reach for an imagery target in front of them and to reach the clock-face target C: Manus robot	passive resistance-free movement of the paretic arm within the exoskeletal arm from the center toward the target displayed on the screen, along with visual feedback.	FMA-UE	1.5 h/d, 3 d/wk, 4 wk, 12 d	No intergroup differences ($p = 0.51$).
Rayegani et al., 2014a [27]	Iran	10/10, RCT	E: con-rehab + BCI-visual feedback MI task: contract the abductor pollicis brevis muscle and perform thumb opposition C: Con-rehab	Patients were provided with visual and audio feedback by watching the contractions on the screen as a game (puzzle).	JHFT	30 min/d, 5 d/wk, 2 wk, 10 d	No intergroup differences.
Ang et al., 2015a [16]	Singapore	10/9, RCT	E: tDCS + BCI- robot MI task: imagine moving their stroke-affected hand toward the target indicated on the 8-point clock-face video game. C: sham tDCS + BCI- robot	Passive resistance-free movement of the paretic arm within the exoskeletal arm from the center toward the target is displayed on the screen, along with visual feedback.	FMA-UE	1 h/d, 5 d/wk, 2 wk	No intergroup differences. Online accuracies of the evaluation part from the tDCS group were significantly higher than those from the sham group.
Pichiorri et al., 2015a [28]	Italy	14/14, RCT	E: con-rehab + BCI-visual feedback MI task: imaging a sustained grasping movement and sustained complete extension of the finger. C: con-rehab+ MI	A simulated hand was projected to demonstrate the imaginary movement as the visual feedback.	FMA-UE, MAS, EEG	30 min/d, 3 d/wk, 4 wk. 12 d	The FMA-UE score improved ($p < 0.03$) in the BCI group.
Kim et al., 2016 [29]	USA Korea	15/15, RCT	E: con-rehab + AOT + BCI-FES ME: Participants performed 18 action observational tasks related to their daily living by watching DVDs of a sequence of movements that should be performed with their own hands including (1) folding a towel, (2) cutting a toilet roll, (3) using scissors, (4) tightening shoelaces, (5) opening and closing a square airtight container, (6) opening a bottle top, (7) turning a faucet, etc. C: con-rehab	If patients correctly imagined the movement and their attention level went up to the attention threshold, FES was triggered and stimulated wrist extensor muscles of the affected upper extremity.	FMA-UE, MAL, MBI	30 min/d, 5 d/wk, 4 wk, 20 d	The FMA-UE was significantly higher in the BCI-FES group ($p < 0.05$).

Table 2. *Cont.*

Study, Year	Country	n(E/C), Study Design	Experimental (E)/Control Group (C)	Feedback	Outcome Measures	Dosage	Main Results
Frolov et al., 2017a [30]	Russia	55/19, RCT	E: Con-rehab + BCI-arm exoskeleton MI task: Kinesthetic imagination of a continuous opening of the right hand and the left hand. C: Con-rehab + sham BCI	The hand exoskeleton helped patients to extend their fingers.	FMA-UE, ARAT	30 min/d, 3 d/wk, 12 d	Both groups improved in FMA-UL. Upon training completion, 21.8% and 36.4% of the patients in the BCI group improved their ARAT and FMA-UE scores respectively.
Biasiucci et al., 2018a [7]	Switzerland	14/13, RCT	E: BCI-FES MA task: attempt to extend the affected hand, fingers, and wrist. C: Sham BCI	If a "movement attempt" was detected, FES was triggered, with which a single bipolar channel is applied on the affected limb to inject current into the extensor digitorum communis muscle.	FMA-UE, MRC, MAS, EEG	1 h/d, 2 d/wk, 5 wk	BCI patients exhibit a significant functional recovery after the intervention. EEG analysis pinpoints significant differences in favor of the BCI group, mainly consisting of an increase in FC between motor areas in the ipsilesional hemisphere.
Ramos-Murguialday et al., 2019a [31]	Germany	16/12, RCT	E: PT rehab + BCI-orthosis MA task: instructed to try to move their paretic upper limb. (1) open and close the fingers or (2) move the paretic upper limb forward and backward. C: PT rehab + Sham BCI	The robotic orthosis was used to open and close the fingers or move the paretic upper limb forward and backward just like the given motor task.	FMA-UE, GAS, MAL, MAS	1 h/d, 5 d/wk, 4 wk, 20 d	The experimental group presented with FMA-UE scores significantly higher in Post2 (13.44 ± 1.96) as compared with the Pre-session (11.16 ± 1.73; $p = 0.015$).
Chen et al., 2020 [32]	China	7/7, RCT	E: BCI + exoskeleton + co-rehab MA task: attempt motion of wrist extension C: co-rehab	The exoskeleton drives the patients' affected hands to complete the wrist extension motion.	FMA-UE	40 min/d, 3 d/wk, 4 wk	Both the BCI group ($p = 0.032$) and the control group ($p = 0.048$) improved in FMA-UE scores.
Miao et al., 2020 [33]	China	8/8, RCT	E: BCI-FES + co-rehab MI task: KMI of wrist dorsiflexion C: co-rehab	Perform the MI task upon the appearance of the cue ("left" or "right"), the avatar would give the subjects visual feedback and the FES would be activated to cause the wrist dorsiflexion of the corresponding side.	FMA-UE	40 min/d, 3 d/wk, 4 wk	The average improvement score of the BCI group was 3.5, which was higher than that of the control group (0.9).
Cheng et al., 2020 [34]	Singapore	5/5, RCT	E: BCI-SRG + Soft Robotic Glove C: Soft Robotic Glove	Imagine ADL movement, like scanning goods, moving an object upward to a cabinet, etc.	FMA-UE, ARAT	120 min/d, 3 d/wk, 6 wk	No intergroup differences.
Chen et al., 2021 [35]	China	16/16, RCT	E: BCI-FES MI task: wrist-extension C: NMES	The electrode slices were attached to the skin above the two ends of the extensor carpi ulnaris	FMA-UE	40 min/d, 4 d/wk, 3 wk.	The FMA-UE was significantly higher than that in the sham group.

Abbr: Brain–computer interfaces, BCI; Functional Electrical Stimulation, FES; Neuromuscular Electrical Stimulation, NMES; the Fugl–Meyer Assessment Upper Extremity Scale, FMA-UE; Action Research Arm Test, ARAT; the Jebsen Hand Function Test, JHFT; the Goal Attainment Scale, GAS; Motor Activity Log, MAL; Modified Ashworth Scale, MAS; Electroencephalogram, EEG; Modified Barthel Index, MBI.

3.1. Motor Task

Detailed information about different kinds of BCI motor tasks such as MI, MA, and ME is listed as follows.

3.1.1. MI Task

The movement of the paretic hand is the main point in the design of the BCIs experiment. Imaging finger movements [25,36–38], including grasping alone, grasping, and opening [39–41], was applied in several experiments. Ang et al. [25] recruited stroke patients to receive hand grasp motor imagery training, and the control group received robot training. Finger extension imagery is still common in trials. Rayegani et al. [27] instructed the experimental group to contract the abductor pollicis brevis muscle and perform thumb opposition. Pichiorri et al. [28] assigned the MI task to imagine a sustained grasping movement and sustained complete extension of the finger. In Frolov et al.'s experiment [30], the experimental group received BCI-arm exoskeleton training, and the patients kinesthetically imagine a continuous opening of the right hand and the left hand.

Motor tasks may also involve movements of multiple joints, including the joints of the shoulder, elbow, and wrist. In several BCI research, patients were instructed to imagine the extension of the wrist [33,35]. Angand Chua et al. [26] instructed patients to imagine their paralyzed hands to reach out and reach the clock-face target on the computer screen. In another experiment [16], patients who were severely injured were enrolled and divided into two groups. The motor task was to imagine moving their affected hand toward the target indicated on the 8-point clock face on the computer screen. Stroke patients were recruited by Li et al. [15] to test the efficacy of MI-based BCIs training. Before treatment, the subjects in the BCI group were trained to complete MI tasks for effectively performing MI. They were trained to practice the experienced task, such as drinking water, and complete the MI task through a video by the unaffected hand. Then during the training course, the subjects were instructed to imagine the upper extremity movements according to the direction of the arrow following the voice "Begin to imagine left/right" and the randomized green arrow with a left or right command showing on the computer screen. In Cheng's study [34], they designed some movements from activities of daily living (ADL), such as scanning goods, moving an object upward to a cabinet, using two hands to move a towel, pouring water into a cup, eating actions, and fine motor movement of picking up a small block using two fingers. The MI task was imagining arm movements and was matched to the performance of the ADL movements that were talked about above.

3.1.2. MA Task

Attempting to extend fingers has also been applied in some experiments. Biasiucci et al. [7] asked the patients to attempt to extend or rest the affected hand (both fingers and wrist). Chen et al. [32] designed a study for subacute stroke patients, in which the BCIs group patients attempted to extend the wrist of the paretic hand. Ramos–Murguialday et al. [17] conducted a randomized controlled clinical trial, and trained patients to move the upper limb and reach forward with the help of arm orthosis. When the patients heard the corresponding auditory cue, they were instructed to try to reach, grasp, and bring an imaginary apple to their lap, and finger extension was involved in the reaching and grasping movement. In another study [31], patients were instructed to try to move their paretic upper limb to open and close the fingers or move forward and backward.

3.2. *Different Feedback for the Motor Tasks*

There are various types of feedback in MI or MA tasks for hand grasping and extension, including visual, auditory, tactile, and proprioceptive feedback.

3.2.1. Visual

Visual feedback is a common choice for the BCIs experiment [16,27,28,34], and it is often presented as a computer screen or projection screen. In practice, patients watch the muscle contractions on the screen [27] as a game or some curtain displaying the simulated hand which demonstrated the imaginary movement [27,28]. In some combination cases, visual and movement feedback was provided by the Manus shoulder–elbow robot, and the exoskeleton assist the paretic arm moved from the center to the target displayed on the screen and back along a predetermined robotic trajectory [16,26].

3.2.2. Proprioception

(1) Orthosis

The orthosis was used to assist the paretic limb to move. In some research, the paretic hand was attached to the orthosis to drive fingers extending (hand opening), and other researchers used arm orthosis (reaching) to assist the upper arm extension. The arm and hand orthoses targeted the patient's ability to open and close the hand [17]. In another study [31], robotic orthosis was used to open and close fingers or move the paretic upper limb forward and backward just like the given motor task. The level of paresis determined the kind of movement to be performed during BCIs training, but all patients performed the movement of opening and closing the fingers. When the mu ERD was detected after the cue instruction to imagine finger extension, the star-shaped cursor moved down on the screen as visual feedback, and then the motor-driven orthosis extended their affected fingers [42].

(2) Robot

The robot used in BCIs is usually in the active-assist mode. The active assist mode likely generates greater proprioceptive sensory signals to the brain than the active non-assist mode does [43]. The Haptic Knob robot helped with the hand-grasping action [25]. They carried out an MI-based BCIs and tactile selective attention experiment. In the MI group, kinesthetic motor imaging (KMI) of the left or right hand was performed according to the direction of the arrow presented on the screen. In the tactile selective attention group, vibration stimulation of the left and right thumbs was implemented. Some KMI movements may be designed with ADL movements, and their feedback from the soft robotic glove is moving the fingers [34].

(3) Exoskeleton

The exoskeleton was also applied in a BCI designed to produce proprioceptive feedback. Frolov et al. [30] instructed patients to imagine the extension of their left or right hand, and the exoskeleton helped them to extend their fingers after receiving the commands. After the BCIs system correctly recognized the intention of the patient's motor attempt, it would output command and manipulate the exoskeleton, driving the patient's affected hands to complete the wrist extension motion [32].

(4) FES

The FES can also be used as feedback in the BCIs system. When patients correctly imagined the movement and their attention level went up the attention threshold, FES was triggered and stimulated wrist extensor muscles of the affected upper extremity. If a "movement attempt" was detected, FES would be triggered, with which a single bipolar channel was applied on the affected limb to inject current into the extensor digitorum communis muscle [7], and the threshold that initiated FES was adjusted after each run for each patient by the therapist, to determine the task difficulty. The FES can act on any muscle as requested, such as extensor carpus radialis muscles [15] or extensor carpi ulnaris [35].

4. Discussion

We summarized the commonly used MI/MA tasks in the BCI experiments. MI [44] refers to mental activity that involves specific movements without actual movement. An example of kinesthetic motor imaging involves imagining the feeling of the hand opening from the perspective of the first person while maintaining muscle relaxation. MA [45] is attempting to move the paralyzed limb while there is still no actual or little movement, and the electromyography (EMG) activities in the affected arm are several times higher during the motion phase than those in the rest phase. MI has been considered a therapy for promoting motor recovery after stroke [46], and they were often connected to the BCIs equipment. BCI has been proven to be effective in subacute and chronic stages of hand recovery of stroke patients. However, patients might encounter kinds of hand recovery difficulties during their rehabilitation courses. In the literature we have referred to, for the MI task, hand-grasping imagery [25,36–38], involving grasping alone, grasping, and opening [39–41], was applied in several BCIs studies. Finger extension imagery is also common in the BCI trials [27,28,30,42]. In some research, patients were instructed to imagine the extension movement of the wrist [33,35]. Grasping and opening are basic functions of a hand, and many motor tasks were designed based on these motions. At the same time, motor tasks may also involve movements of multiple joints, including the joints of the shoulder, elbow, and wrist [15,16,26,34]. As for the motor attempt task, attempting to extend fingers has also been carried out in several experiments [7,17,31,32].

There are various types of feedback in MI or MA tasks for hand grasping and extension, including visual, auditory, tactile, and proprioceptive feedback. Many experiments are designed from their combinations. Proprioception was more frequently used and in a variety of forms, including orthosis [17,25,31,42], robot [16,25,26], exoskeleton [30,32], and functional electrical stimulation (FES) [7,15,29]. We analyzed the specific motor task adopted in BCI experiments. Some researchers trained patients on the MI ability before the treatment to obtain good training effects, some may increase the threshold that initiates the FES to enhance task difficulties, and other experiments set two tasks for hand and arm with the help of a specific robotic orthosis.

As is known to all, motor recovery and functional improvements mainly depend on motor training, and task-based motor relearning is also important for hand rehabilitation after a stroke. After repetitive motor training, the motor function improved following the brain plasticity. Although motor tasks are an essential and non-negligible part of a BCI system, how to choose a motor task of the BCI training system for a stroke patient with hand motor dysfunction remains an unsolved problem, and is of great importance to their clinical outcome. MI and MA tasks are common experimental paradigms in EEG-based BCIs trials. They were used in post-stroke hand function rehabilitation. Patients who received BCIs training were asked to perform motor tasks of different motions. These motions included grasping, fingers extending, and wrist extending. All these motor tasks designed are essential for rehabilitative BCIs. From a meta-analysis published recently [24], we have known that MA in BCIs training appears to be more effective than MI, and we believe that MA may be a better choice in BCIs trials, especially since the task can be referred to the functional status in stroke patients. However, for people with different levels of hand motor impairments, what kind of motor task should be designed for them? As has been mentioned above, the Brunnstrom stage recovery rule for stroke can be an indication for study design. During the recovery, the process from no to mild active movement and segregation movement is a difficult step, so setting the proper task is an urgent need. In Ramos–Murguialday et al. [31] research, they designed two motor tasks for different levels of paresis in stroke patients. Thus, according to the rules, we may mainly focus on patients' difficulties. For patients with no actual movement, we may focus on basic primary functions, such as grasp ability, with the help of embodied BCI feedback, to practice the motion repeatedly.

Different motor tasks may also match different types of feedback. The proprioceptive feedback is provided by an exoskeleton, orthosis, robots, or FES. In addition, virtual feedback can be another type of feedback that directly enters the brain. Feedback is a key element in motor rehabilitation in clinical work, and it has been reported to enhance brain plasticity and promote neural remodeling after rehabilitation training. Thus, varying modalities of feedback have been employed during BCI training. A combination of two or more feedback may create an enriched multi-element environment and be more helpful for stroke rehabilitation. Some studies have demonstrated that proprioceptive feedback is more suitable than visual feedback for entraining the motor network architecture during the interplay between motor imagery and feedback processing [47], and thus, it results in better volitional control of regional brain activity, but the two above are often combined in practice. In Bai et al.'s meta-analysis [24], they made a subgroup analysis, focusing on the relationship between different feedback and effectiveness. They mainly analyzed robot, FES, and visual feedback, and the results indicated that only BCIs triggering the stimulation of FES had a significantly larger effect size on motor function recovery, compared with control interventions. In Xie's meta-analysis [48], they considered BCI combined with FES or visual feedback may be a better combination for functional recovery than a robot.

However, up to now, the mechanism of BCI promotes motor recovery is not very clear. MI-based BCIs involve neural mechanisms that volitionally control the movement of the hand [21], guide nerve plasticity, and enhance the connection between the motor area and the ipsilesional hemisphere [6]. Some studies have shown that after BCI training, the sensorimotor cortex of the ipsilesional hemisphere participates more, which might increase the excitability of the ipsilesional hemisphere [49,50] and change the rhythm of EEG, such as producing stronger ERD [15,28]. Patients with better SMR control may have higher functional improvements [51], and the performance of BCI is related to the improvement of motor function [15,30,52,53]. The proprioceptive sensory signals from these movements reach the motor cortex, the activation or continuous sensory input to the motor cortex of the ipsilesional hemisphere [21,54,55], and increase the afferent feedback, which has been considered useful for improving motor learning [56,57]. The recruitment of muscle spindles and Golgi tendon organs via FES may be effective. Some researchers believed that FES depolarized more motor and sensory axons, sending larger sensory volleys from muscle spindles and Golgi tendon organs into the central nervous system [58], FES or tactile input accompanying MI can produce stronger ERD [59,60], and the monosynaptic excitatory projections from spindles onto motoneurons may activate them concurrently with the presumed descending cortical command, thereby causing Hebbian association.

Facing the current need of patients as well as physicians, we need to design suitable motor tasks and choose corresponding BCI feedback to reach a higher hand function recovery after stroke. If a patient has difficulty extending fingers, the motor task can be designed as an attempt to extend fingers. Then the FES or the robot should assist the patient to extend fingers in an active-assist mode. Similarly, if a patient has difficulty flexing fingers, the motor task can be designed as an attempt to flex fingers and the FES or the robot will also be used as assistance with various feedback. However, there are some limitations to this review. First, our review only focuses on RCT. Thus, more motor tasks could not be presented. Second, the effects of different motor tasks and different feedback were not quantified. Future research should focus on neurophysiological changes and functional improvements and further elaboration on the changes in neurophysiology during the recovery of motor function, which may promote the development of BCI in the neurological field fundamentally.

5. Conclusions

To sum up, we focus on the motor tasks adopted in EEG-based BCIs research, as well as the corresponding feedback adopted in the BCI trial from the very perspective of the clinic. Many motor tasks involve imagining or attempting to grasp or extend the hand and were matched with the BCIs-triggered robot or FES combined with visual feedback. To optimize BCI rehabilitation training, we should focus on patients' difficulties during BCI training to help them to complete grasp motions, finger extension, thumb opposition, and other complex motions with the assistance of the robot or FES, or other combined feedback.

Supplementary Materials: The following supporting information can be downloaded at: https://www.mdpi.com/article/10.3390/brainsci13010056/s1, Supplementary material S1: SEARCH STRATEGY.

Author Contributions: J.F. and S.C. were involved in data collection; J.J. provided ideas and suggestions for the article; J.F. prepared Tables 1 and 2; J.F., S.C. and J.J. were involved in writing and editing the manuscript. All authors have read and agreed to the published version of the manuscript.

Funding: This research was funded by the National Key Research and Development Program Project of China (2018YFC2002300), the National Natural Integration Project (91948302), the National Natural Innovation Research Group Project (82021002), the National Natural Science Foundation of China (82202798), and the Shanghai Sailing Program (22YF1404200).

Institutional Review Board Statement: Not applicable.

Informed Consent Statement: Not applicable.

Data Availability Statement: The original contributions presented in the study are included in the article material, and further inquiries can be directed to the corresponding author.

Conflicts of Interest: The authors declare that they have no competing interest.

References

1. Wu, Y.; Gu, Y.; Rao, X.; Cheng, M.; Chen, P.; He, L. Stroke in China: Advances and challenges in epidemiology, prevention, and management. *Lancet Neurol.* **2019**, *18*, 394–405. [CrossRef] [PubMed]
2. Kwah, L.K.; Harvey, L.A.; Diong, J.; Herbert, R.D. Models containing age and NIHSS predict recovery of ambulation and upper limb function six months after stroke: An observational study. *J. Physiother.* **2013**, *59*, 189–197. [CrossRef] [PubMed]
3. Morris, J.H.; van Wijck, F.; Joice, S.; Donaghy, M. Predicting health related quality of life 6 months after stroke: The role of anxiety and upper limb dysfunction. *Disabil. Rehabil.* **2013**, *35*, 291–299. [CrossRef] [PubMed]
4. McEntire, C.R.; Choudhury, G.R.; Torres, A.; Steinberg, G.K.; Redmond Jr, D.E.; Daadi, M.M. Impaired Arm Function and Finger Dexterity in a Nonhuman Primate Model of Stroke. *Stroke* **2016**, *47*, 1109–1116. [CrossRef] [PubMed]

5. Baricich, A.; Picelli, A.; Santamato, A.; Carda, S.; de Sire, A.; Smania, N.; Cisari, C.; Invernizzi, M. Safety Profile of High-Dose Botulinum Toxin Type A in Post-Stroke Spasticity Treatment. *Clin. Drug. Investig.* **2018**, *38*, 991–1000. [CrossRef]
6. Cervera, M.A.; Soekadar, S.R.; Ushiba, J.; Millán, J.D.R.; Liu, M.; Birbaumer, N.; Garipelli, G. Brain-computer interfaces for post-stroke motor rehabilitation: A meta-analysis. *Ann. Clin. Transl. Neurol.* **2018**, *5*, 651–663. [CrossRef]
7. Biasiucci, A.; Leeb, R.; Iturrate, I.; Perdikis, S.; Al-Khodairy, A.; Corbet, T.; Schnider, A.; Schmidlin, T.; Zhang, H.; Bassolino, M.; et al. Brain-actuated functional electrical stimulation elicits lasting arm motor recovery after stroke. *Nat. Commun.* **2018**, *9*, 2421. [CrossRef]
8. Baniqued, P.D.E.; Stanyer, E.C.; Awais, M.; Alazmani, A.; Jackson, A.E.; Mon-Williams, M.A.; Mushtaq, F.; Holt, R.J. Brain–computer interface robotics for hand rehabilitation after stroke: A systematic review. *J. Neuroeng. Rehabil.* **2021**, *18*, 15. [CrossRef]
9. Abbasi, J. Advanced Brain-Computer Interface for People with Paralysis. *JAMA* **2019**, *321*, 537. [CrossRef]
10. Vansteensel, M.J.; Pels, E.G.; Bleichner, M.G.; Branco, M.P.; Denison, T.; Freudenburg, Z.V.; Gosselaar, P.; Leinders, S.; Ottens, T.H.; Van Den Boom, M.A.; et al. Fully Implanted Brain–Computer Interface in a Locked-In Patient with ALS. *N. Engl. J. Med.* **2016**, *375*, 2060–2066. [CrossRef]
11. Ajiboye, A.B.; Willett, F.R.; Young, D.R.; Memberg, W.D.; Murphy, B.A.; Miller, J.P.; Walter, B.L.; Sweet, J.A.; Hoyen, H.A.; Keith, M.W.; et al. Restoration of reaching and grasping movements through brain-controlled muscle stimulation in a person with tetraplegia: A proof-of-concept demonstration. *Lancet* **2017**, *389*, 1821–1830. [CrossRef] [PubMed]
12. Hochberg, L.R.; Bacher, D.; Jarosiewicz, B.; Masse, N.Y.; Simeral, J.D.; Vogel, J.; Haddadin, S.; Liu, J.; Cash, S.S.; Van Der Smagt, P.; et al. Reach and grasp by people with tetraplegia using a neurally controlled robotic arm. *Nature* **2012**, *485*, 372–375. [CrossRef]
13. Silvoni, S.; Ramos-Murguialday, A.; Cavinato, M.; Volpato, C.; Cisotto, G.; Turolla, A.; Piccione, F.; Birbaumer, N. Brain-computer interface in stroke: A review of progress. *Clin. Eeg. Neurosci.* **2011**, *42*, 245–252. [CrossRef] [PubMed]
14. Sitaram, R.; Ros, T.; Stoeckel, L.; Haller, S.; Scharnowski, F.; Lewis-Peacock, J.; Weiskopf, N.; Blefari, M.L.; Rana, M.; Oblak, E.; et al. Closed-loop brain training: The science of neurofeedback. *Nat. Rev. Neurosci.* **2017**, *18*, 86–100. [CrossRef] [PubMed]
15. Li, M.; Liu, Y.; Wu, Y.; Liu, S.; Jia, J.; Zhang, L. Neurophysiological substrates of stroke patients with motor imagery-based brain-computer interface training. *Int. J. Neurosci.* **2014**, *124*, 403–415. [CrossRef]
16. Ang, K.K.; Guan, C.; Phua, K.S.; Wang, C.; Zhao, L.; Teo, W.P.; Chen, C.; Ng, Y.S.; Chew, E. Facilitating Effects of Transcranial Direct Current Stimulation on Motor Imagery Brain-Computer Interface With Robotic Feedback for Stroke Rehabilitation. *Arch. Phys. Med. Rehab.* **2015**, *96*, S79–S87. [CrossRef]
17. Ramos-Murguialday, A.; Broetz, D.; Rea, M.; Läer, L.; Yilmaz, Ö.; Brasil, F.L.; Liberati, G.; Curado, M.R.; Garcia-Cossio, E.; Vyziotis, A.; et al. Brain-machine interface in chronic stroke rehabilitation: A controlled study. *Ann. Neurol.* **2013**, *74*, 100–108. [CrossRef]
18. Robinson, N.; Thomas, K.P.; Vinod, A.P. Neurophysiological predictors and spectro-spatial discriminative features for enhancing SMR-BCI. *J. Neural Eng.* **2018**, *15*, 66032. [CrossRef]
19. Chang, H.; Yang, J. Genetic-based feature selection for efficient motion imaging of a brain-computer interface framework. *J. Neural Eng.* **2018**, *15*, 56020. [CrossRef]
20. Perry, C.E. Principles and techniques of the Brunnstrom approach to the treatment of hemiplegia. *Am. J. Phys. Med.* **1967**, *46*, 789–815.
21. Remsik, A.; Young, B.; Vermilyea, R.; Kiekhoefer, L.; Abrams, J.; Evander Elmore, S.; Schultz, P.; Nair, V.; Edwards, D.; Williams, J.; et al. A review of the progression and future implications of brain-computer interface therapies for restoration of distal upper extremity motor function after stroke. *Expert Rev. Med. Devic.* **2016**, *13*, 445–454. [CrossRef] [PubMed]
22. Monge-Pereira, E.; Ibañez-Pereda, J.; Alguacil-Diego, I.M.; Serrano, J.I.; Spottorno-Rubio, M.P.; Molina-Rueda, F. Use of Electroencephalography Brain-Computer Interface Systems as a Rehabilitative Approach for Upper Limb Function After a Stroke: A Systematic Review. *PM R* **2017**, *9*, 918–932. [CrossRef] [PubMed]
23. Carvalho, R.; Dias, N.; Cerqueira, J.J. Brain-machine interface of upper limb recovery in stroke patients rehabilitation: A systematic review. *Physiother. Res. Int.* **2019**, *24*, e1764. [CrossRef] [PubMed]
24. Bai, Z.; Fong, K.N.K.; Zhang, J.J.; Chan, J.; Ting, K.H. Immediate and long-term effects of BCI-based rehabilitation of the upper extremity after stroke: A systematic review and meta-analysis. *J. Neuroeng. Rehabil.* **2020**, *17*, 57. [CrossRef]
25. Ang, K.K.; Guan, C.; Phua, K.S.; Wang, C.; Zhou, L.; Tang, K.Y.; Ephraim Joseph, G.J.; Kuah, C.W.K.; Chua, K.S.G. Brain-computer interface-based robotic end effector system for wrist and hand rehabilitation: Results of a three-armed randomized controlled trial for chronic stroke. *Front. Neuroeng.* **2014**, *7*, 30. [CrossRef] [PubMed]
26. Ang, K.K.; Chua, K.S.G.; Phua, K.S.; Wang, C.; Chin, Z.Y.; Kuah, C.W.K.; Low, W.; Guan, C. A Randomized Controlled Trial of EEG-Based Motor Imagery Brain-Computer Interface Robotic Rehabilitation for Stroke. *Clin. EEG Neurosci.* **2014**, *46*, 310–320. [CrossRef]
27. Rayegani, S.M.; Raeissadat, S.A.; Sedighipour, L.; Mohammad Rezazadeh, I.; Bahrami, M.H.; Eliaspour, D.; Khosrawi, S. Effect of Neurofeedback and Electromyographic-Biofeedback Therapy on Improving Hand Function in Stroke Patients. *Top. Stroke Rehabil.* **2014**, *21*, 137–151. [CrossRef]
28. Pichiorri, F.; Morone, G.; Petti, M.; Toppi, J.; Pisotta, I.; Molinari, M.; Paolucci, S.; Inghilleri, M.; Astolfi, L.; Cincotti, F.; et al. Brain-computer interface boosts motor imagery practice during stroke recovery. *Ann. Neurol.* **2015**, *77*, 851–865. [CrossRef]

29. Kim, T.; Kim, S.; Lee, B. Effects of Action Observational Training Plus Brain-Computer Interface-Based Functional Electrical Stimulation on Paretic Arm Motor Recovery in Patient with Stroke: A Randomized Controlled Trial. *Occup. Ther. Int.* **2016**, *23*, 39–47. [CrossRef]
30. Frolov, A.A.; Mokienko, O.; Lyukmanov, R.; Biryukova, E.; Kotov, S.; Turbina, L.; Nadareyshvily, G.; Bushkova, Y. Post-stroke Rehabilitation Training with a Motor-Imagery-Based Brain-Computer Interface (BCI)-Controlled Hand Exoskeleton: A Randomized Controlled Multicenter Trial. *Front. Neurosci.-Switz.* **2017**, *11*, 400. [CrossRef]
31. Ramos-Murguialday, A.; Curado, M.R.; Broetz, D.; Yilmaz, Ö.; Brasil, F.L.; Liberati, G.; Garcia-Cossio, E.; Cho, W.; Caria, A.; Cohen, L.G.; et al. Brain-Machine Interface in Chronic Stroke: Randomized Trial Long-Term Follow-up. *Neurorehabilit. Neural Repair* **2019**, *33*, 188–198. [CrossRef]
32. Chen, S.; Cao, L.; Shu, X.; Wang, H.; Ding, L.; Wang, S.H.; Jia, J. Longitudinal Electroencephalography Analysis in Subacute Stroke Patients During Intervention of Brain-Computer Interface With Exoskeleton Feedback. *Front. Neurosci.-Switz.* **2020**, *14*, 809. [CrossRef] [PubMed]
33. Miao, Y.; Chen, S.; Zhang, X.; Jin, J.; Xu, R.; Daly, I.; Jia, J.; Wang, X.; Cichocki, A.; Jung, T.P. BCI-Based Rehabilitation on the Stroke in Sequela Stage. *Neural Plast.* **2020**, *2020*, 8882764. [CrossRef] [PubMed]
34. Cheng, N.; Phua, K.S.; Lai, H.S.; Tam, P.K.; Tang, K.Y.; Cheng, K.K.; Yeow, R.C.H.; Ang, K.K.; Guan, C.; Lim, J.H. Brain-Computer Interface-Based Soft Robotic Glove Rehabilitation for Stroke. *IEEE. Trans. Biomed. Eng.* **2020**, *67*, 3339–3351. [CrossRef] [PubMed]
35. Chen, L.; Gu, B.; Wang, Z.; Zhang, L.; Xu, M.; Liu, S.; He, F.; Ming, D. EEG-controlled functional electrical stimulation rehabilitation for chronic stroke: System design and clinical application. *Front. Med.* **2021**, *15*, 740–749. [CrossRef] [PubMed]
36. Buch, E.R.; Modir Shanechi, A.; Fourkas, A.D.; Weber, C.; Birbaumer, N.; Cohen, L.G. Parietofrontal integrity determines neural modulation associated with grasping imagery after stroke. *Brain* **2012**, *135*, 596–614. [CrossRef] [PubMed]
37. Darvishi, S.; Gharabaghi, A.; Boulay, C.B.; Ridding, M.C.; Abbott, D.; Baumert, M. Proprioceptive Feedback Facilitates Motor Imagery-Related Operant Learning of Sensorimotor β-Band Modulation. *Front. Neurosci.* **2017**, *11*, 60. [CrossRef] [PubMed]
38. Pichiorri, F.; Fallani, F.D.V.; Cincotti, F.; Babiloni, F.; Molinari, M.; Kleih, S.C.; Neuper, C.; Kübler, A.; Mattia, D. Sensorimotor rhythm-based brain–computer interface training: The impact on motor cortical responsiveness. *J. Neural Eng.* **2011**, *8*, 25020. [CrossRef]
39. Nagai, H.; Tanaka, T. Action Observation of Own Hand Movement Enhances Event-Related Desynchronization. *IEEE. Trans. Neural Syst. Rehabil.* **2019**, *27*, 1407–1415. [CrossRef]
40. Kaiser, V.; Daly, I.; Pichiorri, F.; Mattia, D.; Müller-Putz, G.R.; Neuper, C. Relationship Between Electrical Brain Responses to Motor Imagery and Motor Impairment in Stroke. *Stroke* **2012**, *43*, 2735–2740. [CrossRef]
41. Broetz, D.; Braun, C.; Weber, C.; Soekadar, S.R.; Caria, A.; Birbaumer, N. Combination of Brain-Computer Interface Training and Goal-Directed Physical Therapy in Chronic Stroke: A Case Report. *Neurorehabilit. Neural Repair* **2010**, *24*, 674–679. [CrossRef] [PubMed]
42. Kasashima-Shindo, Y.; Fujiwara, T.; Ushiba, J.; Matsushika, Y.; Kamatani, D.; Oto, M.; Ono, T.; Nishimoto, A.; Shindo, K.; Kawakami, M.; et al. Brain-computer interface training combined with transcranial direct current stimulation in patients with chronic severe hemiparesis: Proof of concept study. *J. Rehabil. Med.* **2015**, *47*, 318–324. [CrossRef] [PubMed]
43. Takahashi, C.D.; Der-Yeghiaian, L.; Le, V.; Motiwala, R.R.; Cramer, S.C. Robot-based hand motor therapy after stroke. *Brain.* **2008**, *131*, 425–437. [CrossRef] [PubMed]
44. Kilteni, K.; Andersson, B.J.; Houborg, C.; Ehrsson, H.H. Motor imagery involves predicting the sensory consequences of the imagined movement. *Nat. Commun.* **2018**, *9*, 1617. [CrossRef]
45. Antelis, J.M.; Montesano, L.; Ramos-Murguialday, A.; Birbaumer, N.; Minguez, J. Decoding Upper Limb Movement Attempt from EEG Measurements of the Contralesional Motor Cortex in Chronic Stroke Patients. *IEEE Trans. Biomed. Eng.* **2017**, *64*, 99–111. [CrossRef]
46. Sharma, N.; Simmons, L.H.; Jones, P.S.; Day, D.J.; Carpenter, T.A.; Pomeroy, V.M.; Warburton, E.A.; Baron, J.C. Motor imagery after subcortical stroke: A functional magnetic resonance imaging study. *Stroke* **2009**, *40*, 1315–1324. [CrossRef] [PubMed]
47. Vukelić, M.; Gharabaghi, A. Oscillatory entrainment of the motor cortical network during motor imagery is modulated by the feedback modality. *Neuroimage* **2015**, *111*, 1–11. [CrossRef]
48. Xie, Y.L.; Yang, Y.X.; Jiang, H.; Duan, X.Y.; Gu, L.J.; Qing, W.; Zhang, B. Brain-machine interface-based training for improving upper extremity function after stroke: A meta-analysis of randomized controlled trials. *Front. Neurosci.* **2022**, *16*, 949575. [CrossRef]
49. Sehle, A.; Stuerner, J.; Hassa, T.; Spiteri, S.; Schoenfeld, M.A.; Liepert, J. Behavioral and neurophysiological effects of an intensified robot-assisted therapy in subacute stroke: A case control study. *J. Neuroeng. Rehabil.* **2021**, *18*, 6. [CrossRef]
50. Singh, N.; Saini, M.; Kumar, N.; Srivastava, M.V.P.; Mehndiratta, A. Evidence of neuroplasticity with robotic hand exoskeleton for post-stroke rehabilitation: A randomized controlled trial. *J. Neuroeng. Rehabil.* **2021**, *18*, 76. [CrossRef]
51. Norman, S.L.; McFarland, D.J.; Miner, A.; Cramer, S.C.; Wolbrecht, E.T.; Wolpaw, J.R.; Reinkensmeyer, D.J. Controlling pre-movement sensorimotor rhythm can improve finger extension after stroke. *J. Neural Eng.* **2018**, *15*, 56026. [CrossRef] [PubMed]
52. Naros, G.; Naros, I.; Grimm, F.; Ziemann, U.; Gharabaghi, A. Reinforcement learning of self-regulated sensorimotor β-oscillations improves motor performance. *Neuroimage* **2016**, *134*, 142–152. [CrossRef] [PubMed]

53. Bundy, D.T.; Souders, L.; Baranyai, K.; Leonard, L.; Schalk, G.; Coker, R.; Moran, D.W.; Huskey, T.; Leuthardt, E.C. Contralesional Brain–Computer Interface Control of a Powered Exoskeleton for Motor Recovery in Chronic Stroke Survivors. *Stroke* **2017**, *48*, 1908–1915. [CrossRef] [PubMed]
54. Ono, T.; Shindo, K.; Kawashima, K.; Ota, N.; Ito, M.; Ota, T.; Mukaino, M.; Fujiwara, T.; Kimura, A.; Liu, M.; et al. Brain-computer interface with somatosensory feedback improves functional recovery from severe hemiplegia due to chronic stroke. *Front. Neuroeng.* **2014**, *7*, 19. [CrossRef] [PubMed]
55. Soekadar, S.R.; Birbaumer, N.; Slutzky, M.W.; Cohen, L.G. Brain–machine interfaces in neurorehabilitation of stroke. *Neurobiol. Dis.* **2015**, *83*, 172–179. [CrossRef] [PubMed]
56. Poon, C.S. Sensorimotor learning and information processing by Bayesian internal models. *Conf. Proc. IEEE Eng. Med. Biol. Soc.* **2004**, *2004*, 4481–4482.
57. Rossini, P.M.; Dal Forno, G. Integrated technology for evaluation of brain function and neural plasticity. *Phys. Med. Rehabil. Clin. N. Am.* **2004**, *15*, 263–306. [CrossRef]
58. Bergquist, A.J.; Clair, J.M.; Lagerquist, O.; Mang, C.S.; Okuma, Y.; Collins, D.F. Neuromuscular electrical stimulation: Implications of the electrically evoked sensory volley. *Eur. J. Appl. Physiol.* **2011**, *111*, 2409–2426. [CrossRef]
59. Shu, X.; Chen, S.; Meng, J.; Yao, L.; Sheng, X.; Jia, J.; Farina, D.; Zhu, X. Tactile Stimulation Improves Sensorimotor Rhythm-based BCI Performance in Stroke Patients. *IEEE Trans. Biomed. Eng.* **2018**, *6*, 1987–1995. [CrossRef]
60. Reynolds, C.; Osuagwu, B.A.; Vuckovic, A. Influence of motor imagination on cortical activation during functional electrical stimulation. *Clin. Neurophysiol.* **2015**, *126*, 1360–1369. [CrossRef]

brain sciences

Article

Application of Multi-Dimensional Intelligent Visual Quantitative Assessment System to Evaluate Hand Function Rehabilitation in Stroke Patients

Yuying Du [1], Yu Shi [1], Hongmei Ma [1], Dong Li [1], Ting Su [1], Ou Zhabayier Meidege [1], Baolan Wang [1,*] and Xiaofeng Lu [2,*]

[1] Department of Rehabilitation Medicine, The First Affiliated Hospital of Xinjiang Medical University, Urumqi 830054, China
[2] School of Communication and Information Engineering, Shanghai University, Shanghai 200444, China
* Correspondence: wbl0308@163.com (B.W.); luxiaofeng@shu.edu.cn (X.L.)

Abstract: Background: Hand dysfunction is one of the main symptoms of stroke patients, but there is still a lack of accurate hand function assessment systems. This study focused on the application of the multi-dimensional intelligent visual quantitative assessment system (MDIVQAS) in the rehabilitation assessment of hand function in stroke patients and evaluate hand function rehabilitation in stroke patients. Methods: Eighty-two patients with stroke and unilateral hand dysfunction were evaluated by MDIVQAS. Cronbach's Alpha coefficient was used to assess the internal consistency of MDIVQAS; the F-test is used to assess the differences in MDIVQAS for multiple repeated measures. Spearman's analysis was used to identify correlations of MDIVQAS with other assessment systems. *t*-tests were used to identify differences in outcomes assessed with MDIVQAS in patients before and after treatment. $p < 0.05$ were considered significant. Results: (1) Cronbach's Alpha coefficient of MDIVQAS in evaluating hand's function > 0.9. (2) There was no significant difference between the other repeated measurements, except for thumb rotation in MDIVQAS. (3) MDIVQAS had a significant correlation with other assessment systems ($r > 0.5$, $p < 0.01$). (4) There were significant differences in the evaluation of hand function in patients before and after treatment using MDIVQAS. Conclusion: The MDIVQAS system has good reliability and validity in the evaluation of stroke hand function, and it can also better evaluate the treatment effect.

Keywords: assessment; rehabilitation; stroke; upper extremity; hand

Citation: Du, Y.; Shi, Y.; Ma, H.; Li, D.; Su, T.; Meidege, O.Z.; Wang, B.; Lu, X. Application of Multi-Dimensional Intelligent Visual Quantitative Assessment System to Evaluate Hand Function Rehabilitation in Stroke Patients. *Brain Sci.* **2022**, *12*, 1698. https://doi.org/10.3390/brainsci12121698

Academic Editors: Jie Jia, Yan Hu, Dingguo Zhang and Konstantin V. Slavin

Received: 7 November 2022
Accepted: 7 December 2022
Published: 10 December 2022

1. Introduction

Stroke is a major noncommunicable disease that harms the health of people all over the world. As of 2019, stroke is the second leading cause of death worldwide and the third leading cause of death caused by disability. From 1990 to 2019, the disability rate caused by stroke increased by 32.0% [1], and 70% to 90% of patients after stroke have upper limb dysfunction [2,3], 60–70% of them with hand dysfunction [1,4]. As one of the most important organs of the human body, the hand is involved in many daily activities, and its function accounts for 90% of the upper limb function. Hand dysfunction seriously affects patients' daily life and social participation ability [5]. Rehabilitation therapy is an important method to restore hand function, and accurate treatment is based on an accurate assessment. At present, the commonly used methods for assessing hand function after stroke are mainly qualitative or semi-quantitative, which mainly include the protractor measurement of Active Range of Motion (AROM), FMA-UE, FMA-W/H, Brunnstrom, ARAT and so on. The above evaluation methods have been widely used in clinical practice for a long time, and their reliability and validity are also widely recognized. However, the actual application is easily influenced by personal experience [6–9]. Therefore, there is great interest in developing an automated system to achieve intelligent, objective and quantitative assessment of hand function rehabilitation after stroke. In the last two decades, significant advances have been made in human motion measurement and analysis, providing the technical basis for automated assessment of upper limb and hand function [10]. In recent years, modern methods for quantitative hand function assessment include the 3D motion capture system, Kinect technology, rehabilitation robots and micro sensors, etc. However, the above instruments are still lacking in large sample studies, and some instruments are too bulky and have not been widely used in clinical practice [11–13].

In clinical rehabilitation work, intelligent, quantitative, accurate and efficient hand function assessment tools are needed to provide a better choice for clinical practice. Therefore, this study uses a newly developed intelligent assessment method, application of multi-dimensional intelligent visual quantitative evaluation system (MDIVQAS) to objectively and quantitatively assess the function of the affected hand after stroke.

MDIVAQAS is the core technology of hand motion calculation jointly developed by Huashan Hospital affiliated with Fudan University and Shanghai University with completely independent intellectual property rights. Through the optical smart capture and the integration of computer vision technology, complete animation action standard hand more guidance, the contralateral national health model and subject to lateral hand evaluation process, belongs to the field initiative, and it can complete the quantitative assessment of hand function. The purpose of this study was to verify the reliability of MDIVQAS, and to observe the evaluation effect of the system in clinical application compared with traditional evaluation methods.

2. Materials and Methods

2.1. General Information

Using the pwr package and WebPower package in R, it is assumed that there is a large effect size, statistical testing power 1-β = 0.8 and significance level a = 0.05, and the minimum sample size required for each stage is calculated. From November 2019 to October 2021, 88 stroke patients who met the inclusion criteria and signed informed consent in the Department of Rehabilitation Medicine, the First Affiliated Hospital of Xinjiang Medical University were selected. Inclusion criteria: ① The diagnosis was in line with the diagnostic criteria for stroke (including cerebral infarction and cerebral hemorrhage) formulated by the Cerebrovascular Department of the Neurology Branch of the Chinese Medical Association in 2019 [14]. ② One-hand dysfunction, and in the hand of Brunnstrom recovery stages (BRS-H) II and above. ③ The National Institute of Health Stroke Scale (NIHSS) score ≤ 4, the nerve damage was mild, the condition was relatively stable. ④ Modified Ashworth Scale (MAS) score < level 2. ⑤ Sitting balance ≥ 2 level and can remain seated for 60 min. ⑥ no serious defects in communication, memory or understanding, and the ability to follow the instructions of the assessor; ⑦ Willing to cooperate with the completion of the subject assessment, signed informed consent.

Exclusion criteria: ① Congenital or prior to the onset of the malformation of the affected hand due to other reasons, limited joint activity, etc. ② Motor dysfunction of both hands; ③ the condition is unstable. ④ Poor compliance, patients or family members refused to participate. This study has received ethics approval of hospital (20200624-11). After recruitment, Figure 1 represents the number of samples in each stage.

2.2. Methods

The rehabilitation physician makes a clear diagnosis and refers the patient to a systematically trained rehabilitation therapist, who explains the purpose of the assessment to the patient, informs the assessment content, demonstrates the specific actions before the assessment, obtains the relevant information of the patient and informs the relevant procedures and precautions before the test, so that the patient can fully understand and cooperate.

Before rehabilitation treatment, the enrolled patients were selected to complete the reliability and validity verification. Fifty-seven males completed the comparison and evaluation of the healthy hand modeling and patient hand of the 10 movements of MDIVQAS, among which twenty-four patients completed three repeated measurements by the same examiner with an interval of no more than 24 h. After the completion of MDIVQAS, all enrolled patients underwent the propiometric measurement of AROM, FMA (FMA-UE, FMA-W/H), Brunnstrom (upper limb, hand) and ARAT assessment, once each, within 24 years in sequence. The above assessment was repeated 2 weeks after rehabilitation.

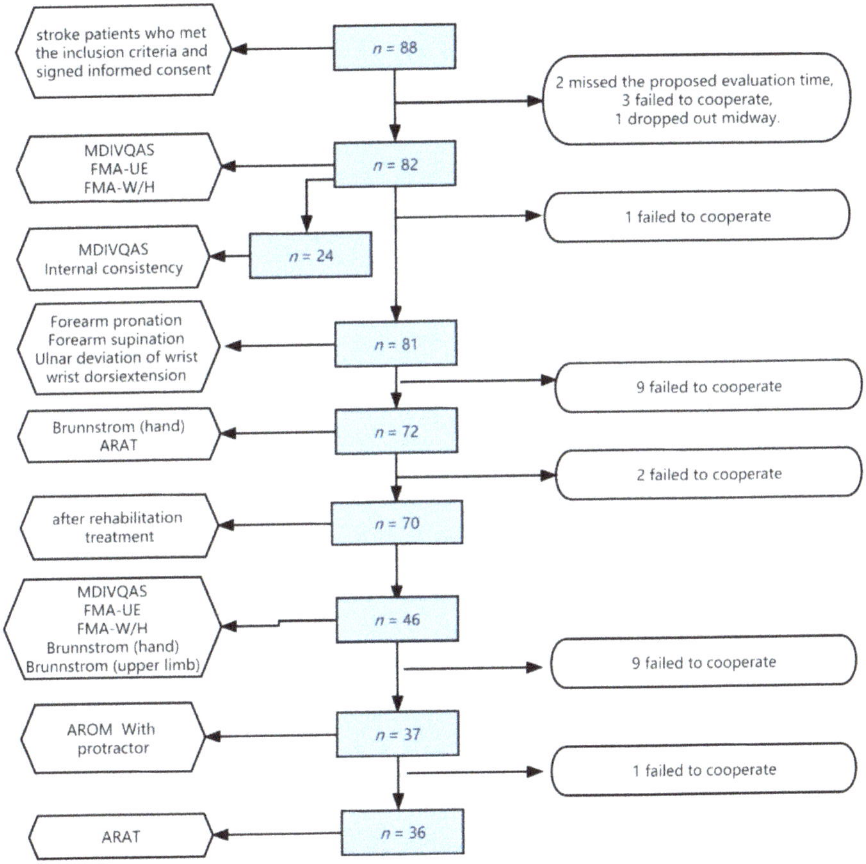

Figure 1. Flow chart of each stage in the study.

Enrolled patients were allowed a short rest between each method of assessment. All patients were required to complete the assessment at the same test site and under the same test conditions. The total assessment time for each patient was approximately 60 min.

The specific assessment methods were as follows:

(1) MDIVQAS: Based on the pathological motor characteristics of hemiplegic hand and a set of post-stroke hand function rehabilitation evaluation actions corresponding to the Brunnstrom scale, Fugl-Meyer Rating Scale and range of motion measurement, it is a computer-aided technology-based assessment tool. Using the comprehensive quantitative evaluation method of healthy hand modeling and comparison evaluation of the affected hand, the 3D spatial position and motion vector information of various joints of the phalanx, metacarpal and wrist were acquired in real time with the help of video equipment, and then various motion parameters of the hand joint were analyzed as the system parameters of the hand function evaluation standard. In order to prevent the ambiguity and subjectivity in the guidance process of the standard movement

demonstration, At the bottom left of the screen, there is a 3D animation of the action being evaluated to achieve a consistent demonstration of standard hand movements. The assessment items included three parts as forearm, wrist and hand, with a total of 10 movements, including ulnar wrist deviation, wrist dorsiextension, five fingers adduction and abduction, forearm pronation, forearm supination, spherical grip, cylindrical grip, thumb flexion and extension, thumb abduction and thumb rotation.

When the patient was seated, the patient information was first input, such as number, name, age, brief medical history, assessment results of common scales, etc. The pathological information of the patient included healthy hand, affected hand, stroke type, stroke brain area, etc. The hospital information includes the name, address and contact information of the hospital. Then, the movements to be evaluated were selected. The patient placed the healthy hand and the affected hand in the evaluation device at the same time, and the same visual and optical acquisition devices were configured for the healthy hand and the affected hand, respectively. In the first step of evaluation, the patient's healthy hand was guided by the standard animated hand to complete the extraction of the motion characteristics and node parameters of the patient's healthy hand and the modeling of the healthy hand model. The 3D animated hand part was captured by Maya software. The standard hand video obtained the foreground hand through the background learning algorithm, and the spatial motion trajectory was tracked by the hand particle filter. In the second step of assessment, the affected hand completed the extraction of motion characteristics and joint parameters in the affected hand working area. In the third step of evaluation, the multi-dimensional hand motion parameters of the patient's affected hand to be evaluated were comprehensively analyzed, and the joint motion of the affected hand, the percentage of joint motion of the affected hand in the healthy hand and the evaluation time were automatically calculated. In the third step of evaluation, the multi-dimensional hand movement parameters of the patient's hand to be evaluated are comprehensively analyzed, and the joint range of motion of the affected hand, the percentage of joint mobility of the affected hand to the healthy hand and the time of evaluation are automatically calculated. Evaluate twice, and the system will automatically select the better angle result for saving. MDIVQAS flow block diagram, see Figure 2.

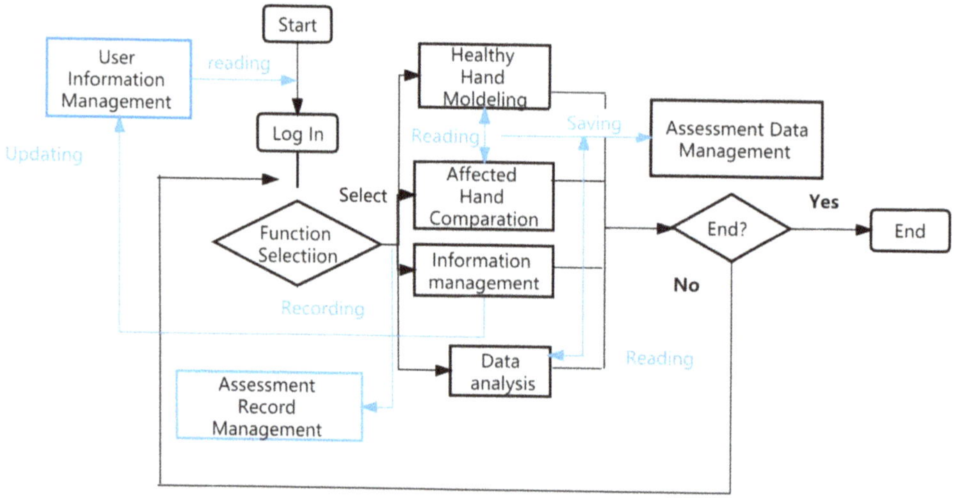

Figure 2. MDIVQAS workflow chart.

(2) Measuring AROM with protractor: A universal protractor was used to measure the forearm pronation, forearm supination, ulnar deviation, wrist dorsiextension and the angle between the fingers of the five fingers [9].

(3) FMA-UE [15,16]: It mainly includes movement, speed, coordination and reflex activities, with a total of 66 points, and each item is scored on a 3-level scale: that is, 0 points, unable to perform; 1 point, partially implemented; 2 points, fully implemented. Among them FMA-W/H is a part of the FMA rating scale, which evaluates the wrist and hand. There are 12 items in total, each item is 0~2 points, full score is 24 points. The higher the score, the better the motor function of the upper limb is indicated.
(4) Brunnstrom Scale [7,17]: upper limb and hand parts; each is divided into stage I–VI, and the higher the level, the better the motor function. Stage I: no exercise; Stage II: slight flexion; Stage III: flexion but not extension; Stage IV: the thumb can be pinched and loosened, and the fingers can be extended semi-randomly in a small area; Stage V: can do spherical or cylindrical grip, and can be free to extend the whole finger, but the range of size is not equal; Stage VI: full range extension of various grips, but with less speed and accuracy than the healthy side.
(5) ARAT [18,19]: Consisting of 4 subscales (grasp, grip, pinch and gross motion), which mainly evaluates the ability of the affected hand to handle objects of different sizes, weights and shapes. ARAT requires a standardized assessment toolbox, consisting of 19 items with a full score of 57, and each item is scored in a 4-point order (0: unable to complete any part of the task within 60 s, 1: complete part of the task within 60 s, 2: The task is completed, but the difficulty is very high or the time is too long (5~60 s), 3 points: the normal completion within 5 s). Each of ARAT's subscales is arranged in a hierarchical order, testing the most difficult items first, then the easiest and then increasing the items in turn. The higher the score, the better the feature.

2.3. *MDIVQAS*

2.3.1. Overall Design Scheme of MDIVQAS

MDIVQAS was a fully independent intellectual property technology jointly developed by Huashan Hospital affiliated with Fudan University and Shanghai University. By collecting video signals and conducting computer vision analysis, the automatic detection and dynamic tracking based on hand position are completed. Then, combined with the intelligent voice prompt module, the real-time hand movements and spatial positions of patients in the process of healthy hand modeling and affected hand assessment are dynamically detected. Through optical intelligent motion capture equipment, real-time acquisition of three-dimensional space information and motion vector data of each joint point of palm, finger and wrist. Aiming at the current hand function rehabilitation training qualitative assessment Brunnstrom scale and other corresponding sets of post-stroke hand function rehabilitation assessment actions such as forearm pronation or supination, wrist radial deviation, wrist ulnar deviation and wrist dorsiextension, thumb adduction and abduction, four fingers (except the thumb) adduction and abduction and other movements, combined with function of this platform hand movements intelligent analysis algorithm software module, feature data dimension reduction and mode matching, analysis of hand joint movement parameters, as the hand function recovery system evaluation parameters of quantitative evaluation criteria. At the same time, through multi-point network connection, a remote management server was set up to achieve quantitative, accurate, standardized and consistent quality management of the evaluation process through data spot check and video monitoring. Using the new idea of unilateral healthy hand to guide the affected hand, the animation standard hand guidance of multiple actions, the modeling of the healthy hand on the healthy side and the assessment of the affected hand on the affected side were completed. A set of standardized and comprehensive quantitative assessment process and implementation methods based on standard hand, patient's healthy hand and patient's affected hand were designed to scientifically and quantitatively solve the problem of phased quantitative assessment of hand function rehabilitation after stroke.

2.3.2. Hardware Platform of MDIVQAS

The platform was mainly composed of the hardware of the operating platform and the computing software of hand function evaluation, which is in line with the characteristics of patient ergonomics and motion. In this study, the industrial design process was used to carry out a complete industrial product-level design through the form frame structure mold opening, the integrated optimization of video and optical motion capture equipment, and the integrated configuration of touch control. The data collected by each hospital can be uploaded to the cloud platform, so as to obtain big data for quantitative evaluation of hand function of different populations for effective data classification and analysis [20]. The evaluation tool has declared a total of 5 patent achievements, of which 3 are invention patents, 1 is design patent and 1 is utility model patents. The project team further developed the identity authentication function based on face recognition, which has been tested in the cloud system, enabling patients to use "face brushing", greatly reducing the complexity of login and other procedures. The core hardware structure frame of this platform was shown in Figure 3.

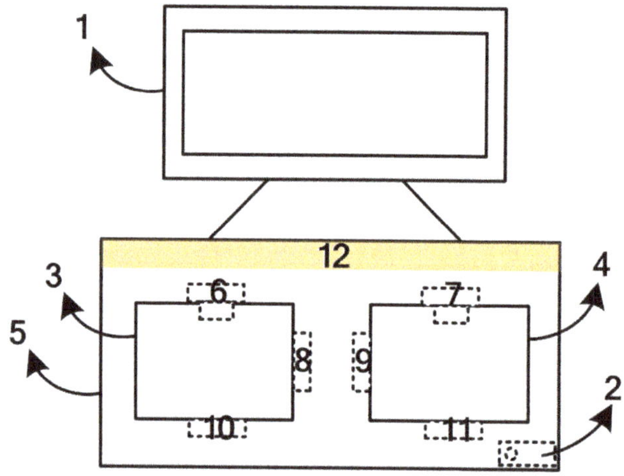

Figure 3. Block diagram of core hardware structure of hardware platform of multi-dimensional intelligent visual quantitative assessment system. 1—Touch display; 2—Computer; 3 and 4—Workspace; 5—External structure frame; 6 and 7—Video capture device; 8, 9, 10 and 11—Optical intelligent motion capture device and 12—Light source.

The touch display was responsible for the input and output of interactive information. Computer was responsible for data processing, logic control, intelligent analysis algorithm and information storage functions. The left and right workspaces were the detection areas of the platform, and patients can complete the functions of modeling the healthy hand and assessing the affected hand. Dual-channel video acquisition equipment could complete video signal acquisition.

A four-way optical motion capture device (developed by Shanghai University, Shanghai, China) was used to obtain real-time 3D spatial data and multiple motion vector information of each joint point of the patient's finger, palm and wrist. The external structure frame was the overall scaffold of the platform. The light source provided a good illumination environment for the working area, reduced noise and improved detection accuracy. A physical photo of the hardware platform prototype of MDIVQAS was shown as Figure 4.

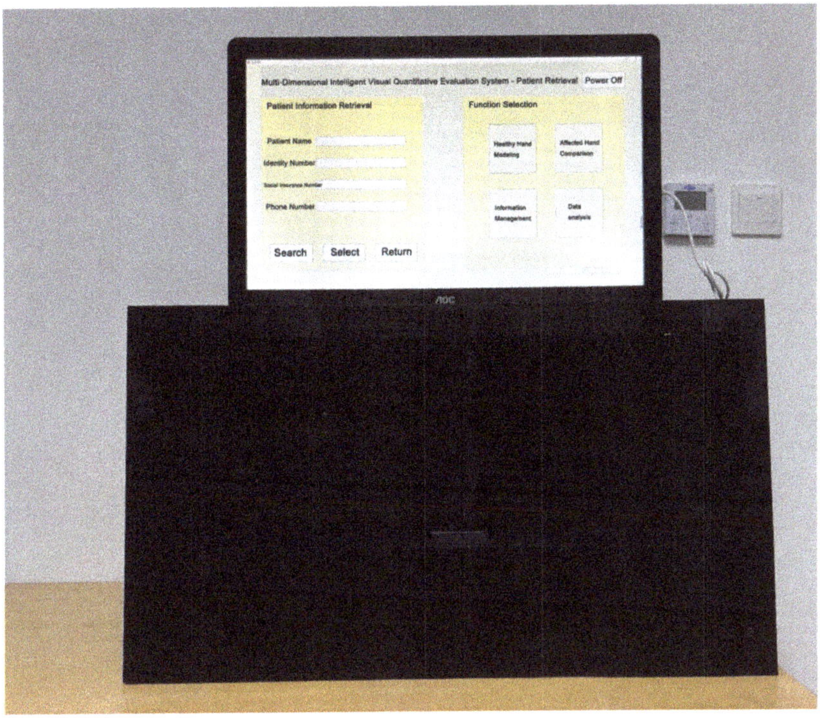

Figure 4. Hardware platform prototype of MDIVQAS.

2.4. Statistical Analysis

SPSS17.0 statistical software was used for statistical processing. Measurement data with normal distribution and homogeneity of variance were expressed as $x \pm$ s. Univariate *t*-test was used for comparison between the two groups, and Pearson coefficient was used for correlation. The data that did not meet the above conditions were described by the median (interquartile range), the comparison between the two groups was performed by Wilcoxon's Kolmogorov–Smirnov Z (K–S) test and the correlation analysis was by Spearman's test. Cronbach's Alpha coefficient and repeated measures were used to analyze the internal consistency of the assessment system. The pwr package in R was used to analyze the required sample size in the study. $p < 0.05$ was considered statistically significant.

3. Results

General data from November 2019 to October 2021: 88 stroke patients who met the inclusion criteria and signed informed consent in the Department of Rehabilitation Medicine, the First Affiliated Hospital of Xinjiang Medical University, were selected, of which six patients were missed (two missed the proposed evaluation time, three failed to cooperate and one dropped out midway). A total of 82 patients, including 57 males (69.5%) and 25 females (30.5%), completed the evaluation of the multi-dimensional intelligent visual quantitative assessment system, with an average age of (54.29 $\pm$ 13.12) years.

3.1. Reliability of MDIVQAS

The consistency test preset large effect size f = 0.4 [21], statistical testing power 1-β = 0.8, significance level a = 0.05 and at least 18 subjects were required. Considering the possibility of sample loss in the process of clinical research, the sample size was appropriately increased by 10% [22], and the results showed that at least 20 subjects were needed. This sample size was used to guide the content consistency test of this study.

The 24 patients enrolled in the group completed 10 movements using MDIVQAS, and each movement was repeated three times by the same examiner. Cronbach's alpha coefficient method was used to analyze the internal consistency of the assessment system. All the 10 actions were greater than 0.9, indicating that the internal homogeneity reliability of MDIVQAS was excellent, and the internal consistency was good. See Table 1 for details.

Table 1. Reliability of MDIVQAS for assessing hand functions.

Movement (n = 24)	Cronbach's Alpha	N of Items
Wrist ulnar deviation	0.989	3
Wrist dorsiextension	0.993	3
Finger adduction and abduction	0.987	3
Forearm pronation	0.998	3
Forearm supination	0.998	3
Cylindrical grip	0.981	3
Spherical grip	0.990	3
Thumb abduction	0.976	3
Thumb flexion and extension	0.989	3
Thumb rotation	0.994	3
Hand function 10 movements overall	0.989	30

Each patient enrolled was completed by MDIVQAS, and each action was evaluated three times within 24 h. Statistical analysis of the internal consistency of the assessment system by repeated measures showed that there was a statistical difference in the consistency test of thumb rotation ($p < 0.05$). However, no statistical difference was found in the repeated measurement of other movements, and there was consistency. See Figure 5 and Supplementary Table S1 for details.

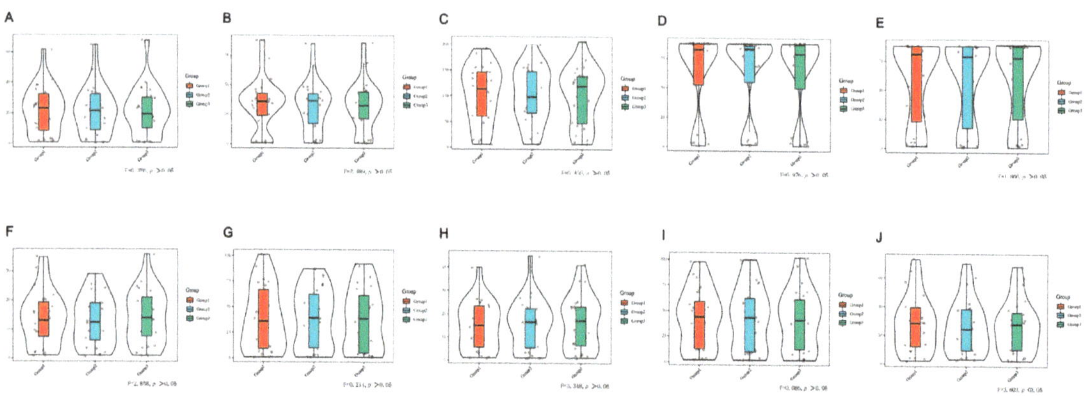

Figure 5. Consistency of the MDIVQAS for repeated measures to assess hand functions. (**A**) Wrist ulnar deviation; (**B**) Wrist dorsiextension; (**C**) Finger adduction and abduction; (**D**) Forearm pronation; (**E**) Forearm supination; (**F**) Cylindrical grip; (**G**) Spherical grip; (**H**) Thumb abduction; (**I**) Thumb flexion and extension; (**J**) Thumb rotation.

3.2. *Validity of MDIVQAS*

3.2.1. Correlation between MDIVQAS, FMA-W/H, Brunnstrom and ARAT Assessment

The correlation had a statistically large effect size $f^2 = 0.35$ [21], statistical test power $1\text{-}\beta = 0.8$ and significance level a = 0.05. At least 30 subjects are needed, considering the possibility of sample loss in the process of clinical study, and the sample size was appropriately increased by 10% on this basis [22], the results showing that at least 33 subjects were needed. This sample size was used to guide the correlation test of this study.

Among the subjects who met the inclusion criteria, Brunnstrom (upper limb) at stage IV or above and Brunnstrom (hand) at stage II or above completed the measurements of the percentage of affected side functions in the healthy side functions of wrist dorsiextension, wrist ulnar deviation, finger adduction and abduction, spherical grip, cylindrical grip, thumb flexion and extension and thumb rotation. Within 24 h, the same patient was given the Fugl-Meyer Assessment of Wrist and Hand (FMA-W/H), which is the wrist–hand assessment part of FMA-UE, Brunnstrom and ARAT scale. Statistical analysis was performed on the correlation between the percentage of the affected hand on the unaffected side measured by MDIVQAS and the various scales. Bivariate Correlations, Pearson's Correlations and two-tailed tests were used for the statistical parameters. The results showed that MDIVQAS was strongly correlated with FMA-W/H, Brunnstrom (hand) and ARAT ($r > 0.5$, $p < 0.01$). See Figure 6 and Supplementary Table S2.

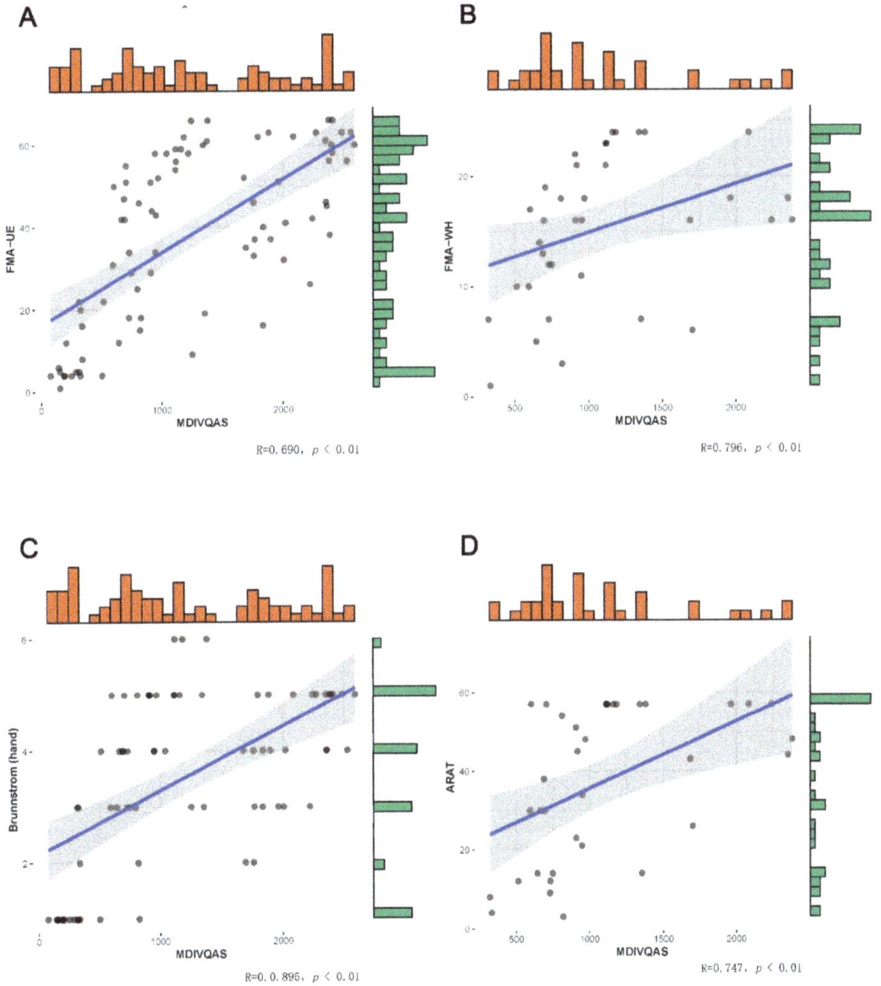

Figure 6. Correlation between MDIVQAS, FMA-W/H, Brunnstrom (hand) and ARAT. (**A**) Correlation between MDIVQAS and FMA-UE. (**B**) Correlation between MDIVQAS and FMA-W/H. (**C**) Correlation between MDIVQAS and Brunnstrom (hand). (**D**) Correlation between MDIVQAS and ARAT.

3.2.2. Correlations MDIVQAS and Protractor Measurement

The patients who met the inclusion criteria used the multi-dimensional intelligent visual quantitative assessment system and the protractor to measure the AROM of joint for the movement of forearm pronation, forearm supination, wrist dorsiextension, wrist ulnar deviation and finger adduction and abduction 1 (angle between the thumb and index finger of the affected hand); finger adduction and abduction 2 (angle between the index finger and the middle finger of the affected hand); finger adduction and abduction 3 (angle between the middle finger and the ring finger of the affected hand) and finger adduction and abduction 4 (angle between the ring finger and the little finger of the affected hand) within 24 h, respectively. Statistical analysis was performed on the correlation of the AROM of joint of the same movement for the two methods. Bivariate Correlations, Spearman's Correlations and two-tailed tests were used to analyze the correlations. The correlation coefficient (r) between MDIVQAS and the protractor measurement in the above actions were all >0.5, indicating a strong correlation. See Figure 7 and Supplementary Table S3.

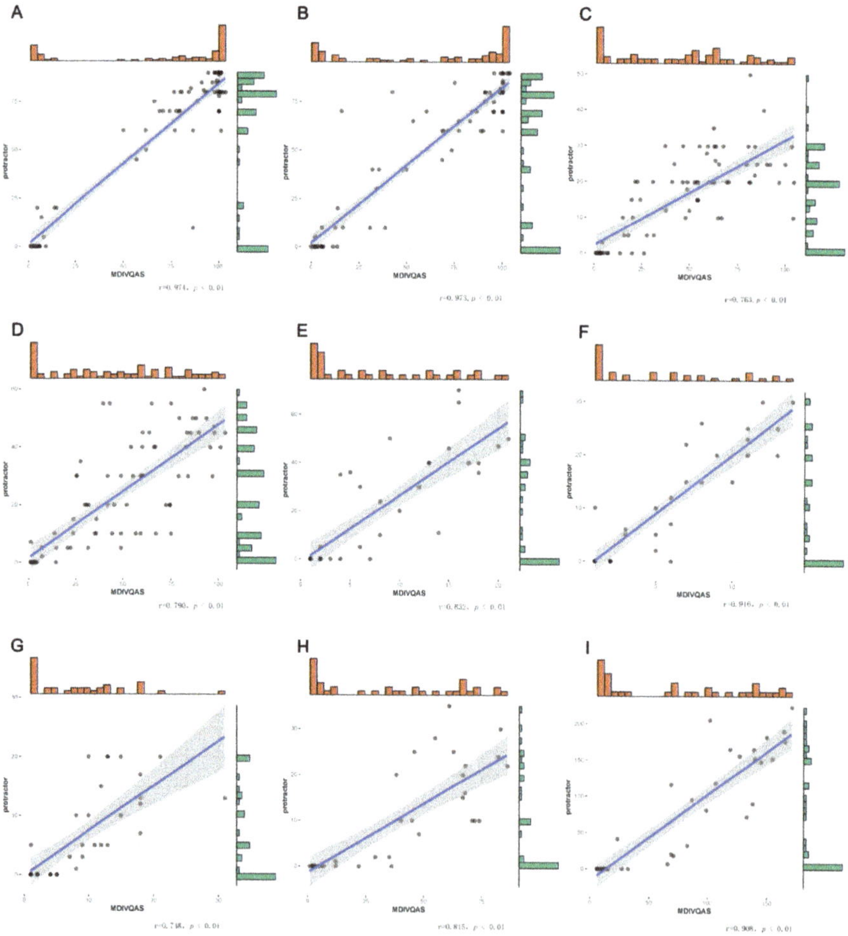

Figure 7. Correlation between MDIVQAS and protractor measurement. (**A**) Forearm pronation; (**B**) Forearm supination; (**C**) Ulnar deviation of wrist; (**D**) wrist dorsiextension; (**E**) Finger adduction and abduction1; (**F**) Finger adduction and abduction2; (**G**) Finger adduction and abduction3; (**H**) Finger adduction and abduction4; (**I**) Sum of finger adduction and abduction.

3.3. Reactivity before and after Treatment

3.3.1. Comparison of Differences of MDIVQAS, FMA-UE, FMA-W/H, Brunnstrom and ARAT before and after Treatment

The difference test between the two groups was presupposed to have a large effect size d = 0.8 [21], statistical testing power 1-β = 0.8 and significance level a = 0.05, and at least 26 subjects were required. Considering the possibility of sample loss in the process of clinical research, the sample size was appropriately increased by 10% [22]. The results showed that at least 29 participants were required.

The enrolled patients used FMA-UE, FMA-W/H, Brunnstrom and ARAT before and 2 weeks after rehabilitation treatment to explore the differences before and after treatment. FMA-UE, FMA-W/H, Brunnstrom and ARAT all met the normality test ($p > 0.05$) and were described as $x \pm$ s. Paired *t*-test was used to analyze the differences between the assessment methods before and after treatment. The results showed that the differences of the above five assessments before and after treatment were statistically significant ($p < 0.05$), suggesting that the results of hand function evaluation of patients after treatment were improved compared with those before treatment. As shown in Figure 8 and Supplementary Table S4.

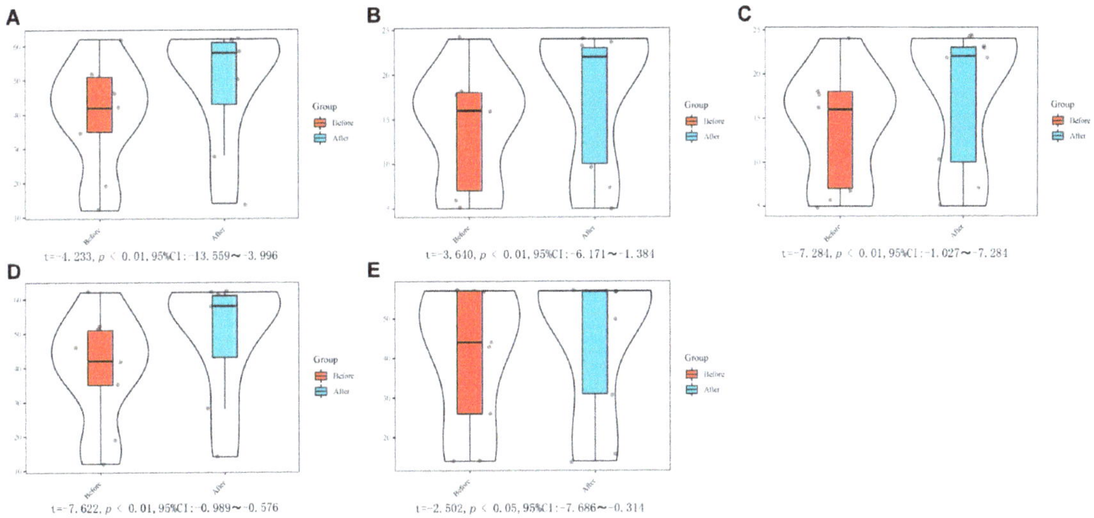

Figure 8. Comparison of differences of FMA-UE, FMA-W/H, Brunnstrom and ARAT before and after treatment. (**A**) FMA-UE; (**B**) FMA-W/H; (**C**) Brunnstrom (hand); (**D**) Brunnstrom (upper limb); (**E**) ARAT.

The patients who met the inclusion criteria were measured with a protractor before and after rehabilitation treatment to measure the AROM in finger adduction and abduction. Nonparametric Tests: Two related samples were used to analyze the differences before and after treatment, and the results showed that there were statistically significant differences in adduction and abduction between the fingers before and after treatment ($p < 0.05$), as shown in Figure 9 and Supplementary Table S5.

The enrolled patients were evaluated by MDIVQA before rehabilitation treatment and 2 weeks after treatment to evaluate the percentage of the affected hand in the healthy hand. The data of wrist ulnar deviation, wrist dorsiextension, finger adduction and abduction, forearm pronation, forearm supination, cylindrical grip, spherical grip, thumb abduction, thumb flexion and extension and thumb rotation did not meet the normality test ($p < 0.05$) and were described by the median (interquartile range). Nonparametric Tests 2: Related samples was used to analyze the differences assessed by MDIVQA before and after rehabilitation treatment, and the results suggested that the above actions had statistical significance before and after treatment ($p < 0.05$). It is suggested that MDIVQA could sensitively assess changes in patients' hand functions, as shown in Figure 10 and Supplementary Table S6.

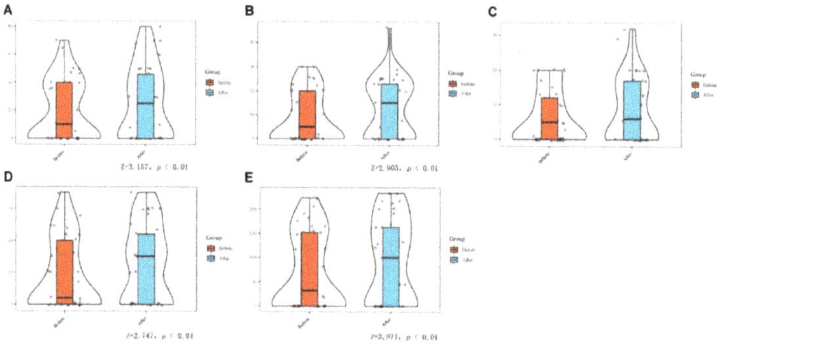

Figure 9. Comparison the differences of the AROM in finger adduction and abduction. With protractor before and after rehabilitation treatment. (**A**) Finger adduction and abduction 1; (**B**) Finger adduction and abduction 2; (**C**) Finger adduction and abduction 3; (**D**) Finger adduction and abduction 4; (**E**) Sum of finger adduction and abduction. Z represents the effect size of the two-sample K-S test (see Methods).

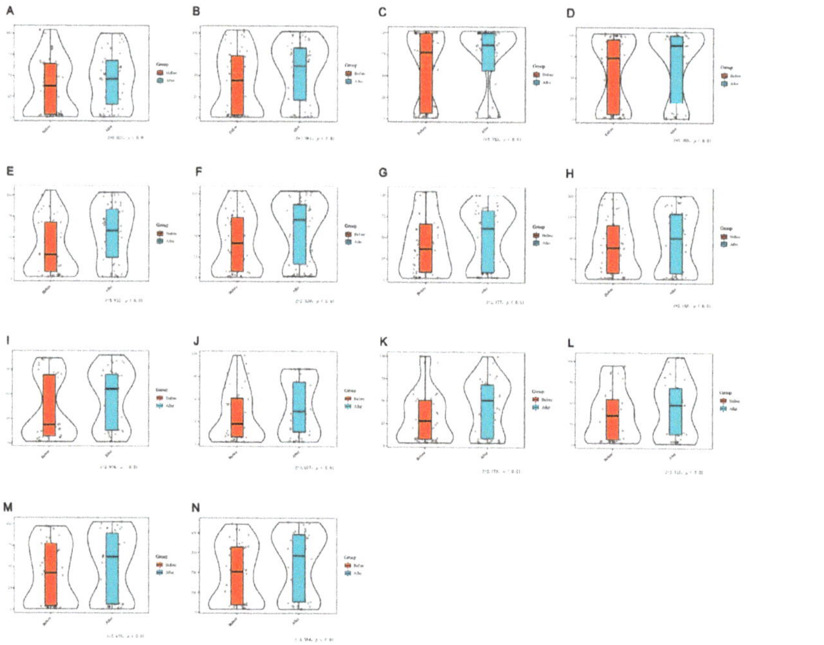

Figure 10. Comparison of differences before and after rehabilitation treatment using MDIVQAS. (**A**) Wrist ulnar deviation; (**B**) Wrist dorsiextension; (**C**) Forearm pronation; (**D**) Forearm supination; (**E**) Cylindrical grip; (**F**) Spherical grip; (**G**) Thumb abduction; (**H**) Thumb flexion and extension; (**I**) Thumb rotation; (**G**) Finger adduction and abduction 1; (**K**) Finger adduction and abduction 2; (**L**) Finger adduction and abduction 3; (**M**) Finger adduction and abduction 4; (**N**) Sum of finger adduction and abduction. Z represents the effect size of the two-sample K–S test (see Methods).

3.3.2. Comparison of the Difference between MDIVQAS and Protractor Measurement of AROM in the Increase of Joint Motion before and after Treatment

The reactivity of the two evaluation methods to the treatment effect was basically the same, and there was no statistical significance in the increase of the range of motion between the two evaluation methods before and after treatment ($p > 0.05$), indicating that the two evaluation methods had the same reactivity to the treatment effect. See Table 2.

Table 2. Comparison of the MDIVQAS and protractor before and after treatment.

Item	n	P25	P50	P75	Z	P
Ulnar deviation increase A	37	0.0	1.0	5.0	−0.184 b	0.854
Ulnar deviation increase B	37	0.0	0.0	6.0		
Forearm pronation increase A	37	−1.5	1.0	11.5	−0.516 b	0.606
Forearm pronation increase B	37	0.0	3.0	10.0		
Forearm supination increase A	37	−0.5	2.0	20.0	−1.034 c	0.301
Forearm supination increase B	37	0.0	0.0	10.0		
Wrist dorsiextension increase A	37	−0.5	3.0	17.5	−0.403 c	0.687
Wrist dorsiextension increase B	37	0.0	3.0	15.0		
Increase in angle between the fingers 1A	37	−0.5	1.0	7.0	−1.267 b	0.205
Increase in angle between the fingers 1B	37	0.0	0.0	12.0		
Increase in angle between the fingers 2A	37	0.0	2.0	5.0	−0.502 b	0.616
Increase in angle between the fingers 2B	37	0.0	0.0	5.0		
Increase in angle between the fingers 3A	37	0.0	1.0	4.0	−0.868 b	0.386
Increase in angle between the fingers 3B	37	0.0	0.0	7.0		
Increase in angle between the fingers 4A	37	0.0	1.0	2.0	−1.783 b	0.075
Increase in angle between the fingers 4B	37	0.0	0.0	5.0		

Note: A: MDIVQAS B: protractor b: Based on the positive rank c: Based on the negative rank. Z represents the effect size of the two-sample K–S test (see methods).

4. Discussion

Hand function plays an important role in people's daily life, affecting people's working, eating, dressing, modifying and other activities. The improvement of hand and upper limb function will maximize the recovery of overall function and improve the quality of life of stroke patients. Effective rehabilitation requires objective, quantitative, effective and reliable rehabilitation assessment [23]. Photoelectric capture technology in intelligent evaluation tools is considered as the gold standard of human motion analysis [24]. MDIVQAS in this study is a newly developed intelligent evaluation method using optical intelligent capture technology. This system is a hand function assessment tool jointly developed by Huashan Hospital affiliated with Fudan University and Shanghai University. It uses optical intelligent motion capture equipment and computer vision technology to conduct hand modeling and hand evaluation and obtain three-dimensional spatial data and motion vector information of each point of fingers, palms and wrists. At present, it has been able to carry out specific intelligent analysis algorithm for the 10 movements of five fingers adduction and abduction, wrist ulnar deviation, wrist dorsiextension, spherical grip, cylindrical grip, thumb flexion and extension, thumb abduction, thumb rotation, forearm pronation and forearm supination, and the exercise parameters of the healthy hand angle value, the affected hand angle value and the affected hand/healthy hand ratio were analyzed. At present, the feasibility study and quantitative evaluation application of the equipment with small samples of normal volunteers have been carried out [25,26]. In the early stage, the research team tested the semi-reliability and duplicate reliability in terms of reliability, and the reliability coefficients are both >0.850, indicating that the system has good reliability, consistency and stability. The reliability of the 10 actions of MDIVQAS showed a statistically significant difference in the reliability of the evaluators ($p < 0.01$), indicating that the reliability of MDIVQAS retest was high, and good and stable results could be obtained by repeating the measurement in a short period of time. In terms of validity test, the content validity test of MDIVQAS in the early stage of our research team showed that all 10 movements were common hand dysfunction after stroke, the I-CVI of the entry level was 1 and each action had a high correlation with the total score ($p < 0.01$), suggesting that it had certain evaluation value. The structural validity test adopts the exploratory factor analysis, a total of one common factor is extracted and the cumulative variance contribution rate is >60%, according to the functional component of the action, indicating that the system has good structural validity and can well reflect the hand motor function, and the structural validity test results show that MDIVQAS is single-dimensional in terms of evaluation content, has strong pertinence and is suitable for quantitative evaluation of hand function. In terms of the convergence validity test, the AVE of the system > 0.500, indicating that it has good convergence validity [27].

The team expanded the sample size of the previous study and, at the same time, used MDIVQAS to test the intra-group consistency of 10 movements of the affected hand of stroke patients, and Cronbach's alpha > 0.9, indicating good internal consistency. The repeatability of 10 actions was measured, and the results showed that the differences in the repeated measurement of nine actions were not statistically significant (all $p > 0.05$), indicating that the system had good repeatability. Only one of the movements (thumb rotation) had a statistically significant difference ($F = 3.603$, $p = 0.045$), indicating that the repeatability of this action needs to be explored. In conclusion, the above evidence shows that MDIVQAS has good confidence in the assessment of hand function after stroke. The consideration of the results of thumb rotation may be related to the fact that the current development of computer vision and pattern recognition algorithms has not reached the level of good recognition of any complex actions. When the dysfunctional hand of stroke patients is the hand, and the Brunnstrom stage $\geq$ IV on this side, the thumb rotation action is more flexible than the healthy hand (the hand that builds the model), the data exceed the modeling range and the data accuracy is reduced. According to the experience of the evaluator, when the hand function is relatively good or recovers to a certain extent, due to the flexibility of the hand, the completion of the action is better than the healthy side, and the accuracy of the data is reduced. It is recommended to debug and rectify the evaluation and measurement methods of the above actions.

At the same time, MDIVQAS was used in this study to test the calibration validity of AROM, FMA-UE, FMA-W/H, Brunnstrom and ARAT, and the results were all > 0.5 and $p < 0.01$, indicating that MDIVQAS was strongly correlated with the above four widely used clinical evaluation methods. It is suggested that MDIVQAS has good validity. Fugl-Meyer, Brunnstrom, ARAT and protractor measurements of AROM are the most commonly used classical methods in clinical evaluation of poststroke motor dysfunction [15,17,18]. Especially, FMA-W/H, FMA-UE and ARAT are the most commonly used scales to evaluate the efficacy of upper limb and hand motor function after stroke and are often used as the gold standard to test the validity of other scales [28]. This study confirmed that all the 10 movements evaluated by MDIVQAS had strong correlation with the above four evaluation methods, so MDIVQAS had good validity.

In this study, the evaluation methods of MDIVQAS and protractor measurement of AROM, Brunnstrom, FMA-W/H, FMA-UE and ARAT were put into clinical practice of stroke hand function rehabilitation, and the effects of hand function rehabilitation before and 2 weeks after treatment were evaluated. The results showed significant differences before and after treatment ($p < 0.01$~0.05), indicating that MDIVQAS could reflect the change of clinical treatment effects such as other classical methods. At the same time, the differences between MDIVQAS and a protractor to measure the increase in AROM before and after treatment were compared, and the results showed that there was no significant difference in the increase in the range of motion before and after treatment between the two evaluation methods ($p > 0.05$), indicating that the responsiveness of MDIVQAS to the treatment effect was consistent with that of the classical methods.

In clinical use, we have found that, first, the spherical grip, cylindrical grip and thumb rotation designed by MDIVQAS can make up for the shortcomings of traditional evaluation methods. Second, based on the automatic detection and dynamic tracking of hand position, combined with intelligent voice prompts and standard 3D animation guidance modules, the system facilitates the dynamic detection of real-time hand movements and spatial positions of patients in the process of healthy hand modeling and affected hand evaluation and realizes real-time dynamic evaluation of hand functions, which is simple to operate, convenient to use and dynamically adjusts and guides rehabilitation treatment plans. Third, the system can also set up a remote management server through a multi-point network connection, and the data collected by each hospital can be uploaded to the cloud platform so as to obtain the big data of the quantitative evaluation of the manual functions of different groups of people and can achieve quantitative, accurate, standardized and consistent evaluation process quality management through data spot checks, video monitoring and other methods. As more data accumulates, MDIVQAS can be optimized gradually. Fourth, the current intelligent quantitative motion evaluation methods for hand function are divided into wearable sensor schemes and noncontact vision schemes [10,29–31]. MDIVQAS is a noncontact evaluation scheme, which avoids the disadvantage that wearable sensor solutions restrict the freedom of movement of patients, especially for the evaluation of fine movements of the hand, which tends to produce large errors. Fifth, the system has certain limitations for subject selection, such as hand dysfunction, critical condition and people who cannot sit for a long time.

5. Conclusions

In conclusion, MDIVQAS has good reliability and validity in the evaluation of hand function in stroke, as well as good evaluation of the treatment effect. However, there are some shortcomings in the application that need to be further studied and improved.

Supplementary Materials: The following supporting information can be downloaded at: https://www.mdpi.com/article/10.3390/brainsci12121698/s1, Table S1: Consistency of the MDIVQAS for repeated measures to assess hand function.Table S2: Correlation between MDIVQAS and FMA-W/H, Brunnstrom (hand), and ARAT. Table S3: Correlations between MDIVQAS and protractor measurement. Table S4: Comparison of differences between FMA-UE, FMA-W/H, Brunnstrom and ARAT before and after treatment. Table S5: Comparison the differences of the AROM in finger adduction and abduction. With protractor before and after rehabilitation treatment. Table S6: Comparison of differences before and after rehabilitation treatment using MDIVQAS.

Author Contributions: Conceptualization, B.W. and X.L.; methodology, Y.S., H.M., D.L., T.S. and O.Z.M.; formal analysis, B.W., X.L. and Y.D.; data curation, Y.S. and H.M.; writing—original draft preparation, Y.D., B.W. and X.L. and writing—review and editing, Y.D. and B.W. All authors have read and agreed to the published version of the manuscript.

Funding: This research was funded by the Xinjiang Uygur Autonomous Region Regional Collaborative Innovation Project, grant number 2019E0283.

Institutional Review Board Statement: This study was approved by the Human Subjects Ethics Subcommittee of the First Affiliated Hospital of Xinjiang Medical University (ethics batch number: 20200624-11).

Informed Consent Statement: Informed consent was obtained from all subjects involved in the study.

Data Availability Statement: Data supporting the results of this study can be available by requesting the first author or corresponding author.

Conflicts of Interest: The authors declare no conflict of interest. The funders had no role in the study design, data collection and analysis, decision to publish or preparation of the manuscript.

References

1. Feigin, V.L.; Stark, B.A.; Johnson, C.O.; Roth, G.A.; Bisignano, C.; Abady, G.G.; Abbasifard, M.; Abbasi-Kangevari, M.; Abd-Allah, F.; Abedi, V.; et al. Global, regional, and national burden of stroke and its risk factors, 1990–2019: A systematic analysis for the Global Burden of Disease Study 2019. *Lancet Neurol.* **2021**, *20*, 795–820. [CrossRef] [PubMed]
2. Pila, O.; Duret, C.; Laborne, F.X.; Gracies, J.M.; Bayle, N.; Hutin, E. Pattern of improvement in upper limb pointing task kinematics after a 3-month training program with robotic assistance in stroke. *J. Neuroeng. Rehabil.* **2017**, *14*, 105. [CrossRef]
3. Franceschini, M.; Goffredo, M.; Pournajaf, S.; Paravati, S.; Agosti, M.; De Pisi, F.; Galafate, D.; Posteraro, F. Predictors of activities of daily living outcomes after upper limb robot-assisted therapy in subacute stroke patients. *PLoS ONE* **2018**, *13*, e193235. [CrossRef] [PubMed]

4. Veldema, J.; Nowak, D.A.; Gharabaghi, A. Resting motor threshold in the course of hand motor recovery after stroke: A systematic review. *J. NeuroEng. Rehabil.* **2021**, *18*, 158. [CrossRef] [PubMed]
5. Pan, B.; Huang, Z.; Jin, T.; Wu, J.; Zhang, Z.; Shen, Y. Motor Function Assessment of Upper Limb in Stroke Patients. *J. Healthc. Eng.* **2021**, *2021*, 6621950. [CrossRef]
6. Hernandez, E.D.; Galeano, C.P.; Barbosa, N.E.; Forero, S.M.; Nordin, Å.; Sunnerhagen, K.S.; Alt Murphy, M. Intra- and inter-rater reliability of Fugl-Meyer Assessment of Upper Extremity in stroke. *J. Rehabil. Med.* **2019**, *51*, 652–659. [CrossRef]
7. Meng, L.; Jiang, X.; Qin, H.; Fan, J.; Zeng, Z.; Chen, C.; Zhang, A.; Dai, C.; Wu, X.; Akay, Y.M.; et al. Automatic Upper-Limb Brunnstrom Recovery Stage Evaluation via Daily Activity Monitoring. *IEEE Trans. Neural Syst. Rehabil. Eng.* **2022**, *30*, 2589–2599. [CrossRef]
8. Nakazono, T.; Takahashi, K.; Suzuki, Y.; Mizuno, K.; Nomura, Y.; Hiraga, Y.; Matsumoto, S.; Nishiyama, K.; Fukuda, M. Reliability and validity of Japanese version of Fugl-Meyer assessment for the lower extremities. *Top. Stroke Rehabil.* **2022**, *29*, 125–132. [CrossRef]
9. van Kooij, Y.E.; Fink, A.; Nijhuis-van der Sanden, M.W.; Speksnijder, C.M. The reliability and measurement error of protractor-based goniometry of the fingers: A systematic review. *J. Hand Ther.* **2017**, *30*, 457–467. [CrossRef]
10. Wang, C.; Peng, L.; Hou, Z.G.; Li, J.; Zhang, T.; Zhao, J. Quantitative Assessment of Upper-Limb Motor Function for Post-Stroke Rehabilitation Based on Motor Synergy Analysis and Multi-Modality Fusion. *IEEE Trans. Neural Syst. Rehabil. Eng.* **2020**, *28*, 943–952. [CrossRef]
11. Sinha, S.; Bhowmick, B.; Chakravarty, K.; Sinha, A.; Das, A. Accurate upper body rehabilitation system using kinect. In Proceedings of the 2016 38th Annual International Conference of the IEEE Engineering in Medicine and Biology Society, Orlando, FL, USA, 16–20 August 2016; Volume 2016, pp. 4605–4609.
12. Antico, M.; Balletti, N.; Laudato, G.; Lazich, A.; Notarantonio, M.; Oliveto, R.; Ricciardi, S.; Scalabrino, S.; Simeone, J. Postural control assessment via Microsoft Azure Kinect DK: An evaluation study. *Comput. Methods Programs Biomed.* **2021**, *209*, 106324. [CrossRef]
13. Xie, C.; Yang, Q.; Huang, Y.; Su, S.W.; Xu, T.; Song, R. A Hybrid Arm-Hand Rehabilitation Robot With EMG-Based Admittance Controller. *IEEE Trans. Biomed. Circuits Syst.* **2021**, *15*, 1332–1342. [CrossRef]
14. Cerebrovascular Disease Group Chinese Association of Neurology; Zeng, J.S.; Liu, M.; Cui, L.Y. Diagnostic criteria of cerebrovascular diseases in China (version 2019). *Chin. J. Neurol.* **2019**, *52*, 710–715.
15. Fugl-Meyer, A.R.; Jääskö, L.; Leyman, I.; Olsson, S.; Steglind, S. The post-stroke hemiplegic patient. 1. a method for evaluation of physical performance. *Scand. J. Rehabil. Med.* **1975**, *7*, 13–31.
16. Lee, S.; Lee, Y.S.; Kim, J. Automated Evaluation of Upper-Limb Motor Function Impairment Using Fugl-Meyer Assessment. *IEEE Trans. Neural Syst. Rehabil. Eng.* **2018**, *26*, 125–134. [CrossRef]
17. Brunnstrom, S. Motor testing procedures in hemiplegia: Based on sequential recovery stages. *Phys. Ther.* **1966**, *46*, 357–375. [CrossRef]
18. Lyle, R.C. A performance test for assessment of upper limb function in physical rehabilitation treatment and research. *Int. J. Rehabil. Res.* **1981**, *4*, 483–492. [CrossRef]
19. Zhao, J.L.; Zhang, T.; Xu, Z.Q.; Ding, M.H.; Leng, Y.; Bian, R.H.; Mao, Y.R.; Huang, D.F. Responsiveness and Predictive Ability of the Chinese Version of the Action Research Arm Test in People with Cerebral Infarction. *BioMed Res. Int.* **2019**, *2019*, 8270187. [CrossRef]
20. Zhao, Z.; Lu, X.; Zhu, M.; Zhao, S.; Zhong, B.; Jie, J.; Chen, S. Post-stroke hand rehabilitation assessment of multi-terminal cloud platform design. *Electron. Meas. Technol.* **2018**, *41*, 10–14.
21. Braitman, L.E. Statistical power analysis in medical research. *Ann. Intern. Med.* **1983**, *99*, 269–271. [CrossRef]
22. Loria, A. Tamaño de muestra de protocolos clínicos. *Gac. Médica México* **2018**, *154*, 409–412. [CrossRef] [PubMed]
23. Murphy, M.A.; Björkdahl, A.; Forsberg-Wärleby, G.; Persson, C.U. Implementation of evidence-based assessment of upper extremity in stroke rehabilitation: From evidence to clinical practice. *J. Rehabil. Med.* **2021**, *53*, m148. [CrossRef] [PubMed]
24. de los Reyes-Guzmán, A.; Dimbwadyo-Terrer, I.; Trincado-Alonso, F.; Monasterio-Huelin, F.; Torricelli, D.; Gil-Agudo, A. Quantitative assessment based on kinematic measures of functional impairments during upper extremity movements: A review. *Clin. Biomech.* **2014**, *29*, 719–727. [CrossRef] [PubMed]
25. Fu, J.; Chen, S.; Qian, Y.; Lu, X.; Long, H.; Cui, X.; Jia, J. Feasibility of Multi-dimensional Visual Hand Function Rehabilitation Quantitative Assessment System in Assess-ing Hand Function for Stroke Patients. *Chin. J. Rehabil. Theory Pract.* **2018**, *24*, 1380–1383.
26. Lu, Y.; Ling, X.; Cong, W.; Zhao, Z.; Jie, J.; Chen, S. Quantitative evaluation method of wrist extension based on hand function evaluation system. *Electron. Meas. Technol.* **2017**, *40*, 127–133.
27. Ma, H.; Shi, Y.; Mu, Y.; Jia, J.; Lu, X.; Fu, J.; Chu, T.; Li, D.; Zhu, L.; Wang, B. The reliability and validity of multi-dimensional, quantitative video evaluation of the hand function of stroke survivors. *Chin. J. Phys. Med. Rehabil.* **2022**, *44*, 116–120.
28. Santisteban, L.; Térémetz, M.; Bleton, J.P.; Baron, J.C.; Maier, M.A.; Lindberg, P.G. Upper Limb Outcome Measures Used in Stroke Rehabilitation Studies: A Systematic Literature Review. *PLoS ONE* **2016**, *11*, e154792. [CrossRef]
29. Öhberg, F.; Bäcklund, T.; Sundström, N.; Grip, H. Portable Sensors Add Reliable Kinematic Measures to the Assessment of Upper Extremity Function. *Sensors* **2019**, *19*, 1241. [CrossRef]

30. Yurkewich, A.; Kozak, I.J.; Hebert, D.; Wang, R.H.; Mihailidis, A. Hand Extension Robot Orthosis (HERO) Grip Glove: Enabling independence amongst persons with severe hand impairments after stroke. *J. Neuroeng. Rehabil.* **2020**, *17*, 33. [CrossRef]
31. Coskunsu, D.K.; Akcay, S.; Ogul, O.E.; Akyol, D.K.; Ozturk, N.; Zileli, F.; Tuzun, B.B.; Krespi, Y. Effects of robotic rehabilitation on recovery of hand functions in acute stroke: A preliminary randomized controlled study. *Acta Neurol. Scand.* **2022**, *146*, 499–511. [CrossRef]

brain sciences

MDPI

Article

FER-PCVT: Facial Expression Recognition with Patch-Convolutional Vision Transformer for Stroke Patients

Yiming Fan [1,†], Hewei Wang [2,†], Xiaoyu Zhu [1], Xiangming Cao [3], Chuanjian Yi [4], Yao Chen [5], Jie Jia [2,*] and Xiaofeng Lu [1,6,*]

1 School of Communication and Information Engineering, Shanghai University, Shanghai 200444, China
2 Department of Rehabilitation, Huashan Hospital, Fudan University, Shanghai 200040, China
3 Department of Oncology, Jiangyin People's Hospital Affiliated to Nantong University, Wuxi 214400, China
4 Department of Rehabilitation, The Affiliated Hospital of Qingdao University, Qingdao 266000, China
5 Department of Rehabilitation, Shanghai Third Rehabilitation Hospital, Shanghai 200436, China
6 Wenzhou Institute, Shanghai University, Wenzhou 325000, China
* Correspondence: luxiaofeng@shu.edu.cn (X.L.); shannonjj@126.com (J.J.)
† These authors contributed equally to this work.

Abstract: Early rehabilitation with the right intensity contributes to the physical recovery of stroke survivors. In clinical practice, physicians determine whether the training intensity is suitable for rehabilitation based on patients' narratives, training scores, and evaluation scales, which puts tremendous pressure on medical resources. In this study, a lightweight facial expression recognition algorithm is proposed to diagnose stroke patients' training motivations automatically. First, the properties of convolution are introduced into the Vision Transformer's structure, allowing the model to extract both local and global features of facial expressions. Second, the pyramid-shaped feature output mode in Convolutional Neural Networks is also introduced to reduce the model's parameters and calculation costs significantly. Moreover, a classifier that can better classify facial expressions of stroke patients is designed to improve performance further. We verified the proposed algorithm on the Real-world Affective Faces Database (RAF-DB), the Face Expression Recognition Plus Dataset (FER+), and a private dataset for stroke patients. Experiments show that the backbone network of the proposed algorithm achieves better performance than Pyramid Vision Transformer (PvT) and Convolutional Vision Transformer (CvT) with fewer parameters and Floating-point Operations Per Second (FLOPs). In addition, the algorithm reaches an 89.44% accuracy on the RAF-DB dataset, which is higher than other recent studies. In particular, it obtains an accuracy of 99.81% on the private dataset, with only 4.10M parameters.

Keywords: facial expression recognition (FER); vision transformer (ViT); convolutional neural networks (CNNs); stroke; rehabilitation

Citation: Fan, Y.; Wang, H.; Zhu, X.; Cao, X.; Yi, C.; Chen, Y.; Jia, J.; Lu, X. FER-PCVT: Facial Expression Recognition with Patch-Convolutional Vision Transformer for Stroke Patients. *Brain Sci.* **2022**, *12*, 1626. https://doi.org/10.3390/brainsci12121626

Academic Editors: Andrew Clarkson and Konstantin V. Slavin

Received: 24 October 2022
Accepted: 23 November 2022
Published: 28 November 2022

1. Introduction

The incidence, mortality, and disability of stroke in China have been higher than those in developed countries such as the United Kingdom, the United States, and Japan in the past 15 years [1]. Most stroke survivors cannot normally live because of suffering from sequelae such as hemiplegia, limb numbness, swallowing disorders, and depression. Brain neurobiology suggests that early training, at the right intensity, will aid recovery [2]. However, physicians need to be aware of patients' feelings in real-time during early rehabilitation to determine whether the training matches their physical recovery, then tailor the most rehabilitation-friendly training for each patient. This existing manual monitoring mode in clinical practice, which causes an enormous burden on medical resources, urgently needs to be improved and optimized.

Deep learning, as one of the powerful medical assistance technologies, has been widely applied in the medical field [3]. These applications include but are not limited to automatic diagnosis of breast cancer based on whole slide imaging [4], accurate measurement of morphological changes in intervertebral discs based on axial spine Magnetic Resonance Image (MRI) [5], detection of fundus lesions based on fundus imaging [6], and segmentation of brain tumors based on T1-weighted MRI [7]. These studies show that deep learning dramatically reduces the heavy and urgent workload of physicians and improves the efficiency of medical care. In particular, deep learning and machine learning also play an important role in stroke prediction, prognostics, and management. Iqram and Se proposed a real-time health monitoring system for stroke prognostics [8] and a cardiac monitoring system for stroke management [9]. These studies provide technical support for early stroke prognostics and have medical practice implications for predicting acute stroke. In addition, emotion classification techniques for stroke patients based on electroencephalography (EEG) [10–12] and facial electromyography (EMG) [13] also provide physicians with meaningful assessment information to replace traditional clinical methods based on observation or scoring.

However, these physiological signal-based approaches to stroke prognostics inevitably require contact with the patient's skin to capture the information. For stroke rehabilitation, wearable devices are likely to interfere with patients' training. In contrast, the facial expression recognition (FER) technique based on computer vision can acquire the state of patients in training without contact, which is more suitable for stroke rehabilitation. At present, although the application of the FER technique in the field of stroke rehabilitation is less than that of other medical fields, such as Down syndrome prediction [14], depression diagnosis [15], and autism spectrum disorder identification [16], it is significantly improving stroke management and quality of stroke care [17,18].

Few studies have published facial expression datasets and FER algorithms for stroke patients because of their privacy and sensitive nature. However, FER for healthy people is one of the mainstream tasks in computer vision. The relevant datasets contain a large number of samples, such as the Facial Expression Recognition 2013 dataset (FER2013, 35,886 images) [19], the Static Facial Expression in the Wild (SFEW, 1766 images) [20], the Real-world Affective Faces Database (RAF-DB, 29,672 images) [21], and AffectNet (400,000 images) [22]. In terms of algorithms, Convolutional Neural Networks (CNNs), such as Visual Geometry Group (VGG) [23], Google Inception Network (GoogleNet) [24], and Residual Network (ResNet) [25], are the most commonly used structures in this field because of their excellent robustness to changes in face position and image scale. With Attention [26] proposed, many studies used it to replace part of CNNs or combine them to improve performance while the model's overall structure remained unchanged [27–29]. In 2020, Vision Transformer (ViT) did not use convolution and outperformed state-of-the-art CNNs on mainstream small- and med-sized image classification datasets [30]. Moreover, in recent years, improved algorithms based on Transformer have continuously surpassed the previous algorithms in performance [31,32]. Fayyaz et al. [33] showed that ViT is more robust than CNNs in handling occluded images, feature transformation, and token reorganization. Nevertheless, the proposers of ViT also illustrated that ViT outperforms ResNet only when trained on enormous datasets (14–300 million images). To address this problem, some studies have combined CNNs and Transformers to model both local and global dependencies for image classification [34,35]. However, these algorithms are designed to achieve higher accuracy, inevitably requiring huge parameters, computational cost, and Giga Floating-point Operations Per Second (GFLOPs), which make them hard to embed into rehabilitation medical equipment.

We aim to design a lightweight FER algorithm for stroke rehabilitation in clinical practice, so as to assist physicians in determining whether the training intensity of stroke patients matches their physical rehabilitation and whether patients are active or focused during training. The key contributions of this paper can be summarized as follows:

- We propose a lightweight FER algorithm named Facial Expression Recognition with Patch-Convolutional Vision Transformer. It requires less memory and computation for model training/inference while ensuring high accuracy.

- The proposed algorithm effectively combines the local perception ability of CNN and the advantages of ViT in extracting global features, which makes the algorithm achieve the highest accuracy on the RAF-DB dataset.
- We treat emotion features as the weighted sum of neutral and V-A-like emotion features at different scales and design a unique classifier, which has been verified that more detailed facial emotion information of stroke patients has been extracted for classification.

2. Materials and Methods

2.1. Data Sources and Data Preprocessing

There are three datasets used in this study: (1) two public datasets for healthy people, RAF-DB [21] and FER+ [36]; (2) a private dataset for stroke patients. Table 1 describes the sample properties of three datasets in detail.

Table 1. Properties of three datasets with data.

Class	FER+		RAF-DB		Private Dataset	
	Simple Size	Proportion (%)	Simple Size	Proportion (%)	Simple size	Proportion (%)
happy	5165	24.41	5957	38.84	141	10.83
surprised	3963	18.73	1619	10.55	62	4.76
sad	3765	17.79	2460	16.04	78	5.99
angry	2594	12.26	867	5.65	44	3.38
neutral	4748	22.44	3204	20.89	509	39.09
fearful	633	2.99	355	2.31	-	-
disgusted	145	0.69	877	5.72	-	-
contempt	148	0.70	-	-	-	-
painful	-	-	-	-	85	6.53
strained	-	-	-	-	298	22.89
tired	-	-	-	-	85	6.53
Min/Max sample size	0.0281	-	0.0596	-	0.0864	-
SUM	21,161	100	15,339	100	1302	100

- RAF-DB dataset

The Real-world Affective Faces Database (RAF-DB) contains a single-label subset with 15,339 images, which can be divided into seven basic emotional classes: happy, sad, surprised, angry, fearful, disgusted, and neutral. These samples are of significant variability in subjects' age, ethnicity, head poses, lighting conditions, occlusions (e.g., glasses, facial hair, or self-occlusion), and post-processing operations (e.g., various filters and effects) [21]. These diverse differences make the trained models have better generalization.

- FER+ dataset

The Face Expression Recognition Plus dataset (FER+) contains 35,887 images of size 48×48 that can be divided into 10-class emotions. Only 21,161 images/8 emotions are used in this experiment: happy, sad, surprised, angry, fearful, disgusted, neutral, and contempt.

- Private dataset

The inclusion criteria were as follows: (1) patients aged 18–85 years old; (2) diagnosed with stroke confirmed by computed tomography (CT) and/or magnetic resonance imaging (MRI); (3) $\geq$2 weeks post-stroke; (4) upper limb of the healthy or affected side can use the upper limb rehabilitation robot for training; (5) patients signed the informed consent. The exclusion criteria were: (1) patients with unstable cerebrovascular disease; (2) patients with sensory aphasia or motor aphasia, and those who were unable to cooperate with assessment and testing; (3) Montreal Cognitive Assessment (MoCA) score $\leq$ 25; (4) patients with severe organ dysfunction or with malignant tumors; (5) House–Brackmann (H-B) grade $\geq$ III.

There were 42 participants in the experiment, of which 37 patients with stroke (25 men and 12 women, 31–87 years old) were confirmed cases from the Shanghai Third rehabilitation hospital and 5 healthy controls (4 physicians and 1 student). All subjects signed an informed consent form before the experiment.

In this study, four basic emotions (happy, sad, surprised, and angry) were used as biomarkers to assess the patient's concentration, and four special emotions (painful, strained, tired, and neutral) were used as biomarkers to determine whether the current training intensity is suitable for the patient. There were two schemes for collecting emotional videos. First, we guided patients to express these four basic emotions through videos and pictures. Second, these four special emotions were collected while patients were training with the upper limb rehabilitation robot. In addition, we asked patients to repeatedly lift the upper extremity and gradually increase the range of motion to capture these desired emotions. In this experiment, each patient participated in collections of two emotions at least, which ensured that each subject's sample had positive and negative labels.

After collecting the emotional videos, data preprocessing is an indispensable step, mainly sampling images, correcting faces, and labeling samples. The DB Face [37], a face detection algorithm, was used to predict the anchor boxes of faces and corresponding confidence scores in emotional videos automatically. Then, we removed face images with low confidence and incomplete from numerous video slices containing facial expressions. These preserved facial images were adjusted by rotating so that the line connecting the eyes' feature points detected by the DB Face algorithm was in the horizontal direction, with the midpoint of the line as the center of rotation. The line's rotation angle $\boldsymbol{\theta}$ is calculated by Equation (1). The transformation matrix $\boldsymbol{M}$ of all pixels in the original image is defined as Equation (2). The coordinates of all original pixels can be transformed into the corrected coordinates using Equation (3).

$$\theta = \tan^{-1}\frac{y_r - y_l}{x_r - x_l} \tag{1}$$

$$A = \begin{bmatrix} \cos\theta & \sin\theta \\ -\sin\theta & \cos\theta \end{bmatrix},\ B = \begin{bmatrix} (1-\cos\theta)\cdot x_c - \sin\theta\cdot y_c \\ \sin\theta\cdot x_c + (1-\cos\theta)\cdot y_c \end{bmatrix},\ M = \begin{bmatrix} A & B \end{bmatrix} \tag{2}$$

$$\begin{bmatrix} x' \\ y' \end{bmatrix} = A\begin{bmatrix} x \\ y \end{bmatrix} + B = M\begin{bmatrix} x \\ y \\ 1 \end{bmatrix} \tag{3}$$

where (x_l, y_l), (x_r, y_r), and (x_c, y_c) are the feature coordinates of the left eye, the right eye, and the midpoint of the line connecting eyes in the original image, respectively. (x', y') is the corrected coordinate.

We labeled the face-aligned images using the Facial Action Coding System (FACS) [38]. First, the emotional label of each sample was initially determined based on the content of the corresponding emotional video of the sample. Then, these images were annotated again according to FACS definitions of eight expressions. Table 2 shows FACS definitions of eight expressions in this experiment. In addition to the five expressions of happy, sad, angry, surprised, and neutral, the other expressions required for this experiment must be clearly defined by FACS. Referring to the PSPI [39], FACS features of painful expressions include lowered brow (AU4), raised cheeks (AU6), tightened lid (AU7), wrinkled nose (AU9), raised upper lip (AU10), and closed eyes (AU43). By comparing the facial features corresponding to each AU, we defined that FACS features of strained expressions are lowered brow (AU4), raised cheeks (AU6), tightened lips (AU23), pressed lips (AU24), and sucked lips (AU28); FACS features of tired expressions are closed eyes (AU43) and downed head (AU54), as shown in Figure 1.

Table 2. FACS definitions of eight expressions.

Emotions	Code *
painful	AU4 + (AU6/AU7) + (AU9/AU10) + AU43
strained	AU4 + AU6 + (AU23/AU24/AU28)
tired	AU43 + AU54
neutral	/
happy	AU6 + AU12
sad	AU1 + AU4 + AU15
surprised	AU1 + AU2 + AU5 + AU26
angry	AU4 + AU5 + AU7 + AU23

* AU1: Inner Brow Raiser; AU2: Outer Brow Raiser; AU4: Brow Lowerer; AU5: Upper Lid Raiser; AU6: Cheek Raiser; AU7: Lid Tightener; AU9: Nose Wrinkler; AU10: Upper Lip Raiser; AU12: Lip Corner Puller; AU15: Lip Corner Depressor; AU23: Lip Tightener; AU24: Lip Pressor; AU26: Jaw Drop; AU28: Lip Suck; AU43: Eyes Closed; AU54: Head down.

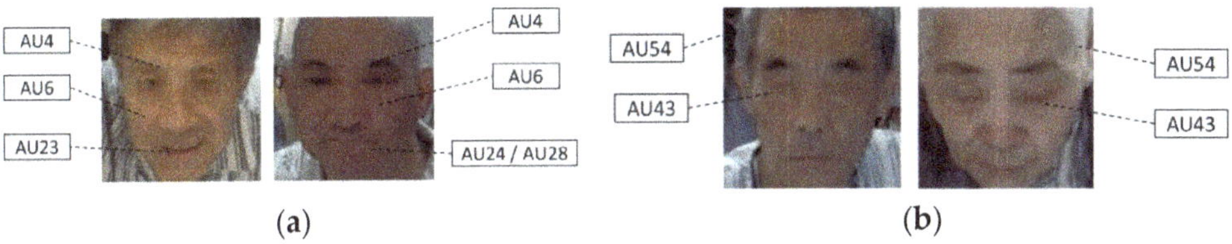

Figure 1. FACS features of strained and tired expressions: (**a**) the strained expressions spontaneously appeared by patients when their limb muscles were tense during training; (**b**) the tired expressions occurred when the patients were resting or undergoing prolonged passive training.

After labeling and collation, the private dataset contains 1302 samples/8 categories, with no sample crossover and duplicates. Some samples of the private dataset are shown in Figure 2.

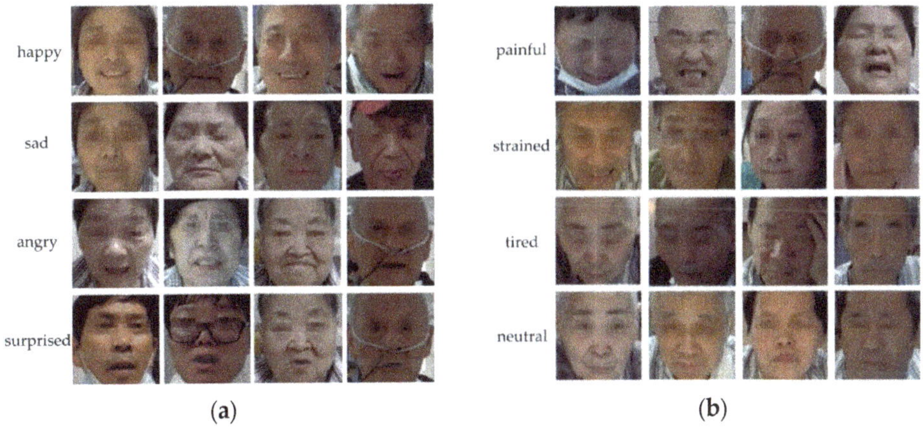

Figure 2. Partial samples of the private dataset: (**a**) these four basic expressions are used to assess training attention and positivity of stroke patients; (**b**) these four special expressions are used to determine whether the training intensity is proper for the patient.

2.2. Model Building

In order to occupy fewer computing resources to identify eight facial expressions of stroke patients accurately, we propose a lightweight FER model shown in Figure 3, named the Facial Expression Recognition with Patch-Convolutional Vision Transformer

(FER-PCVT). The FER-PCVT designed with ViT as the baseline mainly consists of three modules: the Convolutional Patch Embedding (CPE), the Pyramid Transformer (PTF), and the Valence-Arousal-Like Classifier (V-ALC). The first two modules combine to form the backbone network, Patch-Convolutional Vision Transformer (PCVT). The V-ALC is an expression classifier designed based on the Valence-Arousal (V-A) emotion theory [40].

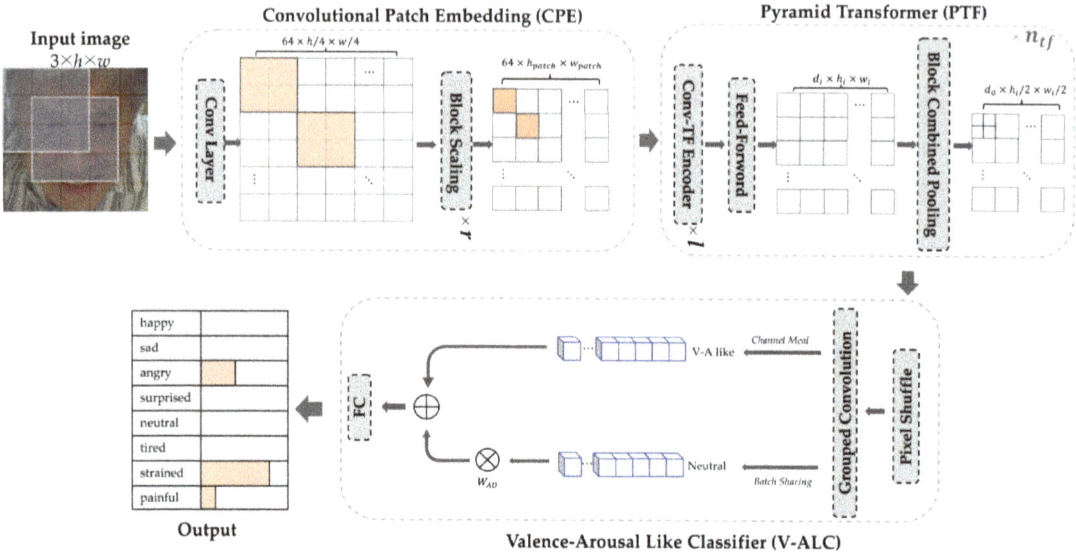

Figure 3. The overall architecture of the FER-PCVT, where r, l, and n_{tf} are the numbers of repetitions of the Block Scaling, the Conv-TF Encoder, and the Pyramid Transformer, respectively. HA: happy; SA: sad; AN: angry; SU: surprised; NE: neutral; TI: tired; ST: strained; PA: painful.

2.2.1. Convolutional Patch Embedding

Compared with the direct processing of pixel information of images using the transformer encoder of ViT, the accuracy will be further improved by using CNNs to extract the feature information from images and then processing them with the transformer encoder [35,41]. Based on this, the convolutional patch embedding module is implemented as a pixel-to-sequence mapping module to extract the feature sequences as the input of the Conv-TF Encoder of the pyramid transformer module. Specifically, the feature information extracted from the image by the convolutional layer and pooling layer is reduced to the patch size by the Block Scaling module. The Block Scaling module, consisting of two convolutional layers (size 2 × 2, stride 2, and size 1 × 1, stride 1), is applied to adjust the dimensions of feature maps entered into the Conv-TF Encoder by varying the number of repetitions. That is, the length and width of the sequence will be shortened to $1/2^r$ of the original size after repeating r times. This method of introducing convolutions into ViT achieves feature mapping from pixel to sequence while preserving the position information between patches. The detailed structure is shown in Figure 4a.

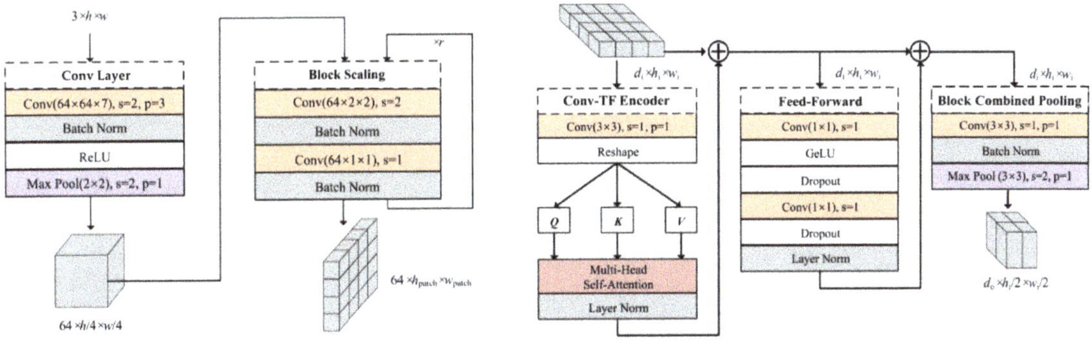

(a) (b)

Figure 4. The pipeline of the PCVT architecture. (**a**) Details of the Convolutional Patch Embedding (CPE). (**b**) Details of the Pyramid Transformer (PTF).

2.2.2. Pyramid Transformer

ViT requires the input and output sequences in the transformer encoder to have the same dimensions. However, the length of sequences output by CNNs is reduced as the network deepens. This pyramidal output mode in the CNNs, significantly reducing the computational cost, has been shown to be beneficial in extracting feature information at different scales [42]. Thus, the PTF designed by introducing this output mode aims to reduce the storage, parameters, and GFLOPs required for computation. Details of the PTF are shown in Figure 4b. We use convolutional mapping instead of the linear mapping in the transformer encoder of ViT to extract the three feature matrices: $\boldsymbol{Q}, \boldsymbol{K}$, and $\boldsymbol{V}$. Then, they are fed into the Multi-Head Self-Attention to be given different weights. In the Feed-Forward module, a bottleneck structure is formed by two convolutional layers with output channels $d_i/2$ and d_i, respectively, which compresses the channel dimension in the model. The activation function GeLU between the two convolutional layers is used to make the model fit data faster, and its expression is Equation (4).

$$GeLU(x) = \frac{1}{2}x\left(1 + erf\left(\frac{x}{\sqrt{2}}\right)\right) \quad (4)$$

where $erf(\cdot)$ is the Gauss Error Function. In the Block Combined Pooling module, d_0 convolution kernels (size 3×3) expand the channel dimension of the input feature map, followed by downsampling with a max pooling window (size 3×3, stride 2). The module allows feature maps to be resized from $d_i \times h_i \times w_i$ to $d_0 \times h_i/2 \times w_i/2$, gradually reducing the feature output, like a pyramid.

In addition, the layer normalization constrains the outputs of the Conv-TF Encoder module and the Feed-Forward module to avoid the vanishing gradient. The inputs and outputs of the above two modules are connected by residual connections to prevent the loss of feature information extracted by the model. At the same time, the batch normalization regularizes the output of the Block Combined Pooling module.

2.2.3. Valence-Arousal-Like Classifier

FACS defines the neutral expression as no AU, meaning that no facial muscle movement can be used as a biomarker. It makes neutral expressions more challenging to identify than other expressions. Especially neutral expressions of some stroke patients are different from those of ordinary people when all facial muscles are completely relaxed. The V-A emotion theory [40] suggests that each emotion is a mixture of arousal and valence in different proportions. Referring to the theory, we design the V-ALC as an expression classifier, considering emotion as a weighted sum of neutral and V-A-like features. Details of the V-ALC are shown in Figure 5.

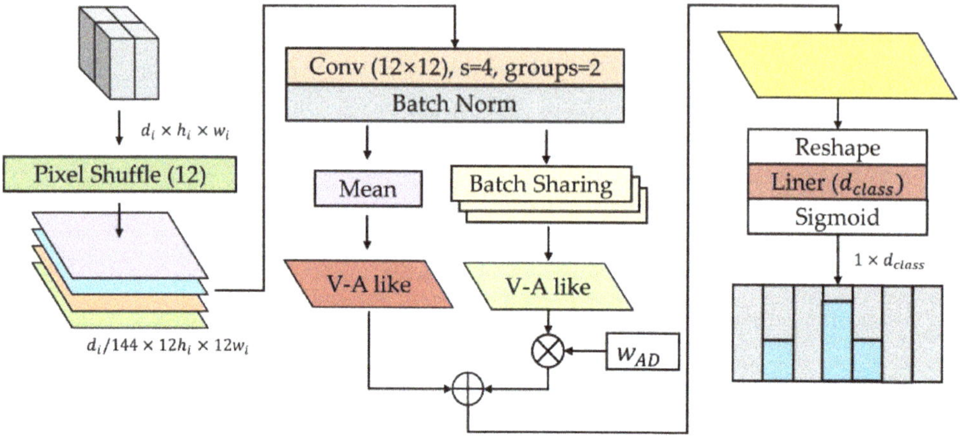

Figure 5. Details of the Valence-Arousal-Like Classifier (V-ALC).

We adopt the pixel shuffle method to reshape low-resolution feature maps into high-resolution ones. That is, the length and width of the input feature map are up-sampled by 12 times, and the result is condensed using a convolution kernel of size 12 × 12. These compressed sequences are grouped into the Channel Mean and the Batch Sharing to obtain the V-A-like and neutral features with one dimension, respectively. The result of multiplying the neutral feature with the adaptive weight w_{AD} is added to the V-A-like feature to output a complete feature map of emotion. Among them, w_{AD} is a parameter learned by the model from many training samples. The Channel Mean means averaging the values of different channels in the same batch, thereby reducing the channel dimension. The Batch Sharing refers to averaging the values in different batches on the basis of the Channel Mean, which aims to extract the most appropriate characteristics of neutral emotions from batches. Their expressions are Equations (5) and (6).

$$Channel\ Meal\ (x_b) = \frac{1}{c}\sum_{i=1}^{c} x_{bi} \tag{5}$$

$$Batch\ Sharing\ (x) = \frac{1}{bc}\sum_{j=1}^{b}\sum_{i=1}^{c} x_{ij} \tag{6}$$

where x is the input feature tensor, x_b is the feature sequence of different batches in the input tensor, i is the ith channel, j is the jth batch, c is the total number of channels, and b is the total number of batches.

After outputting a complete feature map of emotion, considering that emotion may be a composite state, we normalize these sequences using the Sigmoid function to avoid mutually exclusive results using the Softmax function. Finally, the prediction confidence of each category is output, where the expression with the highest confidence is the final result of the model's prediction.

3. Results

3.1. Setup

Table 3 shows the training settings in this experiment, including the selected optimizer, the loss function, and some specific hyperparameters. Table 4 shows the detailed structural parameters for each module combined in this experiment.

Table 3. Training parameter settings.

Parameter	Setting
optimizer	AdamW [43] [1]
loss function	the Cross Entropy Loss
batch size	120
epoch	200
learning rate	0.0003
exponential LR	0.99

[1] The optimizer selected AdamW from the Adam series commonly used in training ViT [44].

Table 4. Structural parameters for each module.

Module	Structural Params	Internal Params	Input Size	Output Size
CPE	$r = 1$	patch size [1] = 8	$3 \times 128 \times 128$	$64 \times 16 \times 16$
PTF1 [2]	$l = 2$	$d_0 = 192$, heads [3] = 8	$64 \times 16 \times 16$	$192 \times 8 \times 8$
PTF2 [2]	$l = 4$	$d_0 = 576$, heads [3] = 4	$192 \times 8 \times 8$	$576 \times 4 \times 4$
V-ALC	-	$d_{class} = 7$	$576 \times 4 \times 4$	1×7

[1] The patch size is the size of each patch when the image is split into patches. [2] The PTF module is repeated twice in the model's overall structure, i.e., $n_{tf} = 2$, so the PTF1 and PTF2 refer to the first and second times, respectively. [3] The heads are the setting of the Multi-Head Self-Attention in the PTF module.

3.2. *Performance Evaluation of PCVT Based on Public Datasets*

We evaluate the learning capabilities of CvT [35], PvT [42], ResNet18 [25], ResNet18*, and PCVT on the RAF-DB dataset, focusing on accuracy and resource consumption. Among them, both CvT and PvT are hybrid variant networks formed by introducing convolution into ViT, which are of the same type as this study. ResNet 18 is the most commonly used convolutional neural network for image classification, and ResNet18* is a pre-trained model of ResNet18. CvT, PvT, ResNet18, and PCVT are retrained from scratch using the same computer to obtain experimental results that are not affected by the device conditions. For ResNet18*, we further trained it using this emotion dataset on top of the parameter weights.

As shown in Figure 6, the iterative curves of these five networks trained and validated on the RAF-DB dataset show that the PCVT proposed in this study performs better on the validation data than other models except for ResNet18*. It means that PCVT has better generalization than PvT, CvT, and ResNet18. Admittedly, as a pre-trained model, ResNet18* predictably shows the best classification ability from the beginning of the iteration. Compare the parameters, GFLOPs, and accuracy of the above five networks on the RAF-DB dataset, as shown in Table 5. The accuracy of PCVT is 84.22%, second only to that of ResNet18* (86.28%). Meanwhile, PCVT has the fewest parameters and GFLOPs.

3.3. *Performance Evaluation of FER-PCVT Based on Public Datasets*

3.3.1. Comparison with State-of-the-Art Methods

The proposed FER-PCVT is compared with the state-of-the-art methods on RAF-DB and FER+ datasets. As shown in Table 6, two FER-PCVT models without pretrained weights trained from scratch on two public datasets achieved 89.44% and 88.21% accuracy, respectively. The FER-PCVT learned on the RAF-DB achieves the highest accuracy, while the FER-PCVT learned on FER+ performs lower than other models.

3.3.2. Analysis Based on Confusion Matrix

The detailed performance of FER-PCVT for each class on the RAF-DB and FER+ datasets is analyzed based on the confusion matrix. As shown in Figure 7, FER-PCVT is sensitive to whether the dataset is balanced. There is no significant deviation in the predicted results on the RAF-DB dataset. However, the model shows significant bias on the FER+ dataset. As shown in Figure 7b, the model's predictions have extreme errors in the "disgust" and "contempt" classes with small samples; conversely, the model has highly accurate for the "happy" and "neutral" classes. Moreover, V-ALV determines the expression baseline based on the features of neutral expressions in the batch, so the imbalance of dataset affected the expression baseline generation. In addition, the Precision, Specificity, Sensitivity, F1-Score, and G-mean of FER-PCVT are also analyzed based on the confusion matrix, as shown in Table 7. We set the Precision and Recall to the same weight to obtain the F1-Score of FER-PCVT for each emotional category. On the RAF-DB dataset, the F1-Score values of FER-PCVT for surprised, fear, disgust, happy, sad, angry, and neutral are 84.2%, 73.3%, 67.9%, 94.5%, 86.7%, 80.4%, and 92.4%, respectively. However, on the FER+ dataset, FER-PCVT only performs well for categories with many samples, such as surprised (86.4%), happy (89.4%), sad (69.1%), and neutral (73.6%). G-mean reflects the contribution of each category to the model's accuracy. Although the model's accuracy reaches 88.21% on the FER+ dataset, the G-mean values of both disgust and contempt are 0%, which means that the accuracy depends on surprised (89.8%), fear (72.3%), happy (94%), sad (75.8%), angry (78.8%), and neutral (86.5%). In contrast, the G-mean values of all categories are higher than 90% in the RAF-DB dataset, and the order from high to low is neutral (96.8%), happy (95.6%), sad (92.1%), surprised (89.4%), anger (85.2%), fear (81.1%), and disgust (81.1%).

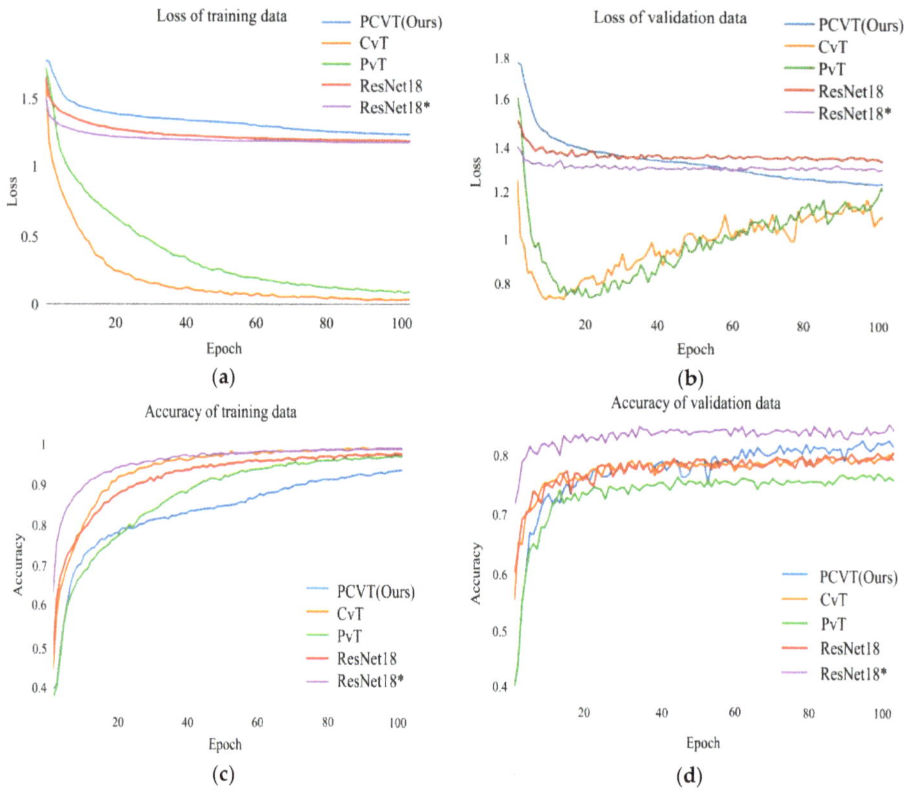

Figure 6. Iterative curves of CvT, PvT, ResNet18, ResNet18*, and PCVT on the RAF-DB dataset. (**a**) Loss plots of these five networks on the training data of RAF-DB. (**b**) Loss plots of these five networks on the validation data of RAF-DB. (**c**) Accuracy plots of these five networks on the training data. (**d**) Accuracy plots of these five networks on the validation data. * It represents a pretrained model.

Table 5. Training results of five networks on the RAF-DB dataset.

Model	Params (M)	GFLOPs	Accuracy (%)
ResNet18	11.20	0.29	81.52
ResNet18 *	11.20	0.29	86.28
CvT	19.55	0.66	81.45
PvT	6.25	0.14	77.80
PCVT(Ours)	2.46	0.12	84.22

* It represents a pretrained model.

Table 6. Performance comparison of FER-PCVT and recent FER models.

Model	Tags	Year	Accuracy	
			FER+	RAF-DB
SPWFA-SE [45]	CNN	2020	-	86.31%
RAN [29]	ResNet	2019	89.16%	86.90%
Ad-Corre [46]	CNN	2022		86.96%
DACL [28]	ResNet	2021	-	87.78%
VTFF [34]	ViT	2022	88.81%	88.14%
SCN [47]	CNN	2020	89.35%	88.14%
FER-VT [48]	ViT	2021	90.04%	88.26%
PSR [49]	VGG-16	2020	-	88.98%
RUL [50]	ResNet	2021	-	88.98%
LResNet50E-IR [51]	ResNet	2020	89.257%	89.075%
FER-PCVT(Ours)	ViT	2022	88.21%	89.44%

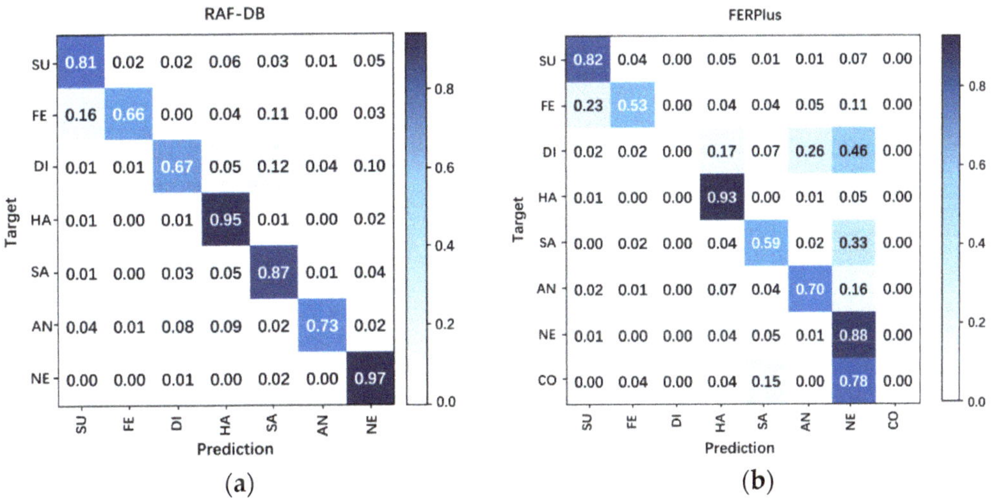

Figure 7. Confusion matrices of FER-PCVT on the RAF-DB dataset (**a**) and the FER+ dataset (**b**). SU: surprise; FE: fear; DI: disgust; HA: happy; SA: sad; AN: angry; NE: neutral; CO: contempt.

Table 7. Precision, Specificity, Sensitivity, F1-score, and G-mean of FER-PCVT on the Raf-DB and FER+ datasets.

Class	RAF-DB					FER+				
	Precision	**Specificity**	**Sensitivity**	**F1-Score**	**G-Mean**	**Precision**	**Specificity**	**Sensitivity**	**F1-Score**	**G-Mean**
surprised	0.877	0.987	0.81	0.842	0.894	0.912	0.982	0.82	0.864	0.898
fear	0.824	0.996	0.66	0.733	0.811	0.555	0.987	0.53	0.542	0.723
disgust	0.688	0.982	0.67	0.679	0.811	0	1	0	0	0
happy	0.941	0.962	0.95	0.945	0.956	0.861	0.951	0.93	0.894	0.940
sad	0.864	0.974	0.87	0.867	0.921	0.835	0.975	0.59	0.691	0.758
angry	0.895	0.995	0.73	0.804	0.852	0.462	0.886	0.70	0.557	0.788
neutral	0.882	0.966	0.97	0.924	0.968	0.632	0.851	0.88	0.736	0.865
contempt	-	-	-	-		0	1	0	0	0

The above parameters for evaluating performance are calculated using the standard formulas shown in Equations (7)–(11):

$$Precision = \frac{TP}{TP + FP} \quad (7)$$

$$Specificity = \frac{TN}{TN + FP} \quad (8)$$

$$Sensitivity = Recall = \frac{TP}{TP + FN} \quad (9)$$

$$F1 - Score = \frac{2 \times Precision \times Recall}{Precision + Recall} \quad (10)$$

$$G_{mean} = \sqrt{Recall \times Specificity} \quad (11)$$

where *TP*, *TN*, *FP*, and *FN* mean the true positive, the true negative, the false positive, and the false negative, respectively.

3.3.3. Visualization of Clustering Ability

The clustering ability of FER-PCVT on the RAF-DB dataset is visualized by the t-SNE plot based on the inputs and outputs of the last linear layer of V-ALC. As shown in Figure 8, the boundaries between the various categories are clear and intuitive, which means that FER-PCVT can distinguish and cluster the seven emotions well.

3.4. *Performance Evaluation of FER-PCVT Based on the Private Dataset*

3.4.1. Accuracy Comparison and Impact of Pretrained Weights

We compare FER-PCVT with ResNet18 and the structure combining PCVT with the Multi-layer Perceptron (MLP) on the private dataset, focusing on the accuracy and parameters of these models with and without pretrained weights. Figure 9 shows the training and validation accuracy curves of ResNet18, PCVT+MLP, and FER-PCVT on the private dataset. As shown in Table 8, the structure formed by PCVT combined with MLP exhibits the worst precision on the private dataset, although it has the lowest number of parameters. FER-PCVT has similar accuracy to ResNet18 on the private dataset with or without pre-trained weights. However, the algorithm proposed in this experiment has only 4.10M parameters, about one-third of the parameters of ResNet18.

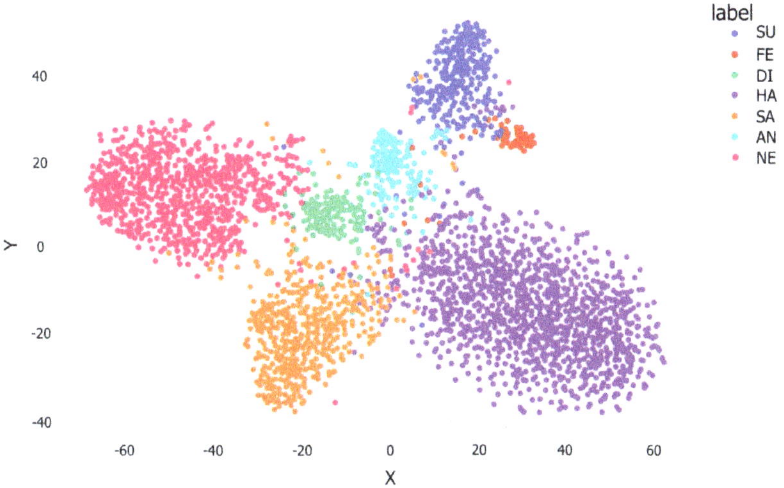

Figure 8. The t−SNE of FER-PCVT on the RAF-DB dataset. SU: surprise; FE: fear; DI: disgust; HA: happy; SA: sad; AN: angry; NE: neutral; CO: contempt.

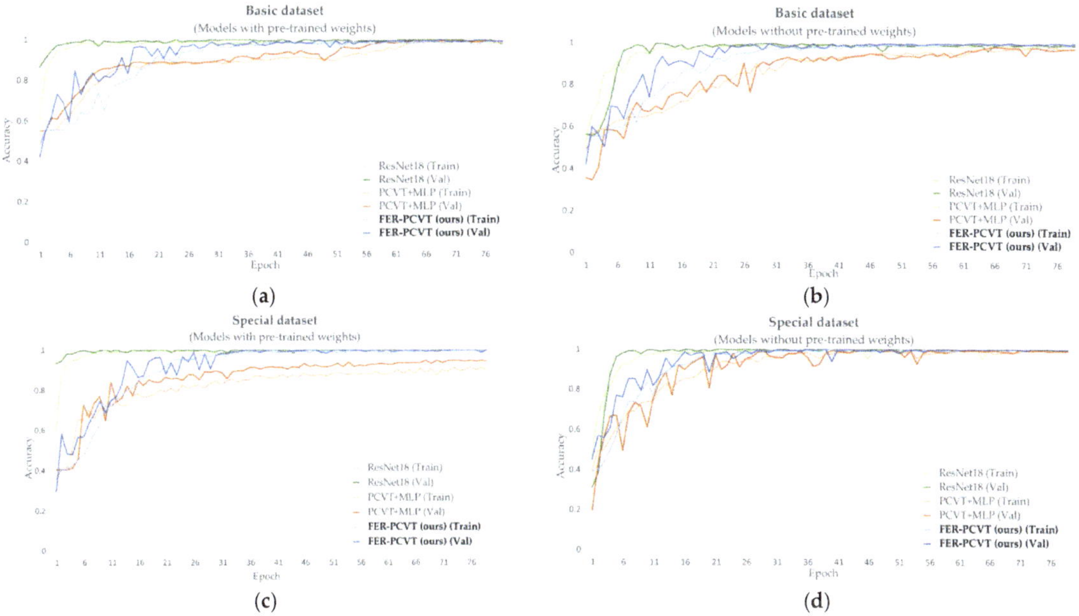

Figure 9. Training and validation accuracy curves of ResNet18, PCVT+MLP, and FER-PCVT on the facial expression dataset of stroke patients. (**a**) Accuracy curves for models with pretrained weights on the basic dataset; (**b**) accuracy curves for models without pretrained weights on the basic dataset; (**c**) accuracy curves for models with pretrained weights on the special dataset; (**d**) accuracy curves for models without pretrained weights on the special dataset. Among them, "Train" means training, and "Val" means validation, and the bold font indicates the algorithm proposed in this study.

Table 8. Accuracy comparison on the facial expression dataset of stroke patients.

Model	Params (M)	Pre-Training	Accuracy (%)		
			Basic Categories [1]	Special Categories [2]	AVG
ResNet18	11.19	✗	98.72	99.66	99.19
		✔	99.58	99.72	99.65
RCVT+MLP	4.06	✗	88.46	97.22	92.84
		✔	98.64	99.21	98.93
PCVT+V-ALC (Ours)	4.10	✗	99.15	99.42	99.29
		✔	99.89	99.72	99.81

[1] The basic categories include surprised, happy, sad, and angry expressions. [2] The special categories include tired, neutral, strained, and painful expressions.

3.4.2. Visualization of Clustering Ability

To visualize the model's ability to classify the eight facial expressions of stroke patients, we plot the t-SNE of FER-PCVT on the private dataset. As shown in Figure 10, the model can cluster the four basic expressions and four special expressions of stroke patients well. Especially in special categories, the distribution of neutral expressions with other expressions is similar to that of the V-A emotion theory.

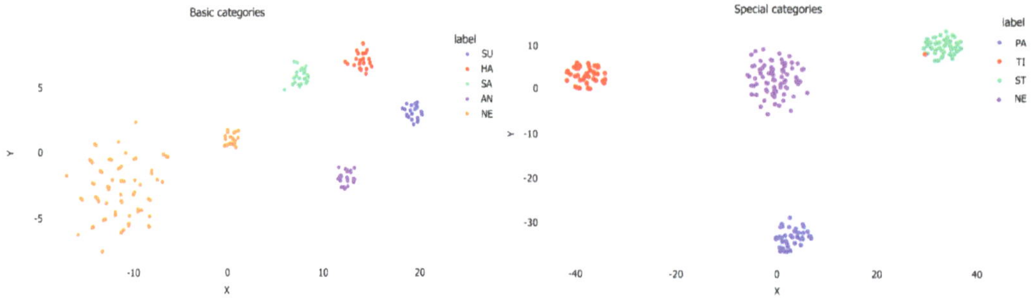

(**a**) (**b**)

Figure 10. The t−SNE of FER-PCVT on the private dataset. (**a**) Visualization of the clustering performance of FER-PCVT for five basic expressions; (**b**) Visualization of the clustering performance of FER-PCVT for four special expressions. SU: surprised; HA: happy; SA: sad; AN: angry; NE: neutral; PA: painful; TI: tired; ST: strained.

3.5. Visual Analysis

We perform a global visual analysis of models to find the regions that models focus on for classification. The Grad-CAM [52] is used to visualize ResNet18*. For ViT and FER-PCVT, visualization is achieved by stacking the attention weights of each layer in order. ResNet18*, ViT, and FER-PCVT have different focus points when identifying the facial emotions of stroke patients, as shown in Figure 11. The part covered in red is the region of the model's most concern when classifying and recognizing expressions. ResNet18* focuses on localized facial regions, while ViT extracts information globally. Although the red regions in the visualization images of ViT appear more on the periphery of the image, ViT also pays attention to the details of the facial features. However, FER-PCVT can focus more on muscle changes due to different expressions while extracting global information. For example, for strained expression, a common emotion when muscles are tense during training, FER-PCVT notices more changes in areas such as eyebrows, eyes, and lips than in other models. Moreover, the facial features of neutral expressions extracted by FER-PCVT are more specific than those of other models. In addition, FER-PCVT also showed a better ability to extract emotional features for these four basic expressions.

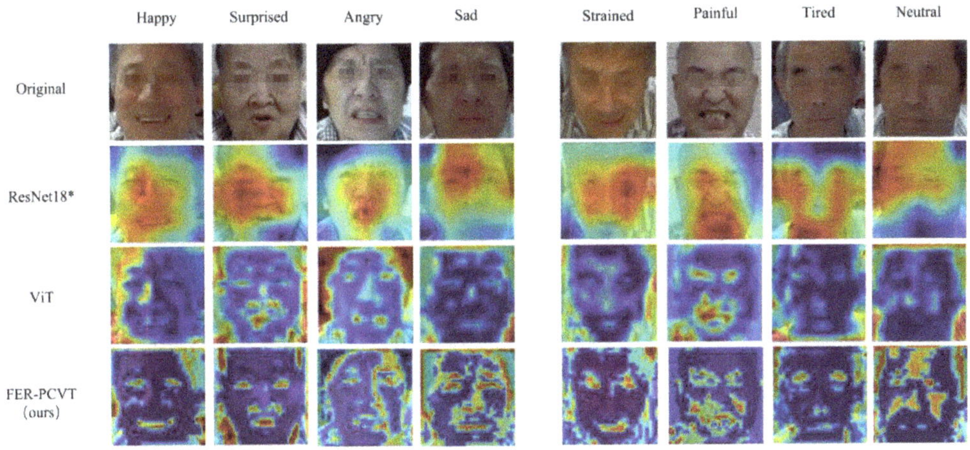

Figure 11. Visualization of ResNet18*, ViT, and FER-PCVT. * It indicates that the model is a pre-trained model.

4. Discussion

Experienced physicians can determine stroke patients' intervention strategies by observing their emotional changes [13]. Similarly, stroke rehabilitation systems based on deep learning/machine learning can also sense the patients' emotions and provide training suggestions according to emotional changes. Currently, more researchers use the patients' physiological signals as the information source of perceived emotion [10–13]. Few studies have designed FER algorithms for stroke rehabilitation. To assist physicians in analyzing the degree of physical recovery and adjusting the training intensity of stroke patients, we use eight common emotions of patients during rehabilitation as biometrics and design a lightweight FER algorithm. By detecting the positive emotions of stroke patients during rehabilitation, such as happy, surprised, and strained, patients' training motivation and interest will be provided to physicians. When painful emotions are detected, it means that the training intensity exceeds the patient's muscle tolerance, and the intensity should be adjusted in time to avoid secondary injuries. In addition, if negative emotions are detected frequently, such as sad, tired, and angry expressions, physicians must pay attention to patients' mental health.

The FER algorithm proposed in this study is an automated assessment technology for stroke rehabilitation, which acquires the training status of patients in a non-contact way. ViT is the basic framework for algorithm design since the global modeling of images using ViT is critical to the emotional classification task, as shown in Figure 11. However, CNNs structures are better at extracting local and detailed information in expression images than ViT. Therefore, introducing the characteristics of CNNs into the ViT structure can improve performance and robustness while maintaining high accuracy and memory efficiency. ViT converts the pixel information (2D) in the patch into the feature sequence (1D) required by the encoder through linear projection and Patch Embedding. The position relationships between patches need to be learned through the Position Embedding module. However, the sequence extracted by convolution contains position information, which is the inductive bias property of convolution. Thus, the CPE module containing convolutional layers and pooling layers is designed to replace the linear projection, the Patch Embedding, and the Position Embedding in ViT. There are some studies that have also introduced convolution into ViT. For example, VTFF [34] extracts the information from the original and local binary pattern images using two ResNet18. Then, it flattens and linearizes feature information to obtain patches with features instead of patches with image blocks in ViT. This network achieves an accuracy of 88.14% on RAF-DB while containing a large number of parameters (51.8M). However, the algorithm proposed in this study performs better on

RAF-DB with 1.3% higher accuracy than VTFF. CvT [35] divides transformers into multiple stages, constituting the transformers' hierarchy. A convolutional token embedding module is added at the beginning of each stage, which is implemented as a convolutional projection to replace the linear projection before each self-attention in ViT. The algorithm proposed in this paper mainly realizes the convolutional mapping between pixels to sequences by combing convolution and pooling instead of linear projection in ViT. At the same time, the location information between patches is preserved. In contrast, we incorporate convolutional features in ViT more concisely. According to the experimental data in Table 5 and Figure 6, PCVT proposed in this study has higher accuracy and lower parameters than CvT on the RAF-DB dataset.

In addition, high accuracy and low parameters are necessary for a model to run well in rehabilitation equipment with less computing power than professional computers. Therefore, we designed the PTF module that introduced a pyramidal feature output mode to reduce parameters and GFLOPs, inspired by PvT [42]. PvT is proposed as a backbone model to serve downstream tasks in various forms, such as image classification, object detection, and semantic segmentation. Similar to this study, both PvT and FER-PCVT have reduced the sequence length of the transformer output as the network deepens, significantly decreasing computational overhead. Regarding implementation details, PvT splits the image/feature map into many patches (size of $P_i \times P_i$, where i is the ith stage), and then feeds each patch into the linear projection to obtain many feature sequences whose dimensions are P_i times shorter than the input. However, we mainly down-sample the feature map by combining convolutional and pooling to get a feature map that the size is reduced by half each time. Validated by the experiments shown in Figure 6 and Table 5, the proposed algorithm has higher accuracy and requires about 3.79M lower parameters than PvT in model training/inference.

Furthermore, considering that some stroke patients have different facial expressions due to impaired facial muscles, we designed a classifier that is more suitable for the emotion classification of stroke patients to improve the accuracy further. We designed the V-ALC classifier based on the V-A emotion theory, treating emotion as the weighted sum of V-A-like and neutral features. The addition of V-ALC improves the model's accuracy from 84.22% to 89.44%, as shown in Tables 5 and 6. According to Table 8, the structure obtained by PCVT splicing V-ALC performs better than that obtained by PCVT splicing MLP in classifying the emotions of stroke patients.

We also visually analyze models to find the attention regions of ViT, ResNet18*, and FER-PCVT in classifying emotions and verify that FER-PCVT combines the advantages of the other two structures well. As shown in Figure 11, ResNet18, a typical CNNs structure, focuses on the facial regions that best represent emotions, similar to the areas humans notice when recognizing the emotions of stroke patients. For example, the tightened and open lips when angry, the wrinkled eyebrows when sad, the raised cheeks when strained, and the relaxed eyes and mouth when tired. Unlike ResNet18, ViT extracts global features while also paying attention to some facial regions located inside the image, especially for surprised and painful expressions. FER-PCVT extracts information globally like ViT but perceives more detailed facial regions than ViT, which means more details about emotions can be captured by FER-PCVT.

However, the algorithm proposed in this study recommends using a dataset with better balance for training, since the designed classifier sums neutral emotion features with weights with other emotion features for classification. Unbalanced sample sizes will affect the model's ability to extract an unbiased emotion baseline. The RAF-DB dataset is more balanced than the FER+ dataset, so the proposed method achieves the highest accuracy on the RAF-DB dataset, as shown in Table 6 and Figure 7. However, its performance on the FER+ dataset is weaker than other FER algorithms, such as RAN [29], VTFF [34], SCN [47], and FER-VT [48].

To summarize, the proposed method has several advantages: (1) It achieves higher recognition accuracy than other existing FER algorithms on the RAF-DB dataset. (2) The network structure successfully combines the local perception of CNNs and the global extraction capability of ViT, which effectively improves the ability of the model to extract feature sequences used to classify patients' emotions. (3) It has fewer parameters and GFLOPs than other algorithms, making it easier to embed in medical rehabilitation equipment with poorer computing performance than professional computers. Although the proposed method has shown lower consumption and better effectiveness on both public datasets and the private dataset, there are still some problems to be improved: (1) The algorithm performs better on the balanced dataset. Therefore, it is necessary to balance the sample size of each category in order to obtain unbiased prediction results. (2) The sample size of the private dataset used in this study is insufficient compared to public datasets, especially for painful and tired expressions. We hope to collect more clinical data to improve the model's generalization. (3) This study only conducted a qualitative analysis of emotions and did not further classify each emotion. For example, painful emotions are divided into severe, moderate, and slight pain in detail. It is hoped that future research can bring more specific and quantitative rehabilitation recommendations for the early training of stroke patients.

5. Conclusions

This study proposes a lightweight FER algorithm, FER-PCVT, which is more conducive to embedding in medical rehabilitation equipment to determine whether the current training intensity received by a stroke patient is most suitable for his physical recovery. To verify the performance of FER-PCVT, we collect and annotate a private dataset of stroke patients containing 1302 samples, which can be divided into 8 classes: painful, strained, tired, neutral, happy, sad, angry, and surprised. This algorithm is compared with other FER algorithms on two public datasets (FER+ and RAF-DB) and a private dataset. The experimental results show that: (1) PCVT, the backbone network of FER-PCVT, achieves an accuracy of 84.22%, parameters of 2.46M, and GFLOPs of 0.12 on the RAF-DB dataset, which is better than CvT, PvT, and ResNet18. (2) FER-PCVT achieves 88.21% and 89.44% on the FER+ and RAF-DB datasets, respectively. Its performance exceeds that of other existing expression recognition algorithms on the RAF-DB dataset. (3) FER-PCVT achieves an accuracy of 99.81% on the private dataset, with only 4.10M parameters. (4) FER-PCVT effectively combines the local perceptual ability and the feature output mode of the CNNs and the global extraction capability of ViT, which significantly reduces the parameters and ensures recognition accuracy. This method has excellent performance on public and private datasets, providing an intuitive and efficient automated assessment technique for stroke patients to receive more suitable early training.

Author Contributions: Conceptualization, Y.F., H.W., X.Z. and X.L.; methodology, Y.F. and X.Z.; software, Y.F. and X.Z.; validation, Y.F. and X.Z.; formal analysis, Y.F. and X.Z.; investigation, Y.F., H.W. and X.Z.; resources, H.W., X.C., Y.C., C.Y. and J.J.; data curation, Y.F.; writing—original draft preparation, Y.F.; writing—review and editing, Y.F. and H.W.; visualization, Y.F.; supervision, X.L. and J.J.; project administration, X.L.; funding acquisition, H.W., Y.C., X.C., J.J. and X.L. All authors have read and agreed to the published version of the manuscript.

Funding: This research was funded by Wuxi Municipal Health Commission Translational Medicine Research Project in 2021 (Wuxi Municipal Health Commission, 100,000, grant No. ZH202102), Scientific and Technological Innovation Plan of Shanghai STC (Shanghai Science & Technology Commission, 300,000, grant No. 21511102605), China National Nature Science Young Foundation (National Natural Science Foundation of China, 300,000, grant No. 82102665), Shanghai Sailing Program (Shanghai Science & Technology Commission, 200,000, grant No. 21YF1404600), Key Subjects Construction Program of the Health System in Jing'an District (Shanghai Municipal Health Commission, 600,000, grant No. 2021PY04) and National Key R&D Program of China (Ministry of Science and Technology of the People's Republic of China, 7,000,000, grant No. 2018YFC2002301).

Institutional Review Board Statement: The study was conducted in accordance with the Declaration of Helsinki and approved by the Ethics Committee of the Third Rehabilitation Hospital of Shanghai, China (SH3RH-2021-EC-001, approved on 29 July 2021).

Informed Consent Statement: Informed consent was obtained from all subjects involved in the study.

Data Availability Statement: Two publicly available datasets FER+ and RAF-DB were analyzed in this study. The FER+ dataset can be found here: Challenges in Representation Learning: Facial Expression Recognition Challenge | Kaggle. The RAF-DB dataset can be found here: Real-world Affective Faces (RAF) Database (whdeng.cn). The private datasets in this study are available from the corresponding authors upon reasonable request.

Conflicts of Interest: The authors declare no conflict of interest. The funders had no role in the design of the study; in the collection, analyses, or interpretation of data; in the writing of the manuscript; or in the decision to publish the results.

References

1. Wang, Y.N.; Wu, S.M.; Liu, M. Temporal trends and characteristics of stroke in China in the past 15 years. *West China Med. J.* **2021**, *36*, 803–807. [CrossRef]
2. Bernhardt, J.; Godecke, E.; Johnson, L.; Langhorne, P. Early rehabilitation after stroke. *Curr. Opin. Neurol.* **2017**, *30*, 48–54. [CrossRef] [PubMed]
3. Budd, S.; Robinson, E.C.; Kainz, B. A survey on active learning and human-in-the-loop deep learning for medical image analysis. *Med. Image Anal.* **2021**, *71*, 102062. [CrossRef] [PubMed]
4. Duggento, A.; Conti, A.; Mauriello, A.; Guerrisi, M.; Toschi, N. Deep computational pathology in breast cancer. *Semin. Cancer Biol.* **2021**, *72*, 226–237. [CrossRef] [PubMed]
5. Lin, L.; Tao, X.; Yang, W.; Pang, S.; Su, Z.; Lu, H.; Li, S.; Feng, Q.; Chen, B. Quantifying Axial Spine Images Using Object-Specific Bi-Path Network. *IEEE J. Biomed. Heal. Inform.* **2021**, *25*, 2978–2987. [CrossRef]
6. Cai, L.; Gao, J.; Zhao, D. A review of the application of deep learning in medical image classification and segmentation. *Ann. Transl. Med.* **2020**, *8*, 713. [CrossRef] [PubMed]
7. Polat, Ö.; Güngen, C. Classification of brain tumors from MR images using deep transfer learning. *J. Supercomput.* **2021**, *77*, 7236–7252. [CrossRef]
8. Hussain, I.; Park, S.J. HealthSOS: Real-Time Health Monitoring System for Stroke Prognostics. *IEEE Access* **2020**, *8*, 213574–213586. [CrossRef]
9. Hussain, I.; Park, S.J. Big-ECG: Cardiographic Predictive Cyber-Physical System for Stroke Management. *IEEE Access* **2021**, *9*, 123146–123164. [CrossRef]
10. Yean, C.; Ahmad, W.W.; Mustafa, W.; Murugappan, M.; Rajamanickam, Y.; Adom, A.; Omar, M.; Zheng, B.; Junoh, A.; Razlan, Z.; et al. An Emotion Assessment of Stroke Patients by Using Bispectrum Features of EEG Signals. *Brain Sci.* **2020**, *10*, 672. [CrossRef]
11. Murugappan, M.; Zheng, B.S.; Khairunizam, W. Recurrent Quantification Analysis-Based Emotion Classification in Stroke Using Electroencephalogram Signals. *Arab. J. Sci. Eng.* **2021**, *46*, 9573–9588. [CrossRef]
12. Bong, S.Z.; Wan, K.; Murugappan, M.; Ibrahim, N.M.; Rajamanickam, Y.; Mohamad, K. Implementation of wavelet packet transform and non linear analysis for emotion classification in stroke patient using brain signals. *Biomed. Signal Process. Control.* **2017**, *36*, 102–112. [CrossRef]
13. Xu, G.; Gao, X.; Pan, L.; Chen, S.; Wang, Q.; Zhu, B.; Li, J. Anxiety detection and training task adaptation in robot-assisted active stroke rehabilitation. *Int. J. Adv. Robot. Syst.* **2018**, *15*, 1729881418806433. [CrossRef]
14. Agbolade, O.; Nazri, A.; Yaakob, R.; Ghani, A.A.; Cheah, Y.K. Down Syndrome Face Recognition: A Review. *Symmetry* **2020**, *12*, 1182. [CrossRef]
15. Wang, Z.; Ma, Z.; Liu, W.; An, Z.; Huang, F. A Depression Diagnosis Method Based on the Hybrid Neural Network and Attention Mechanism. *Brain Sci.* **2022**, *12*, 834. [CrossRef] [PubMed]
16. Rahman, K.K.M.; Subashini, M.M. Identification of Autism in Children Using Static Facial Features and Deep Neural Networks. *Brain Sci.* **2022**, *12*, 94. [CrossRef]
17. Yolcu, G.; Oztel, I.; Kazan, S.; Oz, C.; Palaniappan, K.; Lever, T.E.; Bunyak, F. Deep learning-based facial expression recognition for monitoring neurological disorders. In Proceedings of the 2017 IEEE International Conference on Bioinformatics and Biomedicine (BIBM), Kansas City, MO, USA, 13–16 November 2017.
18. Siddiqi, M.H.; Ali, R.; Sattar, A.; Khan, A.M.; Lee, S. Depth Camera-Based Facial Expression Recognition System Using Multilayer Scheme. *IETE Tech. Rev.* **2014**, *31*, 277–286. [CrossRef]
19. Goodfellow, I.J.; Erhan, D.; Carrier, P.L.; Courville, A.; Mirza, M.; Hamner, B.; Cukierski, W.; Tang, Y.; Thaler, D.; Lee, D.-H.; et al. Challenges in representation learning: A report on three machine learning contests. *Neural Netw.* **2015**, *64*, 59–63. [CrossRef]
20. Gold, J.M.; Barker, J.D.; Barr, S.; Bittner, J.L.; Bromfield, W.D.; Chu, N.; Goode, R.A.; Lee, D.; Simmons, M.; Srinath, A. The efficiency of dynamic and static facial expression recognition. *J. Vis.* **2013**, *13*, 23. [CrossRef]
21. Li, S.; Deng, W.H.; Du, J.P. Reliable Crowdsourcing and Deep Locality-Preserving Learning for Expression Recognition in the Wild. In Proceedings of the IEEE Conference on Computer Vision and Pattern Recognition (CVPR), Honolulu, HI, USA, 21–26 July 2017.
22. Mollahosseini, A.; Hasani, B.; Mahoor, M.H. AffectNet: A Database for Facial Expression, Valence, and Arousal Computing in the Wild. *IEEE Trans. Affect. Comput.* **2017**, *10*, 18–31. [CrossRef]

23. Simonyan, K.; Zisserman, A. Very Deep Convolutional Networks for Large-Scale Image Recognition. *arXiv* **2015**, arXiv:1409.1556. [CrossRef]
24. Mollahosseini, A.; Chan, D.; Mahoor, M.H. Going deeper in facial expression recognition using deep neural networks. In Proceedings of the IEEE Winter Conference on Applications of Computer Vision (WACV), Lake Placid, NY, USA, 7–10 March 2016.
25. He, K.; Zhang, X.; Ren, S.; Sun, J. Deep Residual Learning for Image Recognition. In Proceedings of the IEEE Conference on Computer Vision and Pattern Recognition (CVPR), Las Vegas, NV, USA, 27–30 June 2016.
26. Bahdanau, D.; Cho, K.; Bengio, Y. Neural Machine Translation by Jointly Learning to Align and Translate. *arXiv* **2014**, arXiv:1409.0473. [CrossRef]
27. Wen, Z.; Lin, W.; Wang, T.; Xu, G. Distract Your Attention: Multi-head Cross Attention Network for Facial Expression Recognition. *arXiv* **2021**, arXiv:2109.07270. [CrossRef]
28. Farzaneh, A.H.; Qi, X.J. Facial Expression Recognition in the Wild via Deep Attentive Center Loss. In Proceedings of the IEEE/CVF Winter Conference on Applications of Computer Vision (WACV), Waikoloa, HI, USA, 3–8 January 2021.
29. Wang, K.; Peng, X.J.; Yang, J.F.; Meng, D.B.; Qiao, Y. Region Attention Networks for Pose and Occlusion Robust Facial Expression Recognition. *IEEE Trans. Image Process.* **2020**, *29*, 4057–4069. [CrossRef]
30. Dosovitskiy, A.; Beyer, L.; Kolesnikov, A.; Weissenborn, D.; Zhai, X.; Unterthiner, T.; Dehghani, M.; Minderer, M.; Heigold, G.; Gelly, S.; et al. An Image is Worth 16x16 words: Transformers for Image Recognition at Scale. *arXiv* **2020**, arXiv:2010.11929. [CrossRef]
31. Vaswani, A.; Shazeer, N.; Parmar, N.; Uszkoreit, J.; Jones, L.; Gomez, A.N.; Kaiser, Ł.; Polosukhin, I. Attention Is All You Need. *arXiv* **2017**, arXiv:1706.03762. [CrossRef]
32. Aouayeb, M.; Hamidouche, W.; Soladie, C.; Kpalma, K.; Seguier, R. Learning Vision Transformer with Squeeze and Excitation for Facial Expression Recognition. *arXiv* **2021**, arXiv:2107.03107. [CrossRef]
33. Fayyaz, M.; Koohpayegani, S.A.; Jafari, F.R.; Sengupta, S.; Joze, H.R.V.; Sommerlade, E.; Pirsiavash, H.; Gall, J. Adaptive Token Sampling for Efficient Vision Transformers. *arXiv* **2022**, arXiv:2111.15667. [CrossRef]
34. Ma, F.; Sun, B.; Li, S. Facial Expression Recognition with Visual Transformers and Attentional Selective Fusion. *IEEE Trans. Affect. Comput.* **2021**. [CrossRef]
35. Wu, H.P.; Xiao, B.; Codella, N.; Liu, M.; Dai, X.; Yuan, L.; Zhang, L. CvT: Introducing Convolutions to Vision Transformers. In Proceedings of the IEEE/CVF International Conference on Computer Vision (ICCV), Montreal, QC, Canada, 10–17 October 2021.
36. Barsoum, E.; Zhang, C.; Ferrer, C.C.; Zhang, Z.Y. Training Deep Networks for Facial Expression Recognition with Crowd-Sourced Label Distribution. In Proceedings of the 18th ACM International Conference on Multimodal Interaction (ICMI '16), Tokyo, Japan, 12–16 November 2016.
37. GitHub. Available online: https://github.com/dlunion/DBFace (accessed on 28 March 2022).
38. Ekman, P.E.; Friesen, W.V. Facial Action Coding System (FACS). *Environ. Psychol. Nonverbal Behav.* **1978**. [CrossRef]
39. Lucey, P.; Cohn, J.F.; Prkachin, K.M.; Solomon, P.E.; Matthews, I. Painful data: The UNBC-McMaster shoulder pain expression archive database. In Proceedings of the IEEE international Conference on Automatic Face & Gesture Recognition (FG), Santa Barbara, CA, USA, 21–35 March 2011.
40. Feldman, L.A. Valence focus and arousal focus: Individual differences in the structure of affective experience. *J. Personal. Soc. Psychol.* **1995**, *69*, 153–166. [CrossRef]
41. Xiao, T.; Singh, M.; Mintun, E.; Darrell, T.; Dollár, P.; Girshick, R. Early Convolutions Help Transformers See Better. *Adv. Neural Inf. Process. Syst.* **2021**, *34*, 30392–30400. [CrossRef]
42. Wang, W.H.; Xie, E.Z.; Li, X.; Fan, D.P.; Song, K.; Liang, D.; Lu, T.; Luo, P.; Shao, L. Pyramid Vision Transformer: A Versatile Backbone for Dense Prediction without Convolutions. In Proceedings of the 2021 IEEE/CVF International Conference on Computer Vision (ICCV), Montreal, QC, Canada, 10–17 October 2021.
43. Loshchilov, L.; Hutter, F. Decoupled Weight Decay Regularization. *arXiv* **2017**, arXiv:1711.05101. [CrossRef]
44. Steiner, A.; Kolesnikov, A.; Zhai, X.H.; Wightman, R.; Uszkoreit, J.; Beyer, L. How to train your ViT? Data, Augmentation, and Regularization in Vision Transformers. *arXiv* **2021**, arXiv:2106.10270. [CrossRef]
45. Li, Y.; Lu, G.; Li, J.; Zhang, Z.; Zhang, D. Facial Expression Recognition in the Wild Using Multi-level Features and Attention Mechanisms. *IEEE Trans. Affect. Comput.* **2020**. [CrossRef]
46. Fard, A.P.; Mahoor, M.H. Ad-Corre: Adaptive Correlation-Based Loss for Facial Expression Recognition in the Wild. *IEEE Access* **2022**, *10*, 26756–26768. [CrossRef]
47. Wang, K.; Peng, X.J.; Yang, J.F.; Lu, S.; Qiao, Y. Suppressing Uncertainties for Large-Scale Facial Expression Recognition. In Proceedings of the 2020 IEEE/CVF Conference on Computer Vision and Pattern Recognition (CVPR), Seattle, WA, USA, 13–19 June 2020.
48. Huang, Q.H.; Huang, C.Q.; Wang, X.Z.; Jiang, F. Facial expression recognition with grid-wise attention and visual transformer. *Inf. Sci.* **2021**, *580*, 35–54. [CrossRef]
49. Vo, T.H.; Lee, G.S.; Yang, H.J.; Kim, S.H. Pyramid with Super Resolution for In-the-Wild Facial Expression Recognition. *IEEE Access* **2020**, *8*, 131988–132001. [CrossRef]

50. Zhang, Y.H.; Wang, C.R.; Deng, W.H. Relative Uncertainty Learning for Facial Expression Recognition. *Adv. Neural Inf. Process. Syst.* **2021**, *34*, 17616–17627. Available online: https://openreview.net/forum?id=h1-ilmYbdea&noteId=svNqytjxNmQ (accessed on 25 October 2021).
51. Zhou, H.S.; Meng, D.B.; Zhang, Y.Y.; Peng, X.; Du, J.; Wang, K.; Qiao, Y. Exploring Emotion Features and Fusion Strategies for Audio-Video Emotion Recognition. In Proceedings of the 2019 International Conference on Multimodal Interaction (ICMI'19), Suzhou, China, 14–18 October 2019.
52. Selvaraju, R.R.; Cogswell, M.; Das, A.; Vedantam, R.; Parikh, D.; Batra, D. Grad-CAM: Visual Explanations from Deep Networks via Gradient-Based Localization. In Proceedings of the 2017 IEEE International Conference on Computer Vision (ICCV), Venice, Italy, 22–29 October 2017.

brain sciences

MDPI

Article

A Novel Deep Learning Method Based on an Overlapping Time Window Strategy for Brain–Computer Interface-Based Stroke Rehabilitation

Lei Cao [1,†], Hailiang Wu [1,†], Shugeng Chen [2,†], Yilin Dong [1], Changming Zhu [1], Jie Jia [2,*] and Chunjiang Fan [3,*]

1 Department of Artificial Intelligence, Shanghai Maritime University, Shanghai 201306, China
2 Department of Rehabilitation Medicine, Huashan Hospital, Fudan University, Shanghai 200040, China
3 Department of Rehabilitation Medicine, Wuxi Rehabilitation Hospital, Wuxi 214001, China
* Correspondence: shannonjj@126.com (J.J.); fanchunjiang1980@163.com (C.F.); Tel.: +86-139-1718-0962 (J.J.); +86-136-5619-0701 (C.F.)
† These authors contributed equally to this work.

Abstract: Globally, stroke is a leading cause of death and disability. The classification of motor intentions using brain activity is an important task in the rehabilitation of stroke patients using brain–computer interfaces (BCIs). This paper presents a new method for model training in EEG-based BCI rehabilitation by using overlapping time windows. For this aim, three different models, a convolutional neural network (CNN), graph isomorphism network (GIN), and long short-term memory (LSTM), are used for performing the classification task of motor attempt (MA). We conducted several experiments with different time window lengths, and the results showed that the deep learning approach based on overlapping time windows achieved improvements in classification accuracy, with the LSTM combined vote-counting strategy (VS) having achieved the highest average classification accuracy of 90.3% when the window size was 70. The results verified that the overlapping time window strategy is useful for increasing the efficiency of BCI rehabilitation.

Keywords: brain–computer interface; motor attempt (MA); EEG; deep learning method; overlapping time window

Citation: Cao, L.; Wu, H.; Chen, S.; Dong, Y.; Zhu, C.; Jia, J.; Fan, C. A Novel Deep Learning Method Based on an Overlapping Time Window Strategy for Brain–Computer Interface-Based Stroke Rehabilitation. *Brain Sci.* **2022**, *12*, 1502. https://doi.org/10.3390/brainsci12111502

Academic Editors: Konstantin V. Slavin and Gianluca Di Flumeri

Received: 7 September 2022
Accepted: 31 October 2022
Published: 5 November 2022

1. Introduction

Stroke leads to high rates of disability and death worldwide [1]. To restore brain function affected by stroke, patients need to undergo rigorous rehabilitation. Currently, there are a variety of approaches to help restore motor function after a stroke, including the use of mirror therapy [2], virtual reality [3], aerobic exercise [4], and brain–computer interface (BCI) technology [5–7]. BCI technology can help patients recover independently and perform tasks by efficiently controlling additional devices, making it a good option for patients.

The use of a non-invasive BCI for motor rehabilitation has become a focus of current research and is considered a mainstream experimental method. Patients perform motor imagery (MI) or motor attempt (MA) tasks based on cues from the system. The BCI then decodes and converts the motor intents from the electroencephalogram (EEG) signals into commands and provides feedback according to the experimental protocol [8,9]. However, EEG signals may be unstable or random and show significant individual differences. In addition, EEG signals intended for the same behavior but collected at different times and under different circumstances may also have large differences; hence, it is difficult to classify EEG signals directly. Feature extraction and classification algorithms are needed to extract meaningful information from the multidimensional EEG signals [10].

Based on previous studies, the features extracted by traditional machine learning methods can be classified into three categories: spatial, time, and frequency. In dichotomous BCI tasks, the common spatial pattern (CSP) algorithm is the most common method for extracting spatial features [11], as it is able to extract the spatially distributed components of each class from multichannel EEG signals. Many studies have expanded the CSP algorithm, and the filter bank CSP (FBCSP) developed from the CSP algorithm has achieved very good classification performance in MI-BCI [12]. Analyzing EEG signals in a time series can yield rich statistical features. Geethanjali et al. extracted seven time-domain features from EEG signals and classified them using linear discriminant analysis [13]. As many EEG signal features are reflected in the frequency domain, analysis of frequency domain features is important for BCIs. Furthermore, by converting EEG signals from the time domain to the frequency domain, the distribution and variation of EEG frequencies can be visualized. Chen et al. visualized event-related synchronization and event-related desynchronization in MA and MI tasks in different frequency bands [14]. Although the above method can be applied to MA-BCI and MI-BCI to some extent, they require prior knowledge and manually designed features combined with the use of machine learning for classification, which may present problems of insufficient feature extraction and low adaptability to different patients. Hence, many studies have tried to use deep learning (DL) to automatically learn features gathered from EEG signals for classification.

In contrast to traditional machine learning methods, DL does not require predefined feature vectors, as it can automatically learn latent and highly abstract features from raw EEG signals. The combination of BCI with DL methods has been used in the rehabilitation of patients. Lin et al. developed a convolutional neural network (CNN)-based model for predicting BCI rehabilitation outcomes [15]. Liang et al. used the long short-term memory (LSTM) neural network for generating motor trajectories of the lower-extremity exoskeleton for stroke rehabilitation [16] and a graph embedding-based model, Ego-CNN, for identifying key graph structures during MI [17]. However, BCI systems using DL methods require large amounts of EEG data for training models, which results in a bottleneck in therapy. At present, independent patients experience more difficulty performing control tasks due to tedious experimental steps, which often leads to less data collected and less than optimal accuracy for classification using DL methods.

For smaller datasets, data augmentation techniques have proven to be an effective way to improve the performance of DL models, and the approach is to generate more data from the original data for training the model. In previous studies, some have performed data enhancement by adding noise to the original EEG signals [18]. Sliding time windows are advantageous in augmenting EEG signal data. Hartmann et al. used an overlapping time window to expand a dataset of epileptic patients [19], and Zhang et al. extracted time and frequency domain features from multiple windows for a classification task of left versus right hand movements [20]. In addition, several studies have used generative adversarial network models for generating new data similar to the original EEG signal [21]. This approach can help to compensate for the inability to collect large amounts of EEG signals from patients during motor rehabilitation and further improve the performance of DL methods for classifying EEG signals.

The purpose of this paper was to improve the performance of DL on MA-BCI through data augmentation techniques to contribute to the rehabilitation training of patients. Specifically, we provide more accurate neurofeedback by improving the recognition accuracy of a patient's motor intention. To achieve this aim, we propose a DL method based on overlapping time windows for the classification tasks of MA-BCI. This study compares the classification performance of three different DL models on MA tasks. To investigate the effect of different time periods on BCI classification, we visualized the classification results on a time series and analyzed the differences in EEG signals at different time slices using the power spectral density topography of the brain.

2. Materials and Methods

The data used in our experiment were collected from 7 stroke subjects using BCI interventions. Demographic information and clinical data are reported in Table 1. All subjects typically performed three sessions per week; one session included ninety trials, and each trial corresponded to one type of task: motor attempt (MA) or idle state (IS).

2.1. Experimental Protocol

Figure 1 shows the experimental protocol during rehabilitation training. The experimental setup consists of two components: a BCI module and a force feedback device. The BCI module is responsible for the collection and analysis of EEG signals, and the force feedback device is responsible for providing neurofeedback. The patient's stroke-affected hand was immobilized on the force feedback device that was controlled by the BCI system. When the experimental task was a motor attempt, patients continually attempted wrist extension with the affected hand. When the experimental task was in an idle state, they were ordered to rest and do nothing. The force feedback device drove the patient's stroke-affected hand to complete a wrist extension movement when the BCI system accurately identified the patient's motor intention. For incorrect identification, the device would stay stationary.

Table 1. Demographic information of the subjects.

Subject	Sex	Age	Affected Limb	Stroke Stage
Sub1	Male	31	Right	Subacute
Sub2	Male	40	Left	Subacute
Sub3	Male	42	Right	Subacute
Sub4	Male	47	Right	Subacute
Sub5	Male	36	Right	Subacute
Sub6	Male	30	Right	Subacute
Sub7	Male	65	Left	Subacute
Mean	-	41.6 ± 12.0	-	-

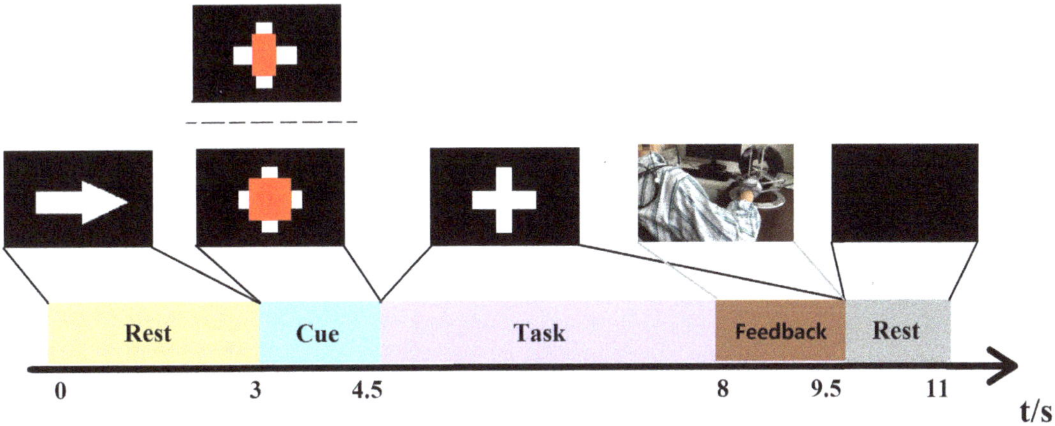

Figure 1. Experimental protocol of rehabilitation training. During the cueing period, a red rectangle is used to alert the user to perform specific tasks. When the cue is a red square, the patient will attempts wrist extension using the stroke-affected hand as hard as possible until the white cross disappears. When the cue is a red rectangle, the patient just needs to stay rested. The patient's stroke-affected hand was passively extended by the force feedback device when the system accurately identified the patient's motor intention.

2.2. Data Acquisition and Preprocessing

According to Figure 1, the EEG signals of each trial were recorded for 11 seconds and started with a white arrow image used to prompt the patient to be prepared. Three seconds later, a task cue (red geometrical shapes) was displayed on the screen, and the patient was asked to perform either a movement attempt or a rest state. After the cue disappeared, the patient was told to continue performing the task following the cue until the white cross disappeared. Then, the patients rested for 1.5 s. The recorded signals were sampled by a 32-channel EEG cap, and the EEG electrodes were placed according to the international 10–20 system. The sampling frequency was 200 Hz. Data from 31 channels were used for calculation, and the filter range was 4 to 40 Hz. Some examples of the preprocessed EEG signals (C3, C4) from the motor function areas of the brain are shown in Figure 2. Five seconds of EEG before the white cross disappeared from each trial were extracted for training the model.

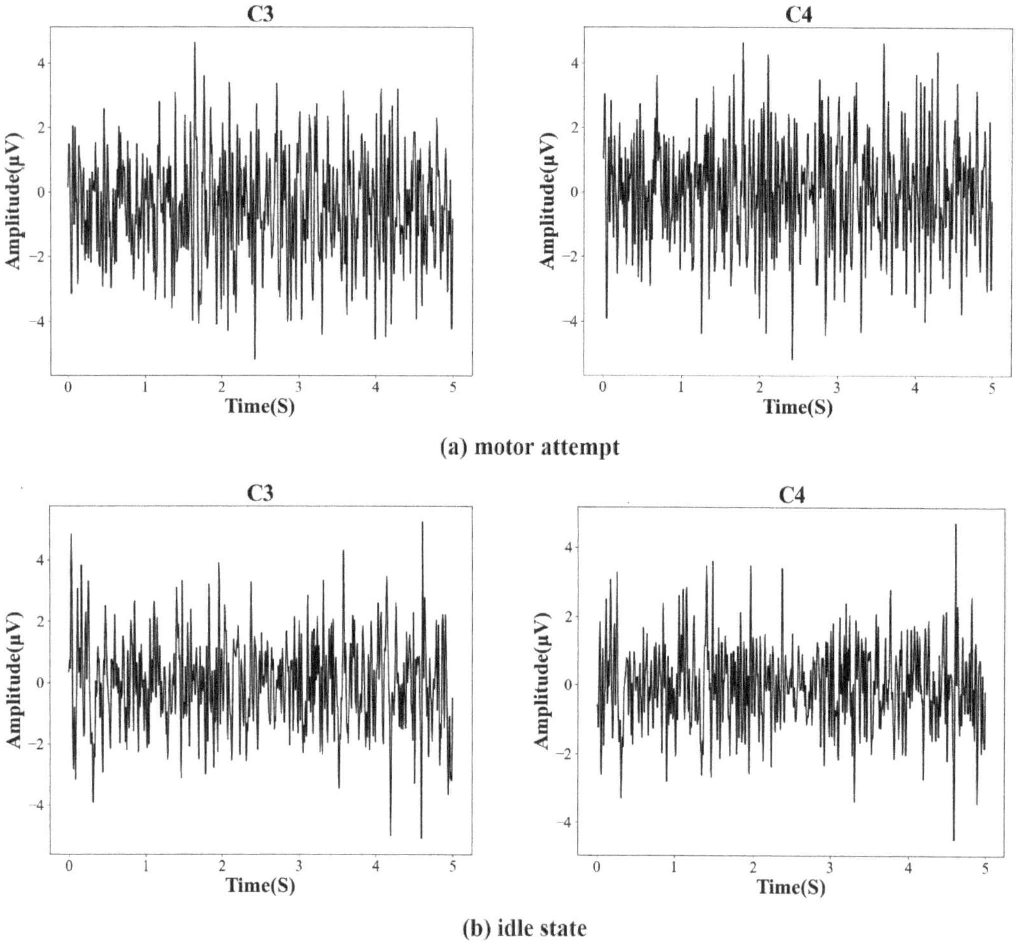

Figure 2. Examples of preprocessed EEG signals from different brain activities.

2.3. *Overlapping Time Window*

The performance of DL models is very heavily dependent on the quantity of data involved in the training. Due to the difficulty of collecting MA data, the amount of data collected for individual patients is small. In existing work, a promising approach is to split the individual signals into multiple subsignals for training the model [19,20,22]. We propose a data augmentation method based on an overlapping time window for increasing the number of instances during training. The raw EEG data were segmented by overlapping windows; each data window served as an independent instance. The number of windows was controlled by two parameters: the time window length L and the overlap rate O. For the original input of experimental data $X^i = [x_1, x_2, \ldots, x_T] \in R^{C^*T}$, i represented the type of task, C represented the channel, and T represented the sampling point; in this experiment, C = 31 and T = 1000. Given the parameters O, L. The raw data were segmented into $D^i_{L,O}$.

$$D^i_{L,O} = \left\{X^i_1, X^i_{2,\ldots,} X^i_{s,} \ldots X^i_n\right\} \in R^{n^*C^*L} \quad (1)$$

$$X^i_s = \{x_t, x_{t+1}, \ldots, x_{t+L} \mid \mathrm{t} = 1 + (\mathrm{s}-1)LO\} \quad (2)$$

$\mathrm{n} = \frac{T-L}{LO} + 1$, which denotes that the original data were sliced into n time segments. The segmented data and the original data had the same task label i. When $n = 1$, the data were not segmented. We divided the original dataset into a training set and a test set. For the training set, each signal X_{train} with a length of 1000 was divided into 32 windows (L = 60, O = 0.5). In this way, the signals in each window were used as instances to train the model. In the testing phase, for each signal X_{test} with a length of 1000 in the test dataset, we divided it into 32 windows using the same approach. The data from these windows were fed into the trained model, and the classification results were obtained on these windows. After that, multiple window classification results of windows were fused into one decision for X_{test} by using the vote-counting strategy (VS). In addition, we also designed another method for classifying X_{test}. We combined the features of different windows from the last hidden layer of the model by summing, and the combined feature was fed into the softmax layer for classification, which is called the feature fusion strategy (FFS) in this paper. "&VS" and "&FFS" refer to strategies for validating trained models on the test set using voting and feature fusion, respectively.

2.4. *Graph Isomorphism Network Model*

2.4.1. Graph Data Construction

The aim of graph neural networks (GNNs) is to use graph structure data and node features as input to learn a representation of the node (or graph) for relevant tasks [23]. Because EEG data are easily converted to graph structure data, several studies have investigated GNNs applied to EEG signal-based tasks [17,24–27]. An important aspect of using a GNN to classify EEG signals is building graph data, the original data first need to be converted into graph structure data. The EEG signal of a window can be defined as $G = (V, E)$, where V and E represent the sets of nodes and edges, respectively. In this experiment, we treated the individual channel as a node and the closed channels as connected edges. Specifically, the average Euclidean distance d between the CZ channel and the other channels was calculated, and the two channels with an electrode distance less than d were treated as connected.

2.4.2. Graph Isomorphism Network

Most GNNs complete the graph classification process through a strategy of aggregating information from neighbors. Formally, node updates and the graph embedding h_G are obtained using the following formula.

$$\mathrm{a}_\mathrm{v}^{(\mathrm{k})} = \mathrm{AGGREGATE}^{(\mathrm{k})}\left(\left\{\mathrm{h}_\mathrm{u}^{(\mathrm{k}-1)} \mid \mathrm{u} \in N(\mathrm{v})\right\}\right) \quad (3)$$

$$\mathrm{h}_\mathrm{v}^{(\mathrm{k})} = \mathrm{COMBINE}^{(\mathrm{k})}\left(\mathrm{h}_\mathrm{v}^{(\mathrm{k}-1)}, \mathrm{a}_\mathrm{v}^{(\mathrm{k})}\right) \quad (4)$$

$$h_G = \mathrm{READOUT}\left(\left\{h_v^{(K)} \mid v \in G\right\}\right) \quad (5)$$

where $h_v^{(k)}$ is the feature vector of node v at the k -th iteration layer, $h_v^{(0)}$ represents node input , and $N(v)$ is a set of nodes adjacent to v. AGGREGATE and COMBINE represent the aggregation of information about neighbors and the aggregation of information about oneself and neighbors, respectively. The choices of $\text{AGGREGATE}^{(k)}(\cdot)$ and $\text{COMBINE}^{(k)}(\cdot)$ in GNNs are crucial. The output h_G aggregates node features via the READOUT function at the final iteration.

In this study, we used a graph isomorphism network (GIN) model for classifying EEG signals. The GIN network is a kind of GNN and uses the summation method to complete AGGREGATE, COMBINE, and READOUT [28]. Following the literature [28], we used the following formula for feature updates of node features:

$$h_v^{(k)} = \text{MLP}^{(k)}\left(\left(1+\epsilon^{(k)}\right)\cdot h_v^{(k-1)} + \sum_{u\in N(v)} h_u^{(k-1)}\right) \quad (6)$$

MLP represents multilayer perceptrons, and ϵ is a parameter that can be trained. We tuned the hyperparameters through a grid search over the training set in this experiment. The search space ranges for the network depth and the number of neurons in GIN were defined as {1, 2, 3, 4} and {32, 64, 128, 256}, respectively. After hyperparameter optimization, the network depth k and the number of neurons were set to 2 and 256, respectively. The learned graph embedding h_G passes through two fully connected layers to output the final feature representation. This experiment focused on the binary classification problem, so the number of neurons in the final fully connected layer was 2. In this study, the output layers of the three models were the softmax layer, and the loss functions were all set to the cross-entropy loss function.

2.5. CNN

Convolutional neural networks (CNNs) are considered to be one of the most successful deep learning models and have been widely used for feature extraction of EEG signals [24,29,30]. The CNN is a deep feed-forward neural network that includes crucial convolutional operations. Compared to traditional neural networks, CNNs reduce the training parameters by local sensing and weight sharing. Each convolutional layer consists of multiple convolutional kernels of the same size for feature extraction. The mathematical description of the convolutional operation is as follows:

$$y_{mn} = f\left(\sum_{j=0}^{J-1}\sum_{i=0}^{I-1} x_{m+i,n+j}w_{ij} + b\right) \quad (7)$$

where x represents the matrix on which the convolution operation is performed, and y is the output of the convolution. I, J corresponds to the size of the convolution kernel w, b represents a bias, and f is the activation function, which was $ReLu$ in this study. The grid search ranges of the parameters were defined as follows: number of convolution layers and max-pooling layers {1, 2, 3, 4}, length of the convolutional kernels {2, 3, 4, 5}, number of convolutional kernels {16, 32, 64, 128}, and number of neurons in the fully connected layer {32, 64, 128, 256}. The optimized model structure in this study consisted of 3 convolutional layers and 3 max pooling layers. The size of the convolutional kernels was $4 * 4$, $2 * 2$, and $2 * 2$, and the number of convolutional kernels was 32, 64, and 128, respectively. After completing the pooling of the final layer, we flattened the extracted features and fed them into a fully connected layer fc_1, which contained 128 neurons. Finally, the output of the fully connected layer fc_1 passed through the $ReLu$ activation function and another fully connected layer fc_2 to output the final 2-dimensional representation feature.

2.6. LSTM

Due to the long duration of the patient performing the task, some useful features still needed to be retained despite the long interval. LSTM can retain the motor intention of EEG signals that are both long and short. LSTM networks are a modified version of recurrent neural networks (RNNs) [31]. Based on RNNs, the LSTM added a multiple gate structure (forget gate f_t, input gate i_t, and output gate o_t) for updating the cell state. The LSTM network layer contains the cell state C_t, which represents the cell information stored at time t. The data features x_t at time t, the hidden features h_{t-1} at moment $t-1$, and the cell state C_{t-1}, were fed into the LSTM nodes, which were processed by gates to output the hidden state and cell state at the next moment. The calculations are as follows.

$$f_t = \text{sigmoid}\left(w_f[x_t, h_{t-1}] + b_f\right) \quad (8)$$

$$i_t = \text{sigmoid}(w_i[h_{t-1}, x_t] + b_t) \quad (9)$$

$$\bar{C}_t = \tanh(w_c[h_{t-1}, x_t] + b_c) \quad (10)$$

$$C_t = f_t * C_{t-1} + i_t * \bar{C}_t \quad (11)$$

where w_f and b_f indicate the weight and bias of the forget gate, respectively. The sigmoid function in the forget gate determines which messages need to be deleted. The corresponding input gate i_t determines which information to retain, and w_i and b_i indicate the weight and bias of the input gate. $\bar{C}_t$ represents the candidate hidden state, and w_c and b_c correspond to the weight and bias, respectively. The output of the forget gate and the input gate are jointly calculated to obtain the cell state value C_t at the current moment.

Finally, the current cell state C_t and the output o_t of the output gate are calculated as follows to obtain the current hidden state h_t.

$$o_t = \text{sigmoid}(w_o[h_{t-1}, x_t] + b_o) \quad (12)$$

$$h_t = o_t * \tanh(C_t) \quad (13)$$

where w_o and b_o are the weight and bias of the output gate, respectively. For a multilayer LSTM model, the hidden state h_t at moment t of the previous layer is used as the input of the next network layer at moment t. The number of LSTM hidden layer units was determined by the time window length, and each time point was a unit. In this study, we employed a two-layer LSTM, and we fed the hidden state at the last moment of the last layer into a fully connected layer to output the final feature representation. The hidden state features of the LSTM perform a grid search in the range {32, 64, 128, 256}, with an optimized feature size of 128.

2.7. Evaluation Procedures

One of the most important aspects of BCI is accuracy. To test the effectiveness of different methods, we used 3-fold cross-validation. For one session, the data were randomly divided into a training set containing 60 trials and a test set containing 30 trials, with a ratio of 2:1. We first optimized hyperparameters on the training set via grid search, with 90% of the data used to train the model and 10% to validate the performance of the hyperparameters and choose the model structure with the highest average accuracy. The data ratio between the two task categories was always 1:1 in the different sets. After completing hyperparameter optimization, we trained the final classification models using all the training data. The average accuracy of each fold was used to evaluate the performance of the model. In addition, we used the information transfer rate (ITR) to evaluate the performance of the BCI [32]. The units of ITR are bits/min, which are calculated from Equation (14). N is the number of task types, which is set to 2 in this study, P is the accuracy rate, and T is the time during the task (60 s).

$$B = \left\{\log_2 N + P\log_2 P + (1-P)\log_2\left[\frac{1-P}{N-1}\right]\right\} \times \frac{60}{T} \quad (14)$$

3. Results and Discussion

3.1. Overall Performance

In this study, the average classification results for seven subjects are reported in Table 2. The results listed include six methods and the accuracies achieved with the same segmentation strategy (L = 60, O = 0.5). The results showed that the LSTM&FFS achieved the highest mean accuracy of 90.1% for all subjects, while the GIN&VS had the lowest accuracy of 81.9%. One of the explanations for differences in accuracy between different methods could be different types of extracted features. To verify that our method is superior to the existing method, we compared our methods with the traditional algorithms [14,33]. After comparison, compared with CSP and FBCSP, the six methods in this study yielded an average improvement of 11.71% and 23.01% in regard to average accuracy. The results indicated that the methods can learn distinctive features of multiple windows for classification and that these features improved classifier performance. To analyze the impact of age on the algorithm, patients were divided into two age groups based on the median age (40 years). Compared to the group aged <40, the group aged ≥40 showed higher accuracy on different algorithms, and the results suggest that the patient's age may be a factor in the accuracy of the classification.

To identify the performance of different models, we recorded the training loss and validation accuracy during model training for Subject 1 in Figure 3. The loss in the CNN and LSTM training set dropped to 0.2 after 100 iterations and the top accuracy of the test sets converged to approximately 93% and 98%, respectively. A faster convergence was observed in GIN, but the accuracy was relatively low. Figure 4 illustrates the training time and the number of training parameters for different models. Although the training parameters of the LSTM model were not the highest, training of the model required more time. This may partially be because of the structure of the LSTM model [34], which could not complete parallel computing in the training process. For real-world applications, the choice of method can consider multiple factors of accuracy and computational complexity.

Paired-sample t-tests were used to determine whether the difference among individual methods was statistically significant. The results are presented in Table 3. Significant differences were found across multiple methods at the 0.05 significance level, and the difference between LSTM&VS and LSTM&FFS was not significant at the 0.01 significance level. Although the performance was different in the six methods, the overall accuracy was high.

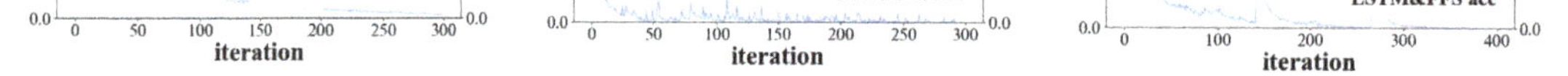

Figure 3. Losses of the training sets for deep learning models and classification accuracies of test sets for different methods.

Table 2. The overall comparison results of average classification performance.

Subjects	Accuracy							
	CSP	FBCSP	GIN&VS	LSTM&VS	CNN&VS	GIN&FFS	LSTM&FFS	CNN&FFS
sub1	0.798 ± 0.079	0.614 ± 0.096	0.914 ± 0.061	0.979 ± 0.025	0.944 ± 0.059	0.931 ± 0.049	0.980 ± 0.017	0.934 ± 0.058
sub2	0.700 ± 0.064	0.578 ± 0.096	0.722 ± 0.069	0.772 ± 0.106	0.741 ± 0.065	0.746 ± 0.060	0.806 ± 0.111	0.757 ± 0.057
sub3	0.771 ± 0.077	0.627 ± 0.094	0.902 ± 0.075	0.938 ± 0.044	0.932 ± 0.047	0.919 ± 0.073	0.949 ± 0.042	0.940 ± 0.046
sub4	0.804 ± 0.072	0.635 ± 0.157	0.938 ± 0.038	0.993 ± 0.011	0.966 ± 0.024	0.952 ± 0.030	0.994 ± 0.010	0.970 ± 0.016
sub5	0.724 ± 0.054	0.644 ± 0.057	0.711 ± 0.066	0.808 ± 0.071	0.762 ± 0.076	0.757 ± 0.073	0.841 ± 0.068	0.769 ± 0.085
sub6	0.687 ± 0.040	0.630 ± 0.053	0.744 ± 0.055	0.801 ± 0.037	0.764 ± 0.058	0.777 ± 0.055	0.825 ± 0.029	0.755 ± 0.050
sub7	0.707 ± 0.082	0.677 ± 0.090	0.798 ± 0.078	0.899 ± 0.066	0.845 ± 0.085	0.842 ± 0.081	0.909 ± 0.062	0.856 ± 0.084
Mean	0.742	0.629	0.819	0.884	0.851	0.846	0.901	0.854
Group1	0.736 ± 0.056	0.629 ± 0.015	0.790 ± 0.108	0.865 ± 0.099	0.823 ± 0.105	0.822 ± 0.095	0.884 ± 0.088	0.820 ± 0.100
Group2	0.746 ± 0.050	0.630 ± 0.041	0.840 ± 0.099	0.901 ± 0.094	0.871 ± 0.101	0.865 ± 0.092	0.915 ± 0.080	0.881 ± 0.096

Group1, age < 40; Group2, age ≥ 40.

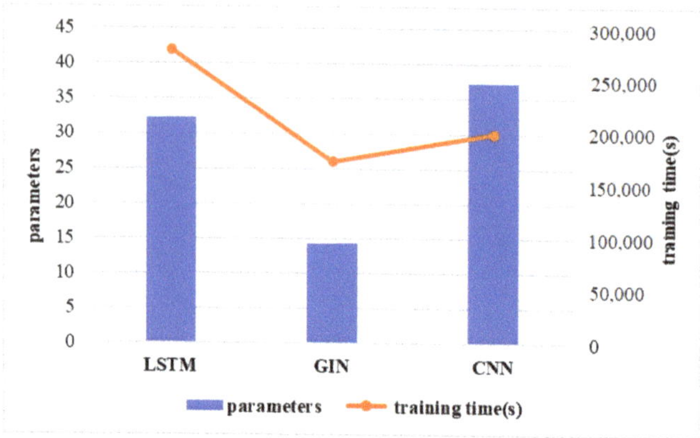

Figure 4. The number of parameters and running times for different models.

Table 3. Paired-sample *t*-test results of different methods.

Method	Comparsion Method	T	df	Sig. (2-Tailed)
GIN&VS	GIN&FFS	−5.451	6	0.002
	CNN&FFS	−5.345	6	0.002
	LSTM&FFS	−7.528	6	<0.001
	CNN&VS	−6.705	6	0.001
	LSTM&VS	−7.140	6	<0.001
CNN&VS	GIN&FFS	1.146	6	0.295
	CNN&FFS	−0.999	6	0.356
	LSTM&FFS	−5.976	6	0.001
	LSTM&VS	−5.805	6	0.001
LSTM&VS	GIN&FFS	6.823	6	<0.001
	CNN&FFS	4.333	6	0.005
	LSTM&FFS	−3.527	6	0.012
GIN&FFS	CNN&FFS	−1.501	6	0.184
	LSTM&FFS	−8.477	6	<0.001
CNN&FFS	LSTM&FFS	−5.400	6	0.002

3.2. Effects of Window Size

To investigate the effect of window size, we experimented with multiple window sizes and evaluated the performances of the models in the corresponding window. The sizes of the comparison time windows were 1000, 200, 100, 90, 80, 70, and 60. Figure 5 presents the average accuracy of the six methods for the different windows. The lowest accuracy was achieved when the window size was 1000, which means without data augmentation. The most likely reason for this phenomenon is probably because the models overfit fewer training data. We illustrate the performance of each method for three window sizes in Table 4. The LSTM&VS accuracy was 90.3% when the window size was 70. However, the LSTM model showed only a classification accuracy of 65.4% without using a time window. The difference in accuracies occurred because the different window sizes changed the lengths of the input time series. In addition, according to the results, when the window size was 70, the average accuracy of each method was higher than that of the method with a window size of 100. This may indicate that relatively small sizes of windows had better performance.

Table 4. Comparison of the accuracies of different methods with time windows of 60, 70, and 1000.

Window Length	Method	Accuracy							
		Sub1	Sub2	Sub3	Sub4	Sub5	Sub6	Sub7	Mean
70	GIN&VS	0.929 ± 0.061	0.764 ± 0.069	0.915 ± 0.075	0.942 ± 0.038	0.760 ± 0.066	0.781 ± 0.055	0.858 ± 0.078	0.850
	GIN&FFS	0.924 ± 0.049	0.755 ± 0.060	0.912 ± 0.073	0.947 ± 0.030	0.755 ± 0.073	0.782 ± 0.054	0.843 ± 0.081	0.845
	CNN&VS	0.94 ± 0.039	0.766 ± 0.076	0.931 ± 0.047	0.967 ± 0.021	0.777 ± 0.059	0.789 ± 0.054	0.871 ± 0.083	0.864
	CNN&FFS	0.939 ± 0.040	0.754 ± 0.079	0.929 ± 0.049	0.960 ± 0.018	0.761 ± 0.053	0.760 ± 0.059	0.856 ± 0.095	0.851
	LSTM&VS	0.985 ± 0.018	0.808 ± 0.101	0.951 ± 0.041	0.997 ± 0.008	0.844 ± 0.072	0.819 ± 0.036	0.917 ± 0.066	0.903
	LSTM&FFS	0.984 ± 0.014	0.801 ± 0.101	0.948 ± 0.038	0.995 ± 0.008	0.842 ± 0.078	0.812 ± 0.047	0.917 ± 0.078	0.900
100	GIN&VS	0.925 ± 0.046	0.764 ± 0.058	0.916 ± 0.065	0.929 ± 0.039	0.746 ± 0.056	0.793 ± 0.053	0.844 ± 0.074	0.845
	GIN&FFS	0.919 ± 0.053	0.755 ± 0.048	0.919 ± 0.069	0.935 ± 0.039	0.745 ± 0.070	0.784 ± 0.056	0.846 ± 0.080	0.843
	CNN&VS	0.938 ± 0.058	0.759 ± 0.057	0.923 ± 0.047	0.941 ± 0.030	0.755 ± 0.052	0.762 ± 0.053	0.852 ± 0.075	0.847
	CNN&FFS	0.925 ± 0.056	0.744 ± 0.064	0.920 ± 0.055	0.946 ± 0.029	0.748 ± 0.053	0.734 ± 0.057	0.830 ± 0.096	0.835
	LSTM&VS	0.982 ± 0.020	0.799 ± 0.095	0.943 ± 0.039	0.995 ± 0.008	0.807 ± 0.077	0.893 ± 0.038	0.816 ± 0.078	0.891
	LSTM&FFS	0.986 ± 0.017	0.792 ± 0.098	0.942 ± 0.040	0.995 ± 0.010	0.814 ± 0.084	0.898 ± 0.046	0.815 ± 0.089	0.892
1000	GIN	0.810 ± 0.057	0.732 ± 0.062	0.814 ± 0.091	0.797 ± 0.051	0.696 ± 0.067	0.700 ± 0.037	0.731 ± 0.057	0.754
	CNN	0.689 ± 0.084	0.625 ± 0.058	0.763 ± 0.013	0.643 ± 0.066	0.634 ± 0.051	0.612 ± 0.062	0.638 ± 0.067	0.658
	LSTM	0.674 ± 0.061	0.630 ± 0.051	0.719 ± 0.111	0.633 ± 0.075	0.644 ± 0.042	0.629 ± 0.042	0.646 ± 0.064	0.654

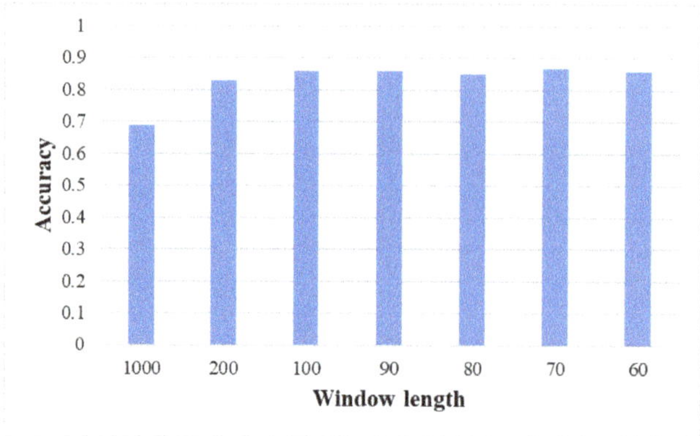

Figure 5. Accuracies for all methods with different window lengths, each column represents the average of the six method accuracies.

3.3. Generic Performance of BCI

It is difficult to compare different BCI systems since there are many aspects that can influence the performance of BCI, such as input, preprocessing, and outputs. The ITR is a widely and generally accepted standard by which the performance of different BCI systems can be compared [35]. Figure 6 illustrates the distribution of ITRs for the sessions. The average ITR for all seven subjects was 10.72 ± 4.82 bits/min. Several subjects (1, 3, 4 and 7) reached the highest ITR with 12 bits/min. Subject 7 had the lowest ITR of 1.73 bits/min. For the ITR of motor attempts, fewer results have been reported. Khalaf et al. obtained an average ITR of 40.83 bits/min for a four-class task [36]. Zeng et al. achieved the highest ITR of 24 bits/min during ankle rehabilitation robot training [37]. In this study, the value of ITR is negatively correlated with T, and the value of ITR is limited by task time.

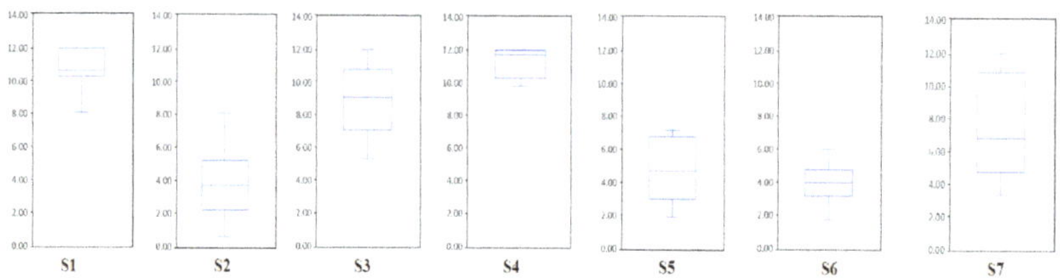

Figure 6. Boxplots represent the ITRs of different sessions for each subject. Each box plot includes 12 sessions of data. The upper and lower lines represent the maximum and minimum ITRs, respectively. The lines in the boxplot represent the median ITR.

3.4. The Visualization of Feature Distribution

To investigate the validity of the time window. A visualization technique called TSNE [38] was used to downscale the learned features for visualization. Figure 7 shows the distribution of features for different time windows. The different colored scatter points in the figure indicate the different task types, and each scatter represents the extracted feature by one window. We observed that the features extracted by methods with time windows were easier to classify. After training, multiple EEG signals of time segments were well identified. However, some EEG signals from different windows were hard to identify. In addition, it was also found that among CNN, GIN, and LSTM, LSTM performed best in feature extraction, which had fewer segments that could not be distinguished. To further observe the LSTM performance, we constructed the LSTM&VS confusion matrices of the seven subjects in Figure 8. The correct classification accuracies are shown on the diagonal cells. It can be seen that the LSTM&VS accuracy in each task was similar for individual subjects. The results demonstrated that LSTM&VS obtained good overall performance.

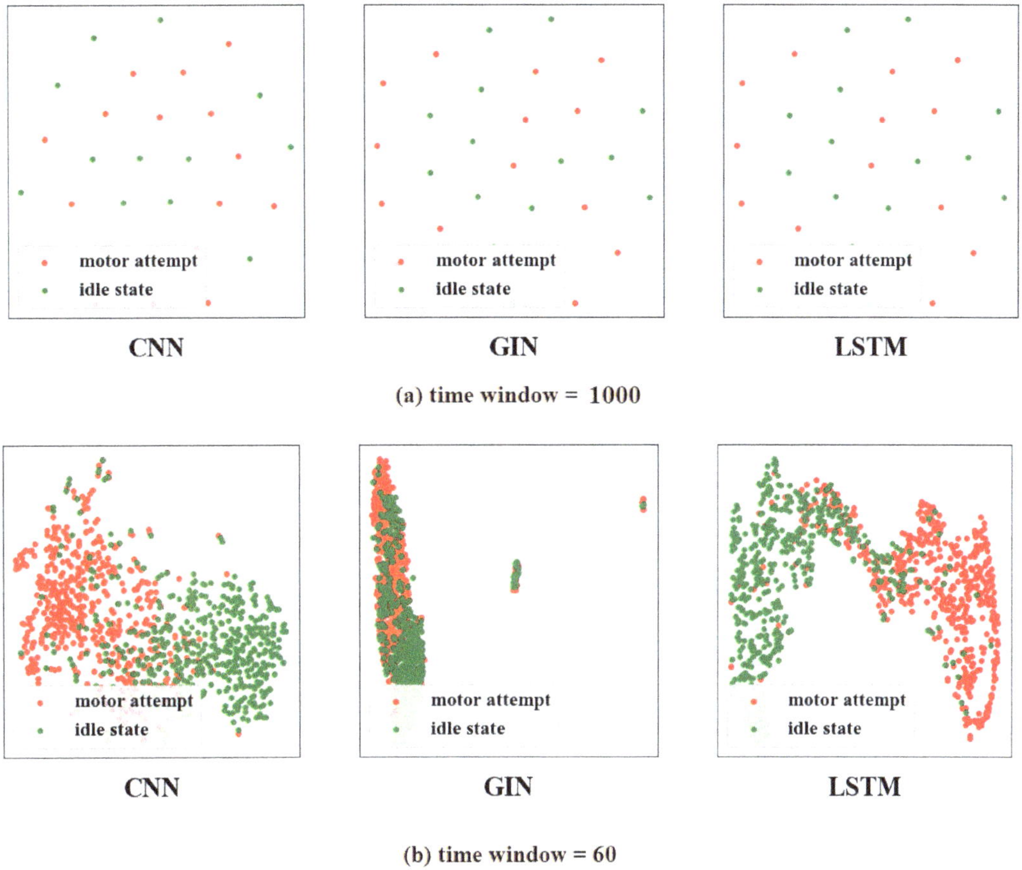

Figure 7. Feature visualization of different models for Subject 1. For time window (**a**), each scatter represents a feature extracted on one trail, and for time window (**b**), each scatter represents a feature extracted on one time window of one trail.

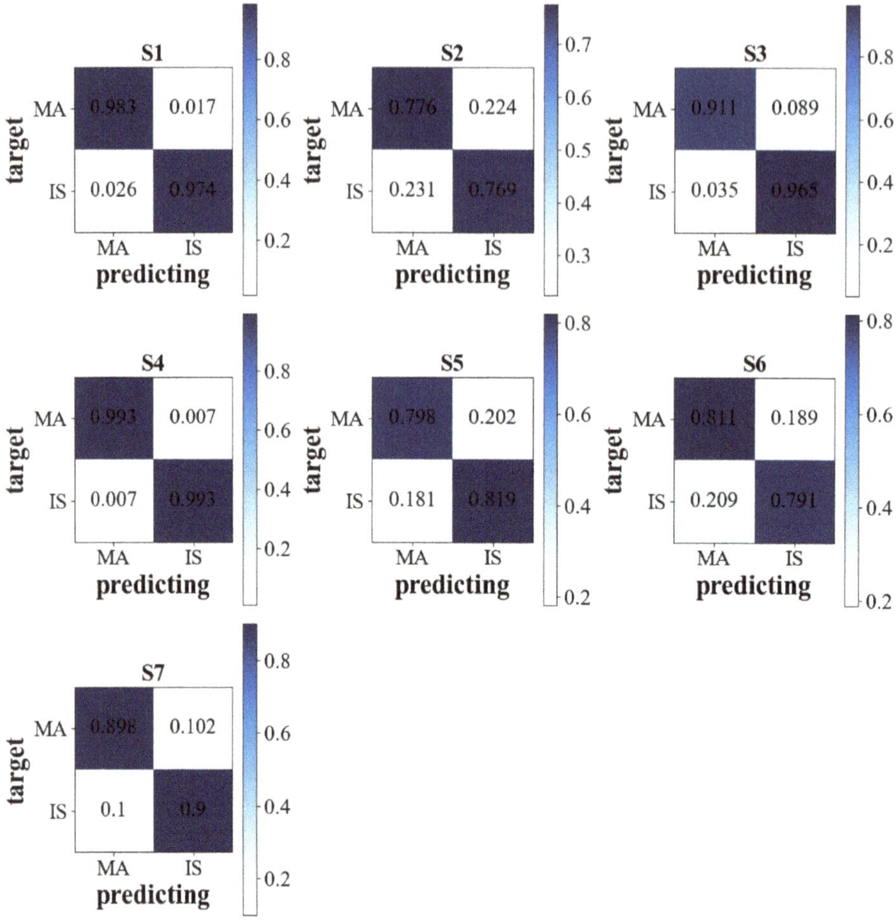

Figure 8. The confusion matrices for all subjects with the LSTM&VS method.

3.5. The Impact of the Number of Network Layers

The number of network layers usually affected the model performance. Table 5 shows the accuracy of models with different numbers of network layers. Compared with other settings, the accuracy of 1 layer was lower. In addition, the accuracies of the CNN&VS and CNN&FFS were more likely to be influenced by the number of network layers, while the accuracies of LSTM&VS and LSTM&FFS were more stable.

Table 5. Accuracy comparison between different numbers of network layers.

Conv Layers	Accuracy					
	GIN&VS	CNN&VS	LSTM&VS	GIN&FFS	CNN&FFS	LSTM&FFS
1 layer	0.803 ± 0.082	0.821 ± 0.091	0.882 ± 0.079	0.834 ± 0.074	0.791 ± 0.072	0.900 ± 0.065
2 layers	**0.819 ± 0.085**	0.844 ± 0.086	**0.884 ± 0.078**	**0.846 ± 0.075**	0.846 ± 0.068	**0.901 ± 0.066**
3 layers	0.816 ± 0.078	**0.851 ± 0.083**	0.883 ± 0.068	0.843 ± 0.082	**0.854 ± 0.080**	0.896 ± 0.069
4 layers	0.806 ± 0.089	0.844 ± 0.088	0.882 ± 0.079	0.821 ± 0.078	0.847 ± 0.069	0.900 ± 0.072
Mean	0.810	0.840	0.882	0.836	0.835	0.900

The highest classification accuracy for a given method are bold marked.

3.6. The Visualization of Accuracy on Time Window

In this section, to analyze the classification differences in each time window, we conducted statistics and visualized the classification results of the EEG signals on the windows by using the LSTM&VS method. Figure 9 shows the sequence of classification results. Each row represents a session, and each column represents the classification statistics of the time window, in which the time windows with higher accuracy are highlighted. As seen in the figure, the distribution of accuracy across the time windows differs in patients. For Subject 3, the time window with higher classification accuracy appeared in the first window, and the window with lower classification accuracy appeared in the last window. The difference in sequence probably occurred because the appearances of the discriminative motor intentions were random during the MA experiment.

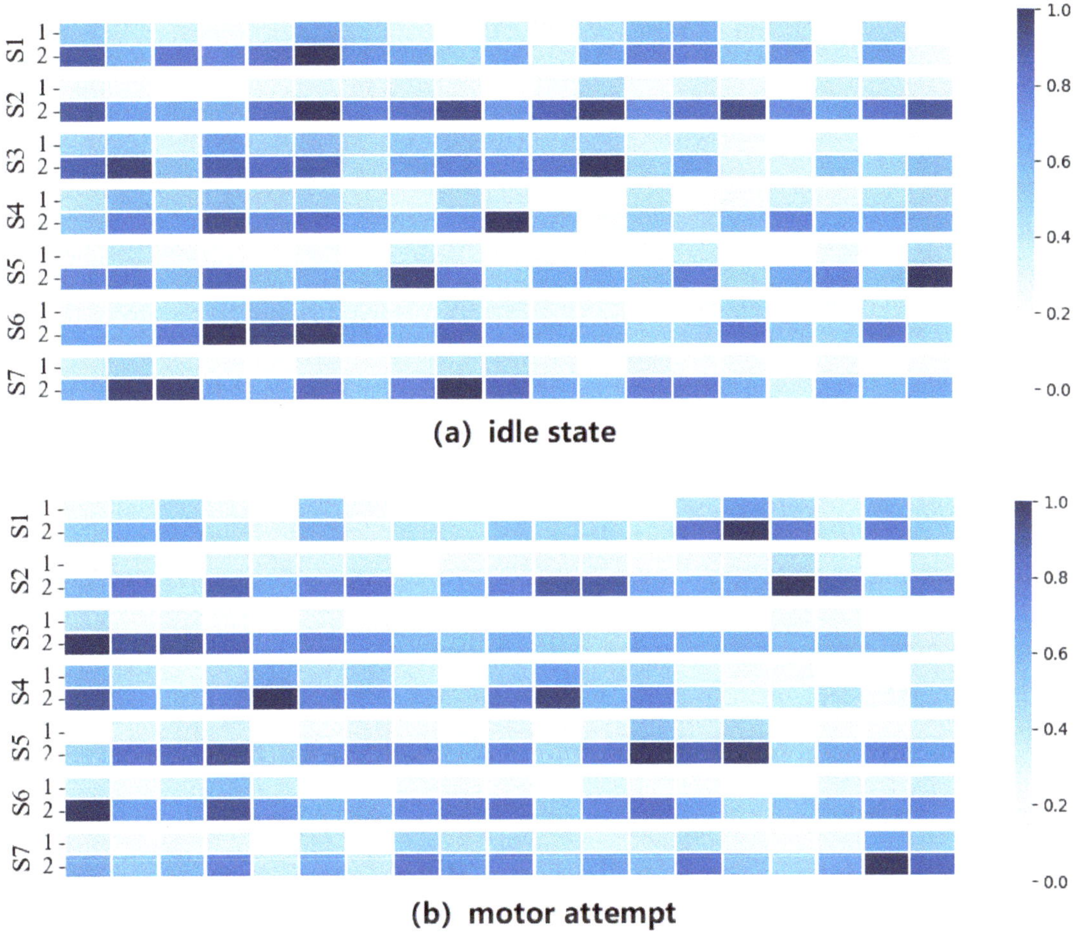

Figure 9. Visualization of classification results learned by LSTM&VS. In each state, two different sessions (1, 2) of seven subjects are visualized. Each row represents a session and each square represents the correct result for classification in a time window.

3.7. Study of Cortical Activity on the Time Window

To further investigate the differences in the EEG signals of time segments with different classification accuracies, we used power spectral density topography to represent the frequency domain information of brain signals. Figure 10 illustrates the topography of alpha power for two tasks. Based on the classification accuracy of the time segments in Figure 9, four different time windows were selected for visualization. For the motor attempt task, the PSD of patients was higher in the frontal lobe. Several studies have indicated that stroke can affect the brain function in the frontal lobe [39,40]. The observations may suggest that motor attempts of patients were associated with the frontal cortical regions, which is consistent with a previous study [41]. Channel information from frontal regions may be important for identifying the brain's motor intentions. When the EEG signals in the frontal lobe are not significant enough, it may contribute to lower classification accuracy.

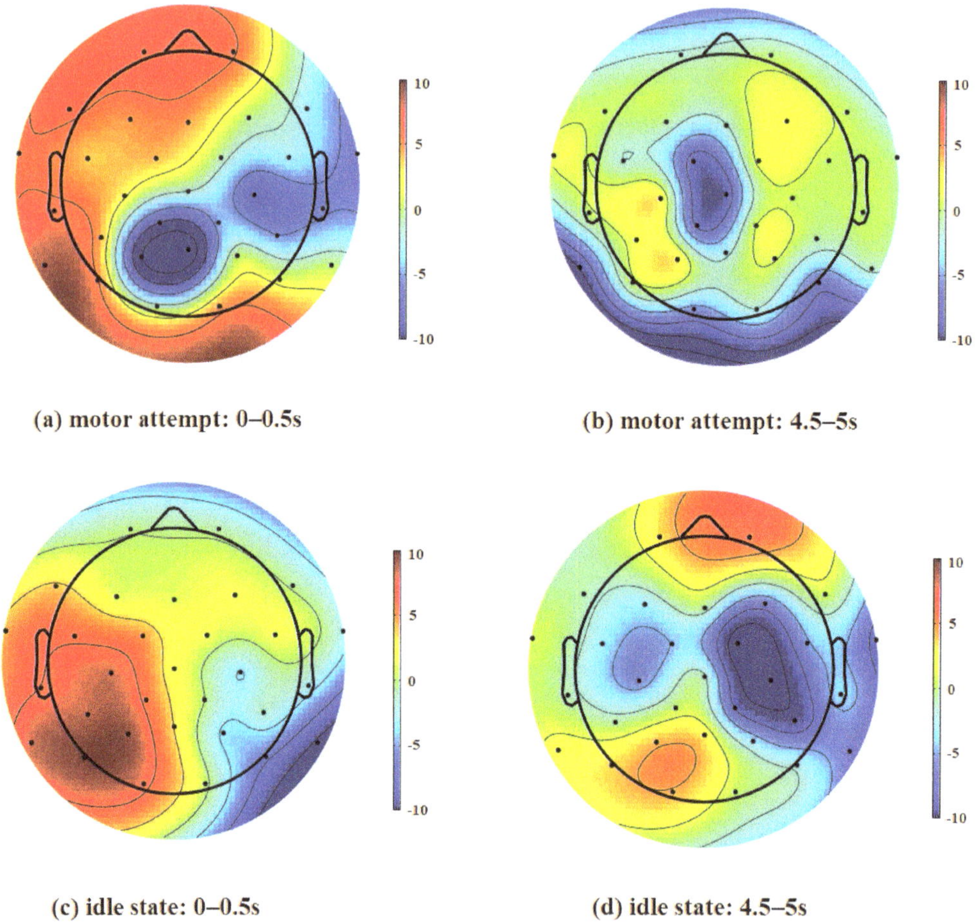

Figure 10. The visualization of the averaged topography of the PSD over the alpha band in different time windows. Session 3 with two task types for Subject 3 is visualized.

3.8. Limitations in Current Work

The findings in this study are limited by the quantity of data collected, and it is difficult to determine the quantity of data that can be classified well without using a time window. In addition, the optimal filter band and model hyperparameters were not selected according to the subjects, which may limit the ability of the models in different patients. In future work, we will investigate the use of feature engineering for reducing the dimensionality of the model inputs. In addition, the fixed starting point for time window sampling may reduce the performance of the BCI system [42]. Therefore, we will optimize the set of time windows by using a window selection algorithm in the feature work.

4. Conclusions

This study showed that for classification tasks during BCI-based stroke rehabilitation, deep learning algorithms based on overlapping time windows achieved good accuracy. It may support improvements in the performance of brain–computer interfaces to generate accurate neurofeedback. One of the more significant findings to emerge from this study is that the distribution of classification results differed across the time windows of the subjects, and it means that there is a possibility of improving classification performance by choosing different windows for classification for different subjects. Therefore, future work can expand on the selection of the time window.

Author Contributions: Conceptualization, L.C.; methodology, L.C., H.W., S.C., C.F. and Y.D.; software, S.C. and J.J.; data curation, S.C.; writing—original draft preparation, L.C. and H.W.; writing—review and editing, L.C., H.W., C.Z. and Y.D.; visualization, L.C. and H.W.; supervision, L.C., C.Z. and Y.D.; project administration, L.C.; L.C., H.W. and S.C. contributed equally. All authors have read and agreed to the published version of the manuscript.

Funding: The work was supported by the National Key R&D Program of China under Grants 2018YFC2002300, 2018YFC2002301, the National Natural Science Young Foundation of China (Grant No. 62102242 & 62103258), Shanghai Education Research Program (Grant No. C2022152), Shanghai Science and Technology Innovation Action Plan (22YF1404200) and Project of Wuxi Health Commission (Grant No. Z2022012, MS201944 and T201906).

Institutional Review Board Statement: The study was conducted in accordance with the Declaration of Helsinki, and approved by the Institutional Review Board of Ethics Committee of Huashan Hospital (Approval no.: 18518-201111KY2017-005).

Informed Consent Statement: Informed consent was obtained from all subjects involved in the study.

Data Availability Statement: The data presented in this study are available on request from the corresponding author.

Conflicts of Interest: The authors declare no conflict of interest.

References

1. Broussalis, E.; Killer, M.; McCoy, M.; Harrer, A.; Trinka, E.; Kraus, J. Current therapies in ischemic stroke. Part A. Recent developments in acute stroke treatment and in stroke prevention. *Drug Discov. Today* **2012**, *17*, 296–309. [CrossRef] [PubMed]
2. Thieme, H.; Mehrholz, J.; Pohl, M.; Behrens, J.; Dohle, C. Mirror therapy for improving motor function after stroke. *Stroke* **2013**, *44*, e1–e2. [CrossRef] [PubMed]
3. Saposnik, G.; Mcilroy, W.E.; Teasell, R.; Thorpe, K.E.; Bayley, M.; Cheung, D.; Mamdani, M.; Hall, J.; Cohen, L.G. Effectiveness of virtual reality using Wii gaming technology in stroke rehabilitation: A pilot randomized clinical trial and proof of principle. *Stroke* **2010**, *41*, 1477. [CrossRef] [PubMed]
4. Rimmer, J.H.; Wang, E. Aerobic Exercise Training in Stroke Survivors. *Top. Stroke Rehabil.* **2005**, *12*, 17–30. [CrossRef]
5. Ang, K.K.; Guan, C.; Phua, K.S.; Wang, C.; Zhou, L.; Tang, K.Y.; Ephraim Joseph, G.J.; Kuah, C.W.K.; Chua, K.S.G. Brain-computer interface-based robotic end effector system for wrist and hand rehabilitation: Results of a three-armed randomized controlled trial for chronic stroke. *Front. Neuroeng.* **2014**, *7*, 30. [CrossRef]
6. Cervera, M.A.; Soekadar, S.R.; Ushiba, J.; Millán, J.D.R.; Liu, M.; Birbaumer, N.; Garipelli, G. Brain-computer interfaces for post-stroke motor rehabilitation: A meta-analysis. *Ann. Clin. Transl. Neurol.* **2018**, *5*, 651–663. [CrossRef]
7. Mane, R.; Chouhan, T.; Guan, C. BCI for stroke rehabilitation: Motor and beyond. *J. Neural. Eng.* **2020**, *17*, 041001. [CrossRef]
8. Pfurtscheller, G.; Neuper, C. Motor imagery activates primary sensorimotor area in humans. *Neurosci. Lett.* **1997**, *239*, 65–68. [CrossRef]
9. Philip, G.R.; Daly, J.J.; Príncipe, J.C. Topographical measures of functional connectivity as biomarkers for post-stroke motor recovery. *J. Neuroeng. Rehabil.* **2017**, *14*, 67. [CrossRef]
10. Xiao, X.; Xu, M.; Jin, J.; Wang, Y.; Jung, T.P.; Ming, D. Discriminative canonical pattern matching for single-trial classification of ERP components. *IEEE Trans. Biomed. Eng.* **2019**, *67*, 2266–2275. [CrossRef]

11. Ramoser, H.; Muller-Gerking, J.; Pfurtscheller, G. Optimal spatial filtering of single trial EEG during imagined hand movement. *IEEE Trans. Rehabil. Eng.* **2000**, *8*, 441–446. [CrossRef] [PubMed]
12. Ang, K.K.; Chin, Z.Y.; Zhang, H.; Guan, C. Filter bank common spatial pattern (FBCSP) in brain-computer interface. In Proceedings of the 2008 IEEE International Joint Conference on Neural Networks (IEEE World Congress on Computational Intelligence), Hong Kong, China, 1–8 June 2008; pp. 2390–2397.
13. Geethanjali, P.; Mohan, Y.K.; Sen, J. Time domain feature extraction and classification of EEG data for brain computer interface. In Proceedings of the 2012 9th International Conference on Fuzzy Systems and Knowledge Discovery, Chongqing, China, 29–31 May 2012; pp. 1136–1139.
14. Chen, S.; Shu, X.; Wang, H.; Ding, L.; Fu, J.; Jia, J. The differences between motor attempt and motor imagery in brain-computer interface accuracy and event-related desynchronization of patients with hemiplegia. *Front. Neurorobot.* **2021**, *15*, 706630. [CrossRef] [PubMed]
15. Lin, P.J.; Jia, T.; Li, C.; Li, T.; Qian, C.; Li, Z.; Pan, Y.; Ji, L. CNN-Based Prognosis of BCI Rehabilitation Using EEG From First Session BCI Training. *IEEE Trans. Neural Syst. Rehabil. Eng.* **2021**, *29*, 1936–1943. [CrossRef]
16. Liang, F.Y.; Zhong, C.H.; Zhao, X.; Castro, D.L.; Chen, B.; Gao, F.; Liao, W.H. Online adaptive and lstm-based trajectory generation of lower limb exoskeletons for stroke rehabilitation. In Proceedings of the 2018 IEEE International Conference on Robotics and Biomimetics (ROBIO), Kuala Lumpur, Malaysia, 12–15 December 2018; pp. 27–32.
17. Jin, J.; Sun, H.; Daly, I.; Li, S.; Liu, C.; Wang, X.; Cichocki, A. A Novel Classification Framework Using the Graph Representations of Electroencephalogram for Motor Imagery Based Brain-Computer Interface. *IEEE Trans. Neural. Syst. Rehabil. Eng.* **2021**, *30*, 20–29. [CrossRef]
18. Wang, F.; Zhong, S.h.; Peng, J.; Jiang, J.; Liu, Y. Data augmentation for eeg-based emotion recognition with deep convolutional neural networks. In *Proceedings of the International Conference on Multimedia Modeling*; Springer: Berlin/Heidelberg, Germany, 2018, pp. 82–93.
19. A, I.U.; B, M.H.; B, E.U.H.Q.; B, H.A. An automated system for epilepsy detection using EEG brain signals based on deep learning approach. *Expert Syst. Appl.* **2018**, *107*, 61–71.
20. Zhang, G.; Davoodnia, V.; Sepas-Moghaddam, A.; Zhang, Y.; Etemad, A. Classification of hand movements from EEG using a deep attention-based LSTM network. *IEEE Sens. J.* **2019**, *20*, 3113–3122. [CrossRef]
21. Hartmann, K.G.; Schirrmeister, R.T.; Ball, T. EEG-GAN: Generative adversarial networks for electroencephalograhic (EEG) brain signals. *arXiv* **2018**, arXiv:1806.01875 .
22. Truong, N.D.; Zhou, L.; Kavehei, O. Semi-supervised Seizure Prediction with Generative Adversarial Networks. In Proceedings of the 2019 41st Annual International Conference of the IEEE Engineering in Medicine and Biology Society (EMBC), Berlin, Germany, 23–27 July 2019.
23. Zhou, J.; Cui, G.; Hu, S.; Zhang, Z.; Yang, C.; Liu, Z.; Wang, L.; Li, C.; Sun, M. Graph neural networks: A review of methods and applications. *AI Open* **2020**, *1*, 57–81. [CrossRef]
24. Zhang, T.; Wang, X.; Xu, X.; Chen, C.P. GCB-Net: Graph convolutional broad network and its application in emotion recognition. *IEEE Trans. Affect. Comput.* **2019**, *13*, 379–388. [CrossRef]
25. Shen, L.; Sun, M.; Li, Q.; Li, B.; Pan, Z.; Lei, J. Multiscale Temporal Self-Attention and Dynamical Graph Convolution Hybrid Network for EEG-Based Stereogram Recognition. *IEEE Trans. Neural. Syst. Rehabil. Eng.* **2022**, *30*, 1191–1202. [CrossRef]
26. Song, T.; Zheng, W.; Song, P.; Cui, Z. EEG emotion recognition using dynamical graph convolutional neural networks. *IEEE Trans. Affect. Comput.* **2018**, *11*, 532–541. [CrossRef]
27. Li, Y. A Survey of EEG Analysis based on Graph Neural Network. In Proceedings of the 2021 2nd International Conference on Electronics, Communications and Information Technology (CECIT), Sanya, China, 27–29 December 2021; pp. 151–155.
28. Xu, K.; Hu, W.; Leskovec, J.; Jegelka, S. How powerful are graph neural networks? *arXiv* **2018**, arXiv:1810.00826.
29. Lun, X.; Yu, Z.; Chen, T.; Wang, F.; Hou, Y. A simplified CNN classification method for MI-EEG via the electrode pairs signals. *Front. Hum. Neurosci.* **2020**, *14*, 338. [CrossRef] [PubMed]
30. Acharya, U.R.; Oh, S.L.; Hagiwara, Y.; Tan, J.H.; Adeli, H. Deep convolutional neural network for the automated detection and diagnosis of seizure using EEG signals. *Comput. Biol. Med.* **2018**, *100*, 270–278. [CrossRef]
31. Pascanu, R.; Gulcehre, C.; Cho, K.; Bengio, Y. How to Construct Deep Recurrent Neural Networks. *arXiv* **2013**, arXiv:1312.6026.
32. Wolpaw, J.R.; Birbaumer, N.; Heetderks, W.J.; McFarland, D.J.; Peckham, P.H.; Schalk, G.; Donchin, E.; Quatrano, L.A.; Robinson, C.J.; Vaughan, T.M. Brain-computer interface technology: A review of the first international meeting. *IEEE Trans. Rehabil. Eng.* **2000**, *8*, 164–173. [CrossRef]
33. Rasheed, S.; Mumtaz, W. Classification of Hand-Grasp Movements of Stroke Patients using EEG Data. In Proceedings of the 2021 International Conference on Artificial Intelligence (ICAI), Islamabad, Pakistan, 5–7 April 2021; pp. 86–90.
34. Gers, F.A.; Schmidhuber, J.; Cummins, F. Learning to forget: Continual prediction with LSTM. *Neural Comput.* **2000**, *12*, 2451–2471. [CrossRef]
35. Huang, X.; Xu, Y.; Hua, J.; Yi, W.; Yin, H.; Hu, R.; Wang, S. A Review on Signal Processing Approaches to Reduce Calibration Time in EEG-Based Brain–Computer Interface. *Front. Neurosci.* **2021**, *15*, 1066. [CrossRef]
36. Khalaf, A.; Sejdic, E.; Akcakaya, M. Common spatial pattern and wavelet decomposition for motor imagery EEG-fTCD brain-computer interface. *J. Neurosci. Methods* **2019**, *320*, 98–106. [CrossRef]

37. Zeng, X.; Zhu, G.; Yue, L.; Zhang, M.; Xie, S. A feasibility study of ssvep-based passive training on an ankle rehabilitation robot. *J. Healthc. Eng.* **2017**, *2017*, 6819056. [CrossRef]
38. Majidov, I.; Whangbo, T. Efficient Classification of Motor Imagery Electroencephalography Signals Using Deep Learning Methods. *Sensors* **2019**, *19*, 1736. [CrossRef]
39. Levine, B.; Schweizer, T.; O'Connor, C.; Turner, G.; Gillingham, S.; Stuss, D.; Manly, T.; Robertson, I. Rehabilitation of Executive Functioning in Patients with Frontal Lobe Brain Damage with Goal Management Training. *Front. Hum. Neurosci.* **2011**, *5*, 9. [CrossRef] [PubMed]
40. Yu, S.; Zeng, Y.; Lei, W.; Wei, L.; Liu, Z.; Zhang, S.; Yang, J.; Wen, W. A Study of the Brain Abnormalities of Post-Stroke Depression in Frontal Lobe Lesion. *Sci. Rep.* **2017**, *7*, 13203.
41. Xu, R.; Jiang, N.; Vuckovic, A.; Hasan, M.; Mrachacz-Kersting, N.; Allan, D.; Fraser, M.; Nasseroleslami, B.; Conway, B.; Dremstrup, K. Movement-related cortical potentials in paraplegic patients: Abnormal patterns and considerations for BCI-rehabilitation. *Front. Neuroeng.* **2014**, *7*, 35. [CrossRef] [PubMed]
42. Feng, J.; Yin, E.; Jin, J.; Saab, R.; Daly, I.; Wang, X.; Hu, D.; Cichocki, A. Towards correlation-based time window selection method for motor imagery BCIs. *Neural. Netw.* **2018**, *102*, 87–95. [CrossRef] [PubMed]

brain sciences

MDPI

Article

A Novel Automated RGB-D Sensor-Based Measurement of Voluntary Items of the Fugl-Meyer Assessment for Upper Extremity: A Feasibility Study

Yue Li [1,†], Chong Li [2,†], Xiaokang Shu [1], Xinjun Sheng [1,*], Jie Jia [2,*] and Xiangyang Zhu [1]

1 State Key Laboratory of Machanical System and Vibration, Shanghai Jiao Tong University, Shanghai 200040, China
2 Department of Rehabilitation Medicine, Huashan Hospital, Fudan University, Shanghai 200040, China
* Correspondence: xjsheng@sjtu.edu.cn (X.S.); shannonjj@126.com (J.J.); Tel.: +86-021-34206547 (X.S.); +86-13617722357 (J.J.)
† These authors contributed equally to this work.

Abstract: Motor function assessment is essential for post-stroke rehabilitation, while the requirement for professional therapists' participation in current clinical assessment limits its availability to most patients. By means of sensors that collect the motion data and algorithms that conduct assessment based on such data, an automated system can be built to optimize the assessment process, benefiting both patients and therapists. To this end, this paper proposed an automated Fugl-Meyer Assessment (FMA) upper extremity system covering all 30 voluntary items of the scale. RGBD sensors, together with force sensing resistor sensors were used to collect the patients' motion information. Meanwhile, both machine learning and rule-based logic classification were jointly employed for assessment scoring. Clinical validation on 20 hemiparetic stroke patients suggests that this system is able to generate reliable FMA scores. There is an extremely high correlation coefficient ($r = 0.981$, $p < 0.01$) with that yielded by an experienced therapist. This study offers guidance and feasible solutions to a complete and independent automated assessment system.

Keywords: stroke rehabilitation; upper limb; automated system; motor function assessment; Fugl-Meyer Assessment

Citation: Li, Y.; Li, C.; Shu, X.; Sheng, X.; Jia, J.; Zhu, X. A Novel Automated RGB-D Sensor-Based Measurement of Voluntary Items of the Fugl-Meyer Assessment for Upper Extremity: A Feasibility Study. *Brain Sci.* **2022**, *12*, 1380. https://doi.org/10.3390/brainsci12101380

Academic Editors: Konstantin V. Slavin and Giovanni Morone

Received: 7 September 2022
Accepted: 5 October 2022
Published: 12 October 2022

1. Introduction

Stroke is one of the leading causes of motor function impairment worldwide, and 30% to 66% of post-stroke hemiplegic patients suffer from permanent upper limb deficits [1]. Restoring upper limb motor function through rehabilitation can considerably improve patients' lives.

As a crucial step in the stroke rehabilitation process [2], assessment contributes much to rehabilitation training guidance and patients' self-confidence enhancement. Traditional clinical assessment relies on the professional therapist observing the patient's behavior based on various scales. According to the International Classification of Functioning, Disability and Health (ICF), these scales can be divided into three main categories [3]: body functions such as Fugl-Meyer Assessment (FMA) and Motor Status Score (MSS), activity ability such as Wolf Motor Function Test (WMFT) and Arm Motor Ability Test (AMAT), and participation such as Stroke Impact Scale (SIS) and EuroQol Quality of Life Scale (QLS). Among them, FMA [4] is probably the most widely used one in both clinical and research applications [5]. It has excellent intra-rater and inter-rater reliability and construct validity [6,7], and is sensitive to change [8]. The FMA upper extremity (FMA-UE) section (Table 1) consists of 33 items, and each item is scored on a 3-point ordinal scale from 0 to 2.

However, the requirement of therapist participation substantially limits the implementation of the assessment. As for patients, especially discharged patients, scientific assessment is not readily available. For therapists, it is time-consuming and laborious. Consequently, automated scale evaluation systems are proposed to solve these problems.

Table 1. Target FMA items and Grouping [1].

Category [2]	Motion [3]	FMA Item	Sensors [4]
Reflex activity		1. Flexors	
		2. Extensors	
Shoulder/Elbow Volitional movement within synergies	I	3. Shoulder elevation	RS
		4. Shoulder retraction	RS
		5. Shoulder abduction(90°)	RS
		6. Shoulder external rotation	RS
		7. Elbow flexion	RS
		8. Forearm supination	RS
		9. Shoulder adduction/internal rotation	RS
		10. Elbow extension	RS
		11. Forearm pronation	RS
Shoulder/Elbow Volitional movement mixing synergies	II	12. Hand to lumbar spine	RS
	III	13. Shoulder flexion 0∼90°	RS
Shoulder/Elbow Volitional movement with little or no synergy	V	15. Shoulder abduction 0∼90°	RS
	III	16. Shoulder flexion 90∼180°	RS
Normal reflex activity		18. Biceps, triceps, finger flexors	
Wrist/Hand	IV + VI_{90}	14. Forearm pronation-supination with elbow 90°	RS + LM
	III + VI_0	17. Forearm pronation-supination with elbow 0°	RS + LM
	VII_{90}	19. Stability at 15° dorsiflexion with elbow 90°	LM
		20. Repeated dorsiflexion/volar flexion with elbow 90°	LM
	VII_0	21. Stability at 15° dorsiflexion with elbow 0°	LM
		22. Repeated dorsiflexion/volar flexion with elbow 0°	LM
	VIII	23. Circumduction	LM
	IX	24. Mass flexion	LM
		25. Mass extension	LM
Grasp	X	26. Hook grasp	FSRs
	XI	27. Thumb adduction	FSRs
	XII	28. Pincer grasp	FSRs
	XIII	29. Cylinder grasp	FSRs
	XIV	30. Sphere grasp	FSRs
Coordination/Speed	XV	31. Tremor	RS
		32. Dysmetria	RS
		33. Time	RS

[1] The gray part indicates the items not included in the automated system, the red part indicates the items scored using random forest classification, and the blue part indicates the items scored using rule-based logic classification. [2] The FMA items involved in the automated system were grouped into four categories (bolded) based on the execution actions and evaluation methods. [3] 30 FMA items were implemented in this automated system with 17 motion tasks, with multiple FMA items corresponding to one motion, or one FMA item split into two motions in some cases. [4] RS means RealSense, LM means Leap Motion, and FSRs means Force Sensitive Resistors.

A few studies on automated evaluation of the upper extremity motor function have been conducted using various sensors. Wearable sensors, including inertial measurement units (IMUs) (or only accelerometers) [9,10], flex sensors, and their combinations [11], have been heavily applied to automate FMA or WMFT [12]. They are portable and accurate. Nevertheless, these sensors are inconvenient for patients to wear and the preparation can take a long time, especially when using the glove sensor to track hand motion. Electromyography (EMG) is a bioelectric signal that reflects neuromuscular behaviors, which is of great significance for understanding motor function levels and guiding rehabilitation [13]. By using EMG, both longitudinal [14] and cross-sectional [15] assessments can be implemented from a more physiological perspective. The multi-camera-based optoelectronic system, such as Vicon (Vicon Motion System, USA) and Impulse (Phase Space, USA) [16], is another commonly used sensor with acute precision for automated assessment system construction. However, their high price and complicated operation limit their use in the laboratory.

Compared with the three kinds of sensors mentioned above, the depth camera, such as Kinect (Microsoft, Redmond, WA, USA), RealSense (Intel, Santa Clara, CA, USA), and Leap Motion (Leap Motion Inc., San Francisco, CA, USA), has the advantages of low cost, convenient installation, and high comfort. These advantages, together with acceptable precision, promote their widespread use in rehabilitation. Kim et al. [17] automated 13 FMA-UE items using Kinect. Bai et al. [18] fused Kinect One and a posture sensor to evaluate 15 FMA items as well as the reachable workspace area. Fang et al. [19] proposed a novel hand assessment framework compliant with Swanson impairment evaluation and FMA based on Leap Motion. Further, Lee et al. [20] combined Kinect v2 and FSRs and achieved the automated evaluation of 26 FMA-UE items. It is worth noting that most of these systems merely consider part of the scale: some aim to evaluate the shoulder and elbow joints [17,18], and others focus on assessing hand function [19,21]. The incompleteness diminishes their practical value. In other words, there is still much room for improvement in these systems for application in independent clinical evaluation.

Aiming to achieve complete, independent, and low-cost assessment without therapists' involvement, this paper proposed an automated evaluation system covering all voluntary FMA-UE items, using no body-worn sensors. Two RGBD cameras (An RGBD camera is a type of depth camera that provides both depth (D) and color (RGB) data) and several force-sensing resistors were included. Both machine learning and rule-based logic classification were applied for score prediction according to different categories. The feasibility of the proposed system was demonstrated with data from 20 hemiparetic stroke patients.

2. Materials and Methods

2.1. Participants

Applying the two-stage sample size approximation method for the Pearson correlation [22], with the estimated correlation coefficient $\tilde{r} = 0.9$, Fisher confidence interval $\omega = 0.3$, and significance level $\alpha = 0.01$ as parameters, a correct sample size $n = 20$ can be obtained. Therefore, twenty stroke patients (fifteen males, five females; age: 58.95 ± 10.58 years) from the Rehabilitation Medicine Department of Huashan Hospital were recruited for this study. The inclusion criteria for participation in the study were: (1) age between 21 and 75 years old; (2) diagnosis of unilateral hemiplegia caused by ischemic or hemorrhagic stroke; (3) absence of apraxia and severe medical complications (including shoulder pain); (4) with no serious cognitive impairment and able to understand and follow instructions (Mini-Mental State Examination (MMSE) score > 20 [23]). The study was pre-approved by the Huashan Hospital Institutional Review Board (KY2018-248) and registered at the Chinese Clinical Trial Registry (ChiCTR1800017568). All participants were provided with and signed the informed consent prior to the experiment.

2.2. *System Design*

2.2.1. FMA Items

The complete scale of FMA-UE is shown in Table 1. All these FMA items except the three reflex ones (item 1, 2, and 18 filled with grey) requiring external forces, were covered in this automated system. It has been suggested that the three reflex items contribute little to volitional movement ability measurement and can be excluded from the FMA-UE evaluation [24,25]. Based on assessment joints and execution actions, the FMA-UE can be divided into four categories: Shoulder/Elbow, Wrist/Hand, Grasp, and Coordination/Speed. Overall, 30 FMA items (33 in total) were implemented in this automated system with 17 motion tasks. According to the scale instruction, item 3–11 only involve one movement, and so do item 24–25, 31–33. For convenience, item 13 and 16 were combined into one action: shoulder flexion 180°. Besides, several minor adjustments have been made in view of the actual application. Item 14 and 17 were broken down into two movements respectively: shoulder/elbow moving to the initial position and forearm pronation/supination at this position. Item 19 and 20 were combined into one action because the automated system could not provide resistance to wrists, and so were item 21 and 22. Each of the rest items corresponded to one indicated action.

2.2.2. Hardware and Software

The sensors used by the system included a RealSense D435, a Leap Motion, and Force Sensitive Resistors (FSRs) (Interlink Electronics, Westlake Village, CA, USA). The hardware layout is shown in Figure 1A.

RealSense D435, a mainstream depth camera having the potential to measure health outcomes [26], was applied to record the movement of the Shoulder/Elbow and Coordination/Speed parts. In this system, RealSense was positioned on a tripod in front of the patient, and data streams were captured at 30 frames per second (fps). The coordinates of 18 joints (Figure 2A) could be extracted from raw data based on skeleton tracking SDK. Leap Motion controller is a depth-sensing camera designed for tracking hand and finger motion at up to 200 fps, which was mainly used in the Wrist/Hand part. At the same time, a support mechanism was specially designed, aiming to fix Leap Motion and human arm comfortably and keep their relative position. The support was placed on the other tripod to achieve the change in pitch angle (Figure 1A). In order to quantitatively measure the interaction force between the hand and the object in the Grasp part, five FSRs were respectively attached to five corresponding grip tools [20]. The detailed information of the raw data collected by the above sensors is summarized in Table 2.

Table 2. Raw data information.

Data Source	RealSense D435	Leap Motion	Force Sensitive Resistors
Sampling frequency	30 fps	200 fps	10 Hz
Experimental protocol	Perform motions I–V, XV	Perform motions VI-IX	Grasp 5 specified tools
Original data format	Color and depth images	Hand tracking data	Voltage and force
Features [1]	3D coordinates of joints ($f \times 18 \times 3$)	Angles ($f \times a$)	Force ($f \times 1$)
Sample Size	20 subjects × 2 repetitions	20 subjects	20 subjects

[1] f is the frame number, and a is the angle number.

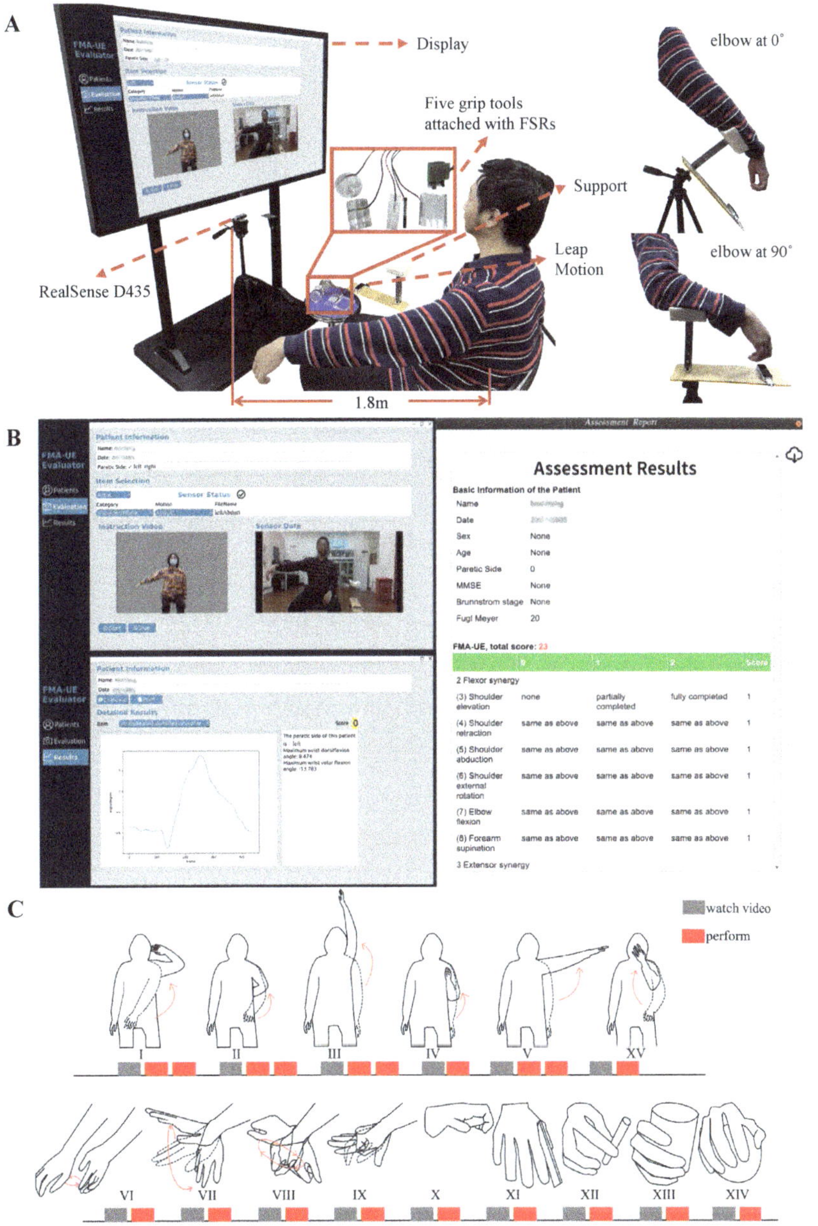

Figure 1. (**A**) The hardware setup and scene of the experiment. On the right are the two initial positions for the Wrist/Hand part. (**B**) The graphical user interface (GUI) of the assessment system. (**C**) The experimental protocol.

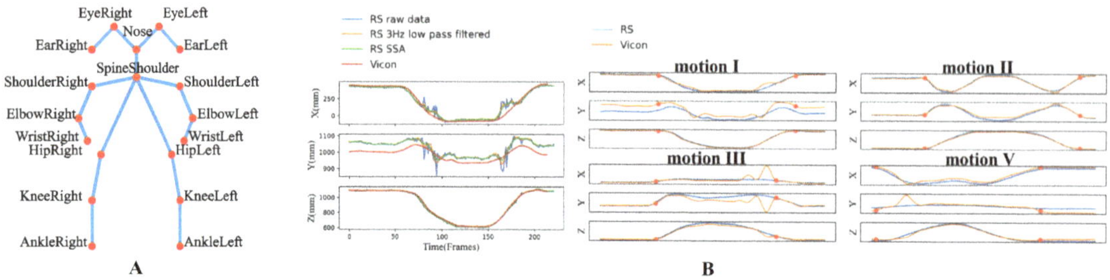

Figure 2. (**A**) 18-joint skeleton of RealSenseD435. (**B**) The 3D coordinates of the wrist joint in the Shoulder/Elbow part motions. Left: The curves of raw RealSense (RS) data, data processed by two denoising methods, and Vicon data of motion I. Right: The SSA-filtered RS data and the Vicon data of four motions, and the red dots mark the motion start and end time.

The automatic administration is also a critical aspect of automated evaluation systems [27], which is mainly embodied in the interaction with the user. Therefore, user-friendly software was also developed (Figure 1B). It has the function of patient information register, data collection, data analysis, and results generation. In the data collection interface (left top of Figure 1B), when an evaluation action is selected, the corresponding instruction video will be played on the left, and the real-time sensor data will be displayed on the right. In the results generation interface (left bottom of Figure 1B), the scores and vital kinematic features of single items are available. Finally, a complete FMA-UE report (right of Figure 1B) from this automated system can be viewed and saved.

2.2.3. Experimental Protocol

As shown in the experimental scene in Figure 1A, the subject sat in a chair facing a display. For each movement, an instruction video was played first, and the subject was asked to try to perform the demonstrated action without assistance (Figure 1C). The four Shoulder/Elbow part motions (I, II, III, V) were performed twice. All other motions were performed once on the less-affected side and paretic sides respectively. At the same time, one experienced therapist also participated to observe and rate each FMA item according to the consistency between patients' performance and the scale instructions.

2.3. Assessment

2.3.1. Data Analysis Procedure

Figure 3A depicts the data analysis procedure of the proposed system, in which the extracted features are listed in Table 3. The data from sensors were first preprocessed, and then specific features were extracted. These features served as inputs to the scoring method. Different scoring methods were applied to different categories. The Shoulder/Elbow part was scored using random forest (RF) classification, an effective machine learning algorithm for estimating scale scores from kinematic features [28,29]. It has the advantages of non-parametric nature, feature importance evaluation capability, and high classification accuracy [30]. The other three were scored using rule-based (RB) logical classification, because the movement evaluation criteria are explicit and concise, suitable to directly abstract logical rules with interpretability for scoring. Meanwhile, it was also found that the RF classification could not achieve better results. The following two sections will separately introduce the automated evaluation process of the Shoulder/Elbow part and the other three parts in detail.

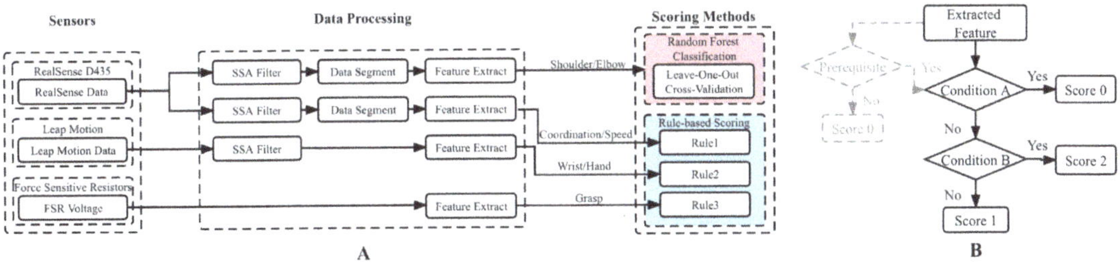

Figure 3. (**A**) Flow chart of data analysis. SSA: singular spectrum analysis. (**B**) The general IF-ELSEIF-ELSE logic model of scoring rules, where the gray part indicates that several items require prerequisites.

2.3.2. The Shoulder/Elbow Part

The RealSense Data consisted of a time series of the 18-key-point 3D positions. Regarding the data with high confidence collected by Vicon as the baseline, it could be found that the raw RealSense data were contaminated by noise (Figure 2B-left). Two algorithms, low pass filter and singular spectrum analysis (SSA) [31], have been compared to attenuate the influence of noise. Finally, SSA was selected because of its stronger smoothing effect. The main steps of SSA include embedding, singular value decomposition, grouping, and reconstruction. It decomposes diverse components (trend, periodic components, noise, etc.) from the initial time series. Selecting the top k components with the largest contribution for reconstruction can achieve the purpose of denoising. Taking the wrist joint in motion I as an example, it can be seen from Figure 2B-left that the data filtered by SSA is highly consistent with the Vicon data. Next, the start time and end time were automatically detected by marking the first and the last frames with higher endpoint velocities than the average one. The preprocessed data (i.e., denoised and segmented data) of the wrist joint are shown in Figure 2B-right, where the red dots represent the motion segmentation points. The wrist joint position offsets (mean Euclid distance between the corresponding joints in each time frame) for the four motions (I, II, III, V) were 54, 43, 138, 150 mm, respectively, with a mean offset of 96mm, which was acceptable and close to that of Kinect V2 (72 mm) [32]. Therefore, the RealSense data processed by SSA could achieve high precision with limited data acquisition conditions.

Before the scoring method was applied, 36 kinematic features in Table 3 were calculated to describe the properties of the preprocessed data, which could be divided into three aspects [33]: endpoint kinematics (6 features, e.g., path length, velocity, smoothness [34]), angular kinematics (24 features, e.g., angles and angular velocity of four degrees of freedoms (DoFs)) and other kinematics (6 features, e.g., inter-joint coordination index (IJCI) [35], time, trunk compensation [36]).The detailed calculation of these features are elaborated in Appendix A. 13 RF classifiers, respectively corresponding to 13 items, were trained, for item 3–13,15,16 (Table 1). The features stated above were used as input and the scores evaluated by one experienced therapist were used as labels.

Comprehensively considering the smoothing effect and computation time, the two main parameters of the SSA filter, the window length L and the reconstruction subsequence number k, were set to 15 and 2, respectively. Additionally, the two main parameters of the RF classifier, the number of trees n and the number of features f, were set to 100 and 6. The parameter n was selected by five-fold cross validation. A sequence of increasing values was applied until the results tended to stabilize.

Table 3. Extracted Features for Each FMA Test Item.

Category	FMA Item	Feature Category/Symbol	Feature
Shoulder/Elbow	3–17 (except 14,17)	Endpoint	Path length of the endpoint
			Max velocity
			Mean velocity
			Velocity variance
			Spectral arc length
			Dimensionless jerk
		Angle (Shoulder flexion, shoulder adduction, shoulder rotation, elbow flexion)	Range of motion (ROM)
			Max angle
			Min angle
			Max angular velocity
			Mean angular velocity
			Angular velocity variance
		Others	Inter-joint coordination index
			Time
			Max shoulder joint displacement (X, Y, Z)
			Trunk compensation
Wrist/Hand	14	δ_{max}, Φ_{max}	Max elbow flexion angle and forearm angle
	17	α_{max}, Φ_{max}	Max shoulder flexion angle and forearm angle
	19–22	$\theta_{max}, \theta_{min}$	Wrist pitch angle (max, min)
	23	θ_{max}, ψ_{max}	Wrist pitch angle and yaw angle (max, min)
	24, 25	$\eta_{i,max}, \rho_{max}$	Finger tip anlge and hand grab strength (max, min)
Grasp	26–30	V_{max}, F_{max}	Max voltage and force
Coordination/Speed	31	$SPARC$	Spectral arc length
	32	$d_{r,min}$	Min relative distance between wrist and nose
	33	T	Time

2.3.3. The Other Three Parts

For the Coordination/Speed part, the parameter L of the SSA algorithm was slightly adjusted so as to avoid removing motion details and maintain the tremor information for item 31. For the Wrist/Hand part, the Leap Motion Data was composed of hand bone vectors and some variables (palm orientation, hand opening, closing degree, etc.) generated by Leap Motion SDK. Data were also first preprocessed using an SSA filter. Then specific features listed in Table 3 were selected for each FMA item for later scoring based on logical rules.

All these rules were based on an IF-ElSEIF-ELSE logic model, as shown in Figure 3B. There was an additional prerequisite for FMA items 14, 17, and 33 (marked gray). For 14 and 17, the prerequisite was whether the subject could move to the initial position, and for 33, the prerequisite was whether the subject could point to the nose with the paretic limb. With regard to item 24 and 25, there was such a logic model for scoring each finger, and finally, the item score was obtained by another model with the total score of four fingers as input. Detailed rules for each item are provided in the Appendix B. The variable with the subscript p represents the feature of the paretic side, with the subscript h represents the less-affected side, and with the subscript N represents the normal reference, which is a constant calculated from the mean value of all subjects' less-affected side features. Notably, the threshold λ_1 and λ_2 in each rule were set as $1/3$ and $2/3$, respectively, achieving the effect of three equal divisions, which were approved by experienced clinicians.

2.4. Data Analysis

The following metrics were calculated in this study. By default, the Leave-One-Out Cross-Validation (LOOCV) method [37] was used for performance evaluation of the RF segment, and the average less-affected-side kinematic features of all subjects were used as the standard references for the RB segment. The LOOCV method uses one subject as the test set and all other subjects as the training set and iterates this step n times (n is the sample size). Then offline scores for each item of each person could be obtained.

1. Total scores: Using Pearson's correlation coefficient, the correlation between the system and therapist scores was investigated. In addition, in order to further prove the system value in practical applications, a simulated online test was also implemented. The 20 participating patients were first ranked in ascending order according to their FMA-UE scores. In order to ensure the involvement of different motor function levels, every other subject was selected to construct a ten-patient training set, and the remaining ten patients made up the test set. For convenience, the result predicted by the automated system was abbreviated as S_FMA and that evaluated by the therapist was abbreviated as T_FMA.
2. Single FMA items: To evaluate the scoring accuracy of the proposed system, both the prediction accuracy and mean absolute error (MAE) of each item were calculated, using scores obtained from the therapist as the gold standard. The consistency between all the scores for a total of 600 items (30 items for each of 20 subjects) obtained by these two assessment methods was estimated by linear weighted Cohen's kappa coefficient. Four additional macro-averaged metrics, including F1-score, sensitivity, specificity, and precision, were also calculated according to the confusion matrix.

All statistical analyses were performed via SPSS (IBM, Chicago, IL, USA).

3. Results

3.1. Participants

A total of 20 patients with stroke participated in this study. Table 4 presents the detailed characteristics of the population.

Table 4. Characteristics of Stroke Subjects.

Index	Age	Sex	Time since Stroke Onset (Month)	Paretic Side	MMSE	Brunnstrom	FMA-UE
P1	54	M	2	Left	28	2	14
P2	70	F	4	Right	29	6	66
P3	51	M	1	Left	30	4	54
P4	61	M	7	Left	28	3	32
P5	43	F	2	Left	29	4	45
P6	70	F	24	Left	27	2	9
P7	69	F	3	Left	29	5	57
P8	58	M	2	Right	30	5	61
P9	58	M	4	Right	28	3	20
P10	54	M	1	Right	28	2	13
P11	73	M	7	Left	24	2	25
P12	68	M	2	Right	28	4	28
P13	33	M	11	Left	28	4	30
P14	56	M	24	Right	29	4	40
P15	74	M	2	Right	27	3	16
P16	61	M	22	Left	27	2	12
P17	70	F	1	Left	28	3	20
P18	58	M	5	Left	28	5	55
P19	51	M	2	Left	27	3	16
P20	47	M	1	Left	28	5	50

3.2. Performance Evaluation on Total Scores

Correlation between S_FMA and T_FMA was particularly high (r = 0.981, $p < 0.01$) (Figure 4), indicating that the system has a strong ability to produce FMA-UE scores consistent with the therapist.

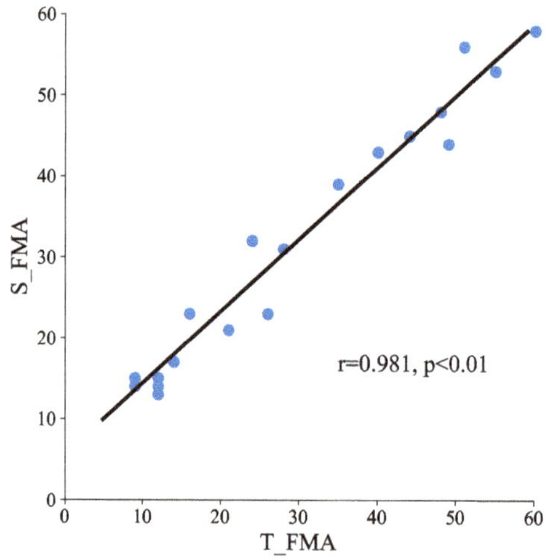

Figure 4. The correlation between the summed scores of the 30 items obtained by the automated system and by a therapist ($n = 20$).

In order to further verify the system value in practical applications, online testing was simulated. The FMA-UE scores of the 20 participating patients in this study are displayed in Figure 5A in ascending order, which are evenly distributed. As shown in the Figure 5B, Pearson's correlation coefficient between S_FMA and T_FMA (r = 0.982, $p < 0.01$) of the simulated online test was equal to the offline test.

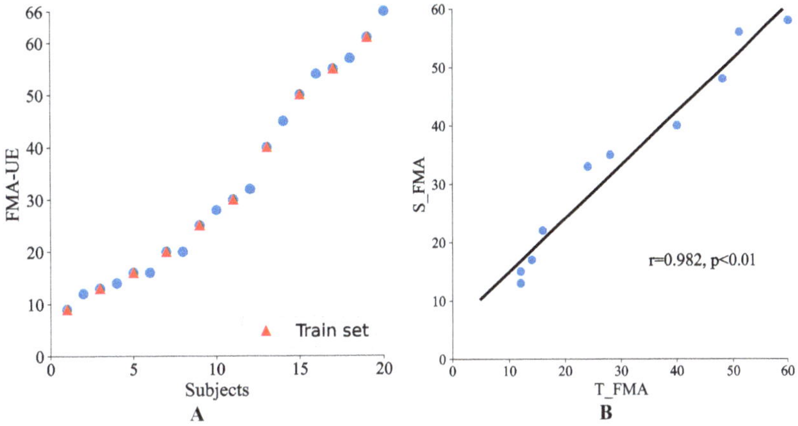

Figure 5. (**A**) The FMA-UE scores of 20 subjects. The subjects with red triangle markers were regarded as the training set in the simulated online test, and other subjects were used as the test set. (**B**) Simulated online test results, the correlation between the total scores of the 30 items obtained by the automated system and by a therapist in the test set (n = 10).

3.3. Performance Evaluation on Single FMA Items

Figure 6A depicts the performance of single FMA items in two indicators: classification accuracy and MAE. Due to different scoring methods and accuracy evaluation approaches, all items were divided into two segments to show the results: the Shoulder/Elbow part and the other three parts, distinguished by two different colors. Item 3, 4, 5, and 7 had the highest accuracy (100%), and item 12 and 23 had the lowest accuracy (60% and 55%, respectively) among each segment. The maximum error (0.55 points) appeared in item 12, which was still far less than the resolution of the scale: 1 point.

Figure 6B shows the confusion matrix of FMA scores assigned by the therapist versus scores estimated by the automated system. The accuracy for score 0 (78.3%) and 2 (90.2%) was higher than that for score 1 (75.1%), implying that the system performed better in extreme cases. Meanwhile, prediction errors mainly occurred in misjudgment of score 0 as 1 (16.3%) and misjudgment of score 1 as 2 (15%), that is, the system tended to overestimate results when it deviated from the therapist assessment. Cohen's kappa coefficient was 0.757, demonstrating a substantial agreement between the two scoring manners.

The mean accuracy, macro-averaged F1-score, precision, sensitivity, and specificity, and MAE for each segment and for all the selected 30 FMA items are shown in Table 5. The average accuracy of the RF classification segment was as high as 88.08% and of all 30 items was over 80.83%. The macro-averaged F1-score, precision, sensitivity, and specificity of all 30 items were 80.97%, 81.11%, 81.22%, and 90.40%, respectively, and there is no significant deviation between precision and sensitivity. It suggests that the system was well behaved under all these performance measures. The average MAE of all 30 items was 0.21.

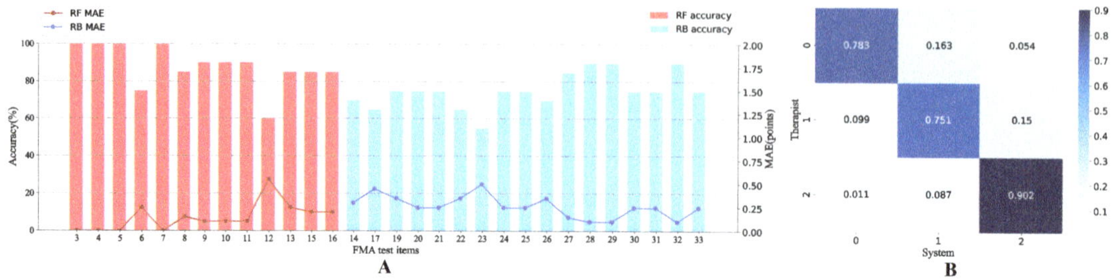

Figure 6. The results of single FMA items. (**A**) Prediction accuracy (%) and mean absolute error (MAE) (points) of each automated FMA item, where the red part denotes the items of the Shoulder/Elbow category scored by random forest classification, and the blue part denotes those of the other three parts scored by rule-based logic methods. The bar graph is the accuracy, while the line graph is the MAE. (**B**) A confusion matrix showing single item scores assigned by a therapist versus estimated by the automated system, with 600 items in total (30 items for each of 20 subjects).

Table 5. Average results of performance metrics for single items.

Indicators	Shoulder/Elbow Part	The Other Three Parts	All Four Parts
Accuracy (%)	88.08	75.30	80.83
F1-score (%)	86.59	74.58	80.97
Precision (%)	88.70	74.27	81.11
Sensitivity (%)	85.81	75.22	81.22
Specificity (%)	93.77	87.72	90.40
Mean absolute error	0.15	0.26	0.21

4. Discussion

In the present study, we proposed a complete automated FMA system to independently assess upper limb motor function in stroke patients and performed preliminary validation. On the whole, the total scores of the system were highly linearly correlated with that of the therapist, which was very close to 1. In terms of single FMA items scores, there was a considerable agreement between these two assessment methods (System and Therapist), as shown in Cohen's kappa coefficient. Meanwhile, detailed scores for each FMA item were also available, though some still had room for improvement in accuracy.

For the Shoulder/Elbow part using RF classification, the accuracy of each item could exceed 75% except for item 12 (hand to lumbar spine). For the other three parts using rule-based logical classification, the accuracy of each item exceeded 65% except for item 23 (wrist circumduction). The highest accuracy 100% occurred in item 3, 4, 5 and 7, which were parsed from one motion. This reveals that the system can successfully evaluate multiple aspects in a comprehensive motion with synergies. Apart from the latent defects in data processing and scoring methods, the motion implementation was also an essential factor contributing to the poor results of item 12 and 23. Item 12 has a short action stroke, enhancing the difficulty of motion distinction. Besides, some patients who could complete this motion well hid their entire forearms behind their backs, causing the misidentification of key skeletal points. For item 23, it was found that some subjects had difficulty understanding and performing the wrist circumduction movement. Even when using the less-affected side, they might perform compensatory movements. This could mislead both the therapist and the system.

In the previous studies of automated FMA, Kim et al. [17] only used Kinect to automate 13 FMA with an average accuracy below 80%. Bai et al. [18] combined Kinect and one posture sensor to automate 15 items and the accuracy rates range from 73% to 92.7%. Song el al. [38] used a cellphone as a wearable sensor and developed a cellphone-based system for 20 items, whose average accuracy is 85%. However, they only recruited 10 patients, and patients with scores between 30–50 were missing. Lee et al. [20] combined Kinect and FSRs to increase the automated items to 25, achieving an average accuracy of 92% in merely 9 subjects. Compared with them, the proposed system had comparable results with more automated items validated in a larger number of subjects.

The single item result of MAE was highly negatively correlated with that of accuracy ($r = -0.976$, $p < 0.01$ for RF classification, $r = -0.961$, $p < 0.01$ for RB classification). The two indicators were almost identical, and most items with the same accuracy rate also had the same error. One possible reason is that the number of cross-level misclassification samples for this system was small. In the confusion matrix of Figure 6B, only 5.4% of 0 points were mistakenly predicted as 2 points, and 1.1% of 2 points were mistakenly predicted as 0 points. This additionally indicates that the system performs well under the comprehensive evaluation of these two indicators. In terms of the accuracy in 600 items, the order from high to low was score 2, 0, and 1. The characteristics of extreme levels tended to be more pronounced and easier to classify accurately. In contrast, the boundaries between median and extreme levels could be ambiguous, thus resulting in a worse result. Additionally, system errors generally occurred in evaluating a level higher than the therapist, which should be paid attention to when patients or physicians utilize the automated system results.

Furthermore, the satisfactory simulated online test result further proved the accuracy and reliability of the system.It also implied that the proposed method could be promoted and applied in practice without difficulty, especially no additional experiments or prior knowledge was needed for the parameter determination.

Compared with other automated assessment systems based on wearable sensors (such as IMUs) and EMG, the proposed system, mainly relying on RGBD cameras, still has limitations. Wearable sensors allow for more accurate motion data collection without occlusion issues. More importantly, their use is not limited by the time and location, i.e., by applying wearable sensors continuous assessment of activities of daily living [39] and assessment performed at the bedside or in bed can be possible [40]. Unlike kinematic data, EMG can be utilized to analyze the neuromuscular differences under different motor functions from a more fundamental perspective, which cannot be obtained by other sensors. Nevertheless, the preliminary validation of the system is promising, and the assessment results are even better [11,15]. In addition, the proposed system can cover a wider assessment scope, and there is no need to calibrate and wear in advance. To conclude, it is more automated, convenient, and low cost.

By promoting strengths and avoiding or compensating for weaknesses, the proposed assessment system can be improved in the following aspects in the future. First, the accuracy of some single items is kind of unsatisfactory, which resulted in the system tending to overestimate patients' motor function. In addition to optimizing data processing methods, refining the instructions and adjusting evaluation paradigms of this automated system may also help improve results. Second, the feasibility of the system has only been preliminarily verified in a small number of subjects. The test-retest reliability will subsequently be measured with more patients participation. Moreover, although the sensors used are all non-wearable sensors, the number of sensor types is relatively large (three types of sensors including RealSense, Leap Motion, and FSRs). This automated system, which is preferably arranged in a separate room, is more suitable for hospitals, local clinics, or communities. There is still room for improvement in its convenience. Future work will focus on using RGB cameras alone to simplify the proposed system. In this way, patients can use a computer or a smartphone with cameras for evaluation at home.

5. Conclusions

This paper proposed an automated FMA system combining software and hardware, which is suitable for use in hospitals and communities. A high correlation coefficient of 0.981 between system and therapist and an average accuracy of over 80% for single

FMA items were achieved, with 20 patients participating. It demonstrates that this system can supplement and has the potential to replace the manual evaluation of the therapist. Compared to previous studies, the completeness of the system eliminates the need for therapists to perform complementary assessment items. This significantly saves their time and reduces their workload, allowing them to focus on rehabilitation training.

Author Contributions: Conceptualization, Y.L., C.L. and X.S. (Xinjun Sheng); methodology, Y.L. and C.L.; software, Y.L.; validation, X.S. (Xiaokang Shu) and X.S. (Xinjun Sheng); formal analysis, Y.L. and X.S. (Xiaokang Shu); investigation, Y.L.; resources, C.L. and J.J.; data curation, Y.L.; writing—original draft preparation, Y.L.; writing—review and editing, C.L., X.S. (Xiaokang Shu), X.S. (Xinjun Sheng) and J.J.; visualization, Y.L.; supervision, X.S. (Xinjun Sheng); project administration, X.S. (Xinjun Sheng) and J.J.; funding acquisition, X.Z. All authors have read and agreed to the published version of the manuscript.

Funding: This research was funded by the National Nature Innovation Research Group Project of China (grant number 82021002), and the National Natural Science Foundation of China (grant numbers 91948302, 9194830003, 51950410602, 52005321).

Institutional Review Board Statement: The study was conducted in accordance with the Declaration of Helsinki, and approved by the Institutional Review Board of the Huashan Hospital (protocol code KY2018-248 and date of approval 21 June 2018).

Informed Consent Statement: Informed consent was obtained from all subjects involved in the study.

Data Availability Statement: Data are available on request due to privacy restrictions.

Acknowledgments: The authors would like to thank all subjects and clinicians who participated in the study.

Conflicts of Interest: The authors declare no conflict of interest.

Appendix A. Detailed Feature Extraction Methods

To construct the kinematic metrics in the endpoint space, the endpoint displacement d_i between two frames is calculated first: $d_i = \|W_i - W_{i-1}\|, i = 1, \cdots, n$ where W_i is the Cartesian 3D coordinates of the wrist in the ith frame and n is the total number of recorded frames. d_i multiplies fps is the velocity and the sum is the path length.

The computable joint angles involved in the moving process include: shoulder flexion/extension angle (α), adduction/abduction angle (β), internal/external rotation angle (γ) and elbow flexion/extension angle (δ). The first three angles were defined by Euler angles from the rotation matrix with XZY sequence, which is further elaborated below.

The coordinate systems of the thorax and the humerus segments for both sides from the 18-joint skeleton of RealSense is shown in Figure A1. Take the right side as an example, and the left side is similar.

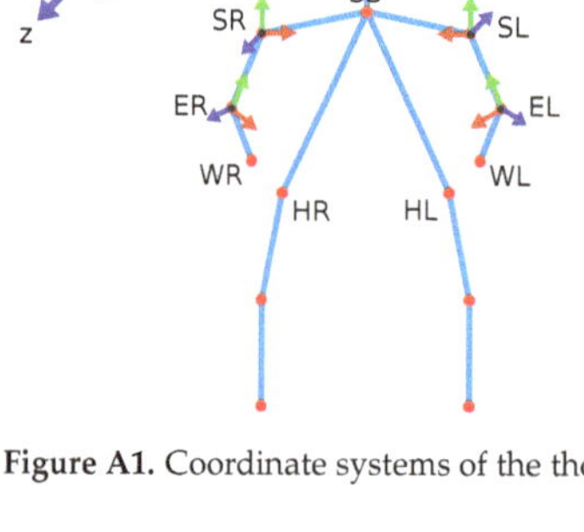

Figure A1. Coordinate systems of the thorax and the humerus segments.

The definition of the thorax segment coordinate system C_1 is as follows: SpineMid (SM) is defined as the midpoint of HR and HL (A1). The y-axis is the unit vector going from SM to SS (A2), the z-axis is the unit vector perpendicular to the the plane formed by y-axis and the vector from SR to SM (A3), and the x-axis is defined by y and z-axes to create a right-hand coordinate system (A4).

$$SM = \frac{1}{2}(HR + HL) \quad \text{(A1)}$$

$$y_{C_1} = \frac{SS - SM}{||SS - SM||} \quad \text{(A2)}$$

$$z_{C_1} = \frac{(SS - SR) \times y_{C_1}}{||(SM - SR) \times y_{C_1}||} \quad \text{(A3)}$$

$$x_{C_1} = \frac{y_{C_1} \times z_{C_1}}{||y_{C_1} \times z_{C_1}||} \quad \text{(A4)}$$

$$C_1 = [x_{C_1}, y_{C_1}, z_{C_1}] \quad \text{(A5)}$$

The definition of the right humerus segment coordinate system C_2 is as follows: the y-axis is the unit vector going from ER to SR (A6), the z-axis is the unit-vector perpendicular to the plane formed by y-axis and the vector from ER to WR (A7), and the x-axis is also defined by y and z-axes to create a right-hand coordinate system (A8).

$$y_{C_2} = \frac{SR - ER}{||SR - ER||} \quad \text{(A6)}$$

$$z_{C_2} = \frac{(WR - ER) \times y_{C_2}}{||(WR - ER) \times y_{C_2}||} \quad \text{(A7)}$$

$$x_{C_2} = \frac{y_{C_2} \times z_{C_2}}{||y_{C_2} \times z_{C_2}||} \quad \text{(A8)}$$

$$C_2 = [x_{C_2}, y_{C_2}, z_{C_2}] \quad \text{(A9)}$$

Then the rotation Matrix R_2^1 can be obtained via the parent coordinate system C_1 and the child coordinate system C_2 (A10). Shoulder flexion/extension, adduction/abduction, and internal/external rotation angles (α, β, γ in order) are Euler angles from R with XZY sequence.

$$R_2^1 = C_1^{-1}C_2 \quad \text{(A10)}$$

Additionally, the elbow flexion/extension angle is defined as:

$$\delta = \frac{\overrightarrow{SE} \cdot \overrightarrow{EW}}{||SE||||EW||} \quad \text{(A11)}$$

where $\overrightarrow{SE} = SR - ER$ or $SL - EL$, and $\overrightarrow{EW} = ER - WR$ or $EL - WL$.

The minimum relative distance between wrist and nose is defined as:

$$d_{r,min} = \min(\frac{||NW||}{||NK||}) \quad \text{(A12)}$$

where $NW = N - WR, NK = N - KR$ or $NW = N - WL, NK = N - KL$.

Appendix B. Scoring Rules

The scoring rules are listed in Tables A1 and A2.

Table A1. Logic Classification Rules.

Category	FMA Item	Rule [1]		Score [2]
Wrist/Hand (Rule2 [3])	14	If Δ		0
		Else	If Φ_1	0
			Else if Φ_2	2
			Else	1
	17	If A		0
		Else	If Φ_1	0
			Else if Φ_2	2
			Else	1
	19, 21	If Θ_1		0
		Else if Θ_2		2
		Else		1
	20, 22	If (Θ_1 AND Θ_3) OR Θ_5		0
		Else if Θ_2 AND Θ_4 AND Θ_6		2
		Else		1
	23	If Θ_5 AND Ψ_1		0
		Else if Θ_6 OR Ψ_2		2
		Else		1
	24	If H_{1i}	$s_i = 0$	
		Else if H_{2i} AND H_{6i}	$s_i = 2$	
		Else	$s_i = 1$	
		If $\sum_{i=2}^{5} s_i < 8\lambda_1$		0
		Else if $\sum_{i=2}^{5} s_i > 8\lambda_2$ AND P_1		2
		Else		1
	25	If H_{3i} OR H_{5i}	$s_i = 0$	
		Else if H_{4i}	$s_i = 2$	
		Else	$s_i = 1$	
		If $\sum_{i=2}^{5} s_i < 8\lambda_1$		0
		Else if $\sum_{i=2}^{5} s_i > 8\lambda_2$ AND P_2		2
		Else		1
Grasp (Rule3)	26–30	If $F_{max,p} = 0$		
			If $V_{max,p} = 0$	0
			Else	1
		Else if $F_{max,p} > \lambda_2 F_{max,h}$		2
		Else		1
Coordination /Speed (Rule1)	31	If $\frac{SPARC_N}{SPARC_p} < \lambda_1$		0
		Else if $\frac{SPARC_N}{SPARC_p} > \lambda_2$		2
		Else		1
	32	If $d_{r,min,h} > \lambda_2$		0
		Else if $d_{r,min,h} < \lambda_1$		2
		Else		1
	33	If $d_{r,min,p} > \lambda_2$		0
		Else	If $T_p - T_h > 6$	0
			Else if $\lvert T_p - T_h \rvert < 2$	2
			Else	1

[1] $\lambda_1 = 1/3, \lambda_2 = 2/3$. [2] Score 0 = cannot perform, 1 = partially completed, 2 = fully completed. [3] The meanings of symbols in Rule2 are explained in Table A2.

Table A2. Symbol meanings in Rule2.

Symbol	Logic Operation [1]
A	$\alpha_{max,p} < 30°$
Δ	$\delta_{max,p} < 90°$
Φ_1	$\phi_{max,p} < \lambda_1 \phi_{max,N}$
Φ_2	$\phi_{max,p} > \lambda_2 \phi_{max,N}$
Θ_1	$\theta_{max,p} < \lambda_1 \theta_{max,N}$
Θ_2	$\theta_{max,p} > \lambda_2 \theta_{max,N}$
Θ_3	$-\theta_{min,p} < -\lambda_1 \theta_{min,N}$
Θ_4	$-\theta_{min,p} > -\lambda_2 \theta_{min,N}$
Θ_5	$(\theta_{max,p} - \theta_{min,p}) < \lambda 1(\theta_{max,N} - \theta_{max,N})$
Θ_6	$(\theta_{max,p} - \theta_{min,p}) > \lambda 2(\theta_{max,N} - \theta_{max,N})$
Ψ_1	$(\psi_{max,p} - \psi_{min,p}) < \lambda 1(\psi_{max,N} - \psi_{max,N})$
Ψ_2	$(\psi_{max,p} - \psi_{min,p}) > \lambda 2(\psi_{max,N} - \psi_{max,N})$
H_{1i}	$\eta_{min,pi} > \frac{\eta_{min,Ni}}{\lambda_1}$
H_{2i}	$\eta_{min,pi} < \frac{\eta_{min,Ni}}{\lambda_2}$
H_{3i}	$\eta_{max,pi} < \lambda_1 \eta_{max,Ni}$
H_{4i}	$\eta_{max,pi} > \lambda_2 \eta_{max,Ni}$
H_{5i}	$\eta_{max,pi} - \eta_{min,pi} < \lambda_1(\eta_{max,Ni} - \eta_{min,Ni})$
H_{6i}	$\eta_{max,pi} - \eta_{min,pi} > \lambda_2(\eta_{max,Ni} - \eta_{min,Ni})$
P_1	$\rho_{max,p} == 1$
P_2	$\rho_{min,p} == 0$

[1] $\lambda_1 = 1/3, \lambda_2 = 2/3$.

References

1. Veerbeek, J.M.; Langbroek-Amersfoort, A.C.; Van Wegen, E.E.; Meskers, C.G.; Kwakkel, G. Effects of robot-assisted therapy for the upper limb after stroke: A systematic review and meta-analysis. *Neurorehabilit. Neural Repair* **2017**, *31*, 107–121. [CrossRef]
2. Warlow, C.P.; Van Gijn, J.; Dennis, M.S.; Wardlaw, J.M.; Bamford, J.M.; Hankey, G.J.; Sandercock, P.A.; Rinkel, G.; Langhorne, P.; Sudlow, C.; et al. *Stroke: Practical Management*, 3rd ed.; Peter, L., Martin, D., Eds.; John Wiley & Sons: Hoboken, NJ, USA, 2008.
3. Sivan, M.; O'Connor, R.J.; Makower, S.; Levesley, M.; Bhakta, B. Systematic review of outcome measures used in the evaluation of robot-assisted upper limb exercise in stroke. *J. Rehabil. Med.* **2011**, *43*, 181–189. [CrossRef]
4. Fugl-Meyer, A.R.; Jääskö, L.; Leyman, I.; Olsson, S.; Steglind, S. The post-stroke hemiplegic patient. 1. A method for evaluation of physical performance. *Scand. J. Rehabil. Med.* **1975**, *7*, 13–31.
5. Lin, J.H.; Hsueh, I.P.; Sheu, C.F.; Hsieh, C.L. Psychometric properties of the sensory scale of the Fugl-Meyer Assessment in stroke patients. *Clin. Rehabil.* **2004**, *18*, 391–397. [CrossRef]
6. Gladstone, D.J.; Danells, C.J.; Black, S.E. The Fugl-Meyer assessment of motor recovery after stroke: A critical review of its measurement properties. *Neurorehabilit. Neural Repair* **2002**, *16*, 232–240. [CrossRef]
7. Kim, H.; Her, J.; Ko, J.; Park, D.s.; Woo, J.H.; You, Y.; Choi, Y. Reliability, concurrent validity, and responsiveness of the Fugl-Meyer Assessment (FMA) for hemiplegic patients. *J. Phys. Ther. Sci.* **2012**, *24*, 893–899. [CrossRef]
8. Poole, J.L.; Whitney, S.L. Assessments of motor function post stroke: A review. *Phys. Occup. Ther. Geriatr.* **2001**, *19*, 1–22. [CrossRef]
9. Wang, J.; Yu, L.; Wang, J.; Guo, L.; Gu, X.; Fang, Q. Automated Fugl-Meyer assessment using SVR model. In Proceedings of the 2014 IEEE International Symposium on Bioelectronics and Bioinformatics (IEEE ISBB 2014), Chung Li, Taiwan, 11–14 April 2014; pp. 1–4.
10. Park, S.J.; Hussain, I.; Hong, S.; Kim, D.; Park, H.; Benjamin, H.C.M. Real-time gait monitoring system for consumer stroke prediction service. In Proceedings of the 2020 IEEE International Conference on Consumer Electronics (ICCE), Las Vegas, NV, USA, 4–6 January 2020; pp. 1–4.
11. Yu, L.; Xiong, D.; Guo, L.; Wang, J. A remote quantitative Fugl-Meyer assessment framework for stroke patients based on wearable sensor networks. *Comput. Methods Programs Biomed.* **2016**, *128*, 100–110. [CrossRef]
12. Li, H.T.; Huang, J.J.; Pan, C.W.; Chi, H.I.; Pan, M.C. Inertial sensing based assessment methods to quantify the effectiveness of post-stroke rehabilitation. *Sensors* **2015**, *15*, 16196–16209. [CrossRef]
13. Hussain, I.; Park, S.J. Prediction of myoelectric biomarkers in post-stroke gait. *Sensors* **2021**, *21*, 5334. [CrossRef]

14. Hesam-Shariati, N.; Trinh, T.; Thompson-Butel, A.G.; Shiner, C.T.; McNulty, P.A. A longitudinal electromyography study of complex movements in poststroke therapy. 2: Changes in coordinated muscle activation. *Front. Neurol.* **2017**, *8*, 277. [CrossRef] [PubMed]
15. Li, Y.; Zhang, X.; Gong, Y.; Cheng, Y.; Gao, X.; Chen, X. Motor function evaluation of hemiplegic upper-extremities using data fusion from wearable inertial and surface EMG sensors. *Sensors* **2017**, *17*, 582. [CrossRef]
16. Olesh, E.V.; Yakovenko, S.; Gritsenko, V. Automated assessment of upper extremity movement impairment due to stroke. *PLoS ONE* **2014**, *9*, e104487.
17. Kim, W.S.; Cho, S.; Baek, D.; Bang, H.; Paik, N.J. Upper extremity functional evaluation by Fugl-Meyer assessment scoring using depth-sensing camera in hemiplegic stroke patients. *PLoS ONE* **2016**, *11*, e0158640. [CrossRef] [PubMed]
18. Bai, J.; Song, A. Development of a novel home based multi-scene upper limb rehabilitation training and evaluation system for post-stroke patients. *IEEE Access* **2019**, *7*, 9667–9677. [CrossRef]
19. Fang, Q.; Mahmoud, S.S.; Gu, X.; Fu, J. A novel multistandard compliant hand function assessment method using an infrared imaging device. *IEEE J. Biomed. Health Inform.* **2018**, *23*, 758–765. [CrossRef] [PubMed]
20. Lee, S.; Lee, Y.S.; Kim, J. Automated evaluation of upper-limb motor function impairment using Fugl-Meyer assessment. *IEEE Trans. Neural Syst. Rehabil. Eng.* **2017**, *26*, 125–134. [CrossRef] [PubMed]
21. Li, C.; Cheng, L.; Yang, H.; Zou, Y.; Huang, F. An Automatic Rehabilitation Assessment System for Hand Function Based on Leap Motion and Ensemble Learning. *Cybern. Syst.* **2020**, *52*, 3–25. [CrossRef]
22. Bonett, D.G.; Wright, T.A. Sample size requirements for estimating Pearson, Kendall and Spearman correlations. *Psychometrika* **2000**, *65*, 23–28. [CrossRef]
23. Folstein, M.F.; Folstein, S.E.; McHugh, P.R. "Mini-mental state": A practical method for grading the cognitive state of patients for the clinician. *J. Psychiatr. Res.* **1975**, *12*, 189–198. [CrossRef]
24. Woodbury, M.L.; Velozo, C.A.; Richards, L.G.; Duncan, P.W.; Studenski, S.; Lai, S.M. Dimensionality and construct validity of the Fugl-Meyer Assessment of the upper extremity. *Arch. Phys. Med. Rehabil.* **2007**, *88*, 715–723. [CrossRef] [PubMed]
25. Woytowicz, E.J.; Rietschel, J.C.; Goodman, R.N.; Conroy, S.S.; Sorkin, J.D.; Whitall, J.; Waller, S.M. Determining levels of upper extremity movement impairment by applying a cluster analysis to the Fugl-Meyer assessment of the upper extremity in chronic stroke. *Arch. Phys. Med. Rehabil.* **2017**, *98*, 456–462. [CrossRef]
26. Siena, F.L.; Byrom, B.; Watts, P.; Breedon, P. Utilising the intel realsense camera for measuring health outcomes in clinical research. *J. Med Syst.* **2018**, *42*, 53. [CrossRef] [PubMed]
27. Simbaña, E.D.O.; Baeza, P.S.H.; Huete, A.J.; Balaguer, C. Review of automated systems for upper limbs functional assessment in neurorehabilitation. *IEEE Access* **2019**, *7*, 32352–32367. [CrossRef]
28. Patel, S.; Hughes, R.; Hester, T.; Stein, J.; Akay, M.; Dy, J.G.; Bonato, P. A novel approach to monitor rehabilitation outcomes in stroke survivors using wearable technology. *Proc. IEEE* **2010**, *98*, 450–461. [CrossRef]
29. Del Din, S.; Patel, S.; Cobelli, C.; Bonato, P. Estimating Fugl-Meyer clinical scores in stroke survivors using wearable sensors. In Proceedings of the 2011 Annual International Conference of the IEEE Engineering in Medicine and Biology Society, Boston, MA, USA, 30 August–3 September 2011; pp. 5839–5842.
30. Rodriguez-Galiano, V.F.; Ghimire, B.; Rogan, J.; Chica-Olmo, M.; Rigol-Sanchez, J.P. An assessment of the effectiveness of a random forest classifier for land-cover classification. *ISPRS J. Photogramm. Remote Sens.* **2012**, *67*, 93–104. [CrossRef]
31. Golyandina, N.; Nekrutkin, V.; Zhigljavsky, A.A. *Analysis of Time Series Structure: SSA and Related Techniques*; CRC Press: Boca Raton, FL, USA, 2001.
32. Wang, Q.; Kurillo, G.; Ofli, F.; Bajcsy, R. Evaluation of pose tracking accuracy in the first and second generations of microsoft kinect. In Proceedings of the 2015 International Conference on Healthcare Informatics, Dallas, TX, USA, 21–23 October 2015; pp. 380–389.
33. Sheng, B.; Wang, X.; Hou, M.; Huang, J.; Xiong, S.; Zhang, Y. An automated system for motor function assessment in stroke patients using motion sensing technology: A pilot study. *Measurement* **2020**, *161*, 107896. [CrossRef]
34. Balasubramanian, S.; Melendez-Calderon, A.; Burdet, E. A robust and sensitive metric for quantifying movement smoothness. *IEEE Trans. Biomed. Eng.* **2011**, *59*, 2126–2136. [CrossRef] [PubMed]
35. Ozturk, A.; Tartar, A.; Huseyinsinoglu, B.E.; Ertas, A.H. A clinically feasible kinematic assessment method of upper extremity motor function impairment after stroke. *Measurement* **2016**, *80*, 207–216. [CrossRef]
36. Scano, A.; Molteni, F.; Molinari Tosatti, L. Low-cost tracking systems allow fine biomechanical evaluation of upper-limb daily-life gestures in healthy people and post-stroke patients. *Sensors* **2019**, *19*, 1224. [CrossRef] [PubMed]
37. Ma, Y.; Liu, D.; Cai, L. Deep learning-based upper limb functional assessment using a single Kinect v2 sensor. *Sensors* **2020**, *20*, 1903. [CrossRef] [PubMed]
38. Song, X.; Chen, S.; Jia, J.; Shull, P.B. Cellphone-Based Automated Fugl-Meyer Assessment to Evaluate Upper Extremity Motor Function After Stroke. *IEEE Trans. Neural Syst. Rehabil. Eng.* **2019**, *27*, 2186–2195. [CrossRef] [PubMed]
39. Held, J.P.; Klaassen, B.; Eenhoorn, A.; Beijnum, B.J.F.v.; Buurke, J.H.; Veltink, P.H.; Luft, A.R. Inertial sensor measurements of upper-limb kinematics in stroke patients in clinic and home environment. *Front. Bioeng. Biotechnol.* **2018**, *6*, 27. [CrossRef] [PubMed]
40. Formstone, L.; Huo, W.; Wilson, S.; McGregor, A.; Bentley, P.; Vaidyanathan, R. Quantification of Motor Function Post-stroke using Novel Combination of Wearable Inertial and Mechanomyographic Sensors. *IEEE Trans. Neural Syst. Rehabil. Eng.* **2021**, *29*, 1158–1167. [CrossRef] [PubMed]

brain sciences

MDPI

Article

The Facial Skin Blood Flow Change of Stroke Patients with Facial Paralysis after Peripheral Magnetic Stimulation: A Pilot Study

Yongli Zhang [1,2,3,†], Shugeng Chen [2,†], Yinglu Ruan [4], Jiaying Lin [1,2], Chengdong Li [5], Chong Li [2,3], Shuo Xu [2], Zhijie Yan [2], Xiangyun Liu [3], Peng Miao [5] and Jie Jia [1,2,4,6,7,8,*]

1 School of Rehabilitation Medicine, Fujian University of Traditional Chinese Medicine, Fuzhou 350122, China
2 Department of Rehabilitation Medicine, Huashan Hospital, Fudan University, Shanghai 200040, China
3 School of Kinesiology, Shanghai University of Sport, Shanghai 200438, China
4 Department of Rehabilitation Medicine, Shanghai Jing'an District Central Hospital, Shanghai 200040, China
5 School of Biomedical Engineering, Shanghai Jiaotong University, Shanghai 200030, China
6 National Clinical Research Center for Aging and Medicine, Huashan Hospital, Fudan University, Shanghai 200040, China
7 National Center for Neurological Disorders, Shanghai 200040, China
8 National Regional Medical Center, Fuzhou 350200, China
* Correspondence: shannonjj@126.com
† These authors contributed equally to this work.

Abstract: Background: Facial paralysis (FP) is a common symptom after stroke, which influences the quality of life and prognosis of patients. Recently, peripheral magnetic stimulation (PMS) shows potential effects on peripheral and central nervous system damage. However, the effect of PMS on FP after stroke is still unclear. Methods: In this study, we applied PMS on the facial nerve of nine stroke patients with FP. At the same time, laser speckle contrast imaging (LSCI) was used to explore the facial skin blood flow (SkBF) in 19 healthy subjects and nine stroke patients with FP before and after the PMS intervention. The whole face was divided into 14 regions to compare the SkBF in different sub-areas. Results: In baseline SkBF, we found that there were no significant differences in the SkBF between the left and right faces in the healthy subjects. However, there was a significant difference in the SkBF between the affected and unaffected faces in Region 7 (Chin area, $p = 0.046$). In the following five minutes after the PMS intervention (Pre_0–5 min), the SkBF increased in Region 5 ($p = 0.014$) and Region 7 ($p = 0.046$) and there was an increasing trend in Region 3 ($p = 0.088$) and Region 6 ($p = 0.069$). In the five to ten minutes after the intervention (Post_6–10 min), the SkBF increased in Region 5 ($p = 0.009$), Region 6 ($p = 0.021$) and Region 7 ($p = 0.023$) and there was an increasing trend in Region 3 ($p = 0.080$) and left and right whole face ($p = 0.051$). Conclusions: These pilot results indicate that PMS intervention could increase facial skin blood flow in stroke patients with FP. A further randomized controlled trial can be performed to explore its possible clinical efficacy.

Keywords: facial paralysis; peripheral magnetic stimulation; blood flows; laser speckle; stroke

Citation: Zhang, Y.; Chen, S.; Ruan, Y.; Lin, J.; Li, C.; Li, C.; Xu, S.; Yan, Z.; Liu, X.; Miao, P.; et al. The Facial Skin Blood Flow Change of Stroke Patients with Facial Paralysis after Peripheral Magnetic Stimulation: A Pilot Study. *Brain Sci.* **2022**, *12*, 1271. https://doi.org/10.3390/brainsci12101271

Academic Editors: Simona Lattanzi and Konstantin V. Slavin

Received: 16 August 2022
Accepted: 10 September 2022
Published: 21 September 2022

1. Introduction

Central facial paralysis (CFP) is the common sequela for people who suffer from stroke, which affects about 45% of stroke patients according to a previous study [1]. CFP patients often present facial muscle dysfunction in the lower part of the face, which refers to the regions of the face below the eye clefts. It not only affects the facial appearance of patients but also causes some relevant deficits such as dysphagia and dysarthria [2,3]. Furthermore, patients with facial paralysis are more likely to have negative emotions like anxiety and depression than those who do not have facial paralysis [4]. Obviously, it may affect the training motivation of the CFP patients, which has a negative impact on clinical treatments.

Thus, paying attention to facial paralysis after a stroke is important, as it influences the quality of life and prognosis of stroke patients [5].

In clinical practice, the common modalities for treating facial paralysis include orofacial exercises [6], mirror therapy [7], acupuncture [8], electrical stimulation [9], and cupping [10]. Training in which the patient actively activates his facial muscles is called active rehabilitation, such as orofacial training. Training in which the patient accepts stimulation passively is called passive rehabilitation, such as acupuncture. Unlike skeletal muscles of limbs, facial muscles contain smaller motor units [11,12]. It seems difficult for patients to control facial movements precisely. Thus, applying active rehabilitation training alone might not achieve satisfactory efficacy. A passive and effective method as a complementary therapy is needed in treating facial paralysis better [13,14].

In recent years, neurostimulation techniques have been widely used for stroke patients in motor and sensory function rehabilitation [15]. For example, electrical stimulation is a common-used technique for facial paralysis in stroke patients [2]. Lee et al. [16] tried to determine the positive effect of neuromuscular electrical stimulation (NMES) on the masseter muscle in acute stroke patients. The results showed that it had a therapeutic effect on oral dysfunction in post-stroke patients. OH et al. [17] applied NMES to stroke patients on their orbicularis oris muscle and they found the lip strength and lip closure function of patients were significantly improved. Choi [2] et al. verified the effect of NMES on improving facial muscle strength and oral function in stroke patients with facial paralysis. However, the potential for painful feelings and allergic reactions to the electrodes during treatment limits the further application of electrical stimulation [18,19]. Peripheral magnetic stimulation (PMS) has been proposed as an alternative to electrical stimulation [20] as it generates a magnetic field and causes eddy currents inside the body, which is similar to the operating principle of electrical stimulation. It could directly penetrate deeper structures and tissues [21] with a less painful sensation of the skin [22] and no risk of inducing allergic reactions.

As a noninvasive treatment method, PMS induces muscle contractions and sensory afferents and it is considered to be an effective treatment in individuals with stroke or other nerve disorders [23–25]. The underlying mechanism of PMS in stroke rehabilitation has been explored for years. There were studies [26,27] speculating that by using PMS on hemiplegia limbs, the activation of frontoparietal loops promoted the improvement of patients' motor function. Besides, it was found that the increased corticomotor excitability of the lesioned hemisphere might be one of the key points [28]. Although PMS has been shown to improve the motor function of the upper and lower limbs in post-stroke patients [14,29], it has not yet been used in treating the facial dysfunction of stroke patients.

Most post-stroke patients suffer from motor dysfunction and it is mostly manifested as increased muscle tension, decreased muscle strength, and decreased blood flow [30,31]. Blood flow is one of the most important objective indicators for motor recovery. Several studies have demonstrated that motor function is related to tissue perfusion or blood flow in stroke patients [32,33]. As a general evaluation tool, laser speckle contrast imaging (LSCI) technology is recognized as a useful tool to determine skin blood flow (SkBF). It is a method of using the speckle pattern created after a laser strikes the moving red blood cells [34]. A unique edge of LSCI is that it provides real-time imaging to monitor near-continuous flow and it is a non-invasive method [35]. According to the previous study, LSCI is recommended for use as an important quantitative tool in clinical studies [36].

As a pilot study, this study aims to compare the facial skin blood flow of healthy subjects and stroke patients with facial paralysis. As for stroke patients, the whole face was divided into 14 regions to explore the SkBF characteristics of different facial areas. The pre-intervention SkBF and post-intervention SkBF were compared to reflect the peripheral effects of a single peripheral magnetic stimulation. Moreover, a customized questionnaire was offered to patients and it was a window to reflect the patients' real feelings and acceptance of PMS. We hypothesized that the blood flow would increase on the affected face of stroke patients after the PMS intervention.

2. Materials and Methods

2.1. Patients Recruitment

This study was performed from March 2022 to April 2022. Nine stroke patients (male, $n = 5$) with central facial paralysis and 19 healthy subjects (male, $n = 5$) without organic diseases were enrolled in the Department of Rehabilitation Medicine, Shanghai Jing'an District Central Hospital. The inclusion criteria of stroke patients were: (1) diagnosed with first unilateral hemispheric stroke confirmed by computed tomography (CT), and/or magnetic resonance imaging (MRI); (2) stroke onset after two weeks; (3) with unilateral central facial paralysis; (4) have not been administered drugs like corticosteroids for facial paralysis. The exclusion criteria were: (1) obvious wounds on faces; (2) diseases that affect blood flow except for hypertension (e.g., metabolic diseases or limb edema); (3) without enough cognitive ability to complete the study. Table 1 lists the patients' demographic and baseline clinical characteristics.

Table 1. The demographic and baseline clinical characteristics of the stroke patients with facial paralysis.

Patients	Sex	Age (y)	Type of Injury	Affected Face	Time Post-Stroke (Month)	House-Brackmann
S1	Male	46–50	hemorrhage	Right	11	IV
S2	Male	66–70	ischemia	Right	4	III
S3	Male	51–55	ischemia	Right	4	II
S4	Male	46–50	hemorrhage	Left	52	IV
S5	Female	66–70	ischemia	Left	6	III
S6	Female	71–75	hemorrhage	Right	2	II
S7	Female	66–70	ischemia	Right	1	II
S8	Female	51–55	hemorrhage	Right	105	II
S9	Male	71–75	ischemia	Left	5	IV

The study received approval from the Ethics Committee of Shanghai Jing'an District Central Hospital (KY2022-06), and each participant or his/her authorized representatives provided written informed consent for study participation. This study was registered in the Chinese Clinical Trial Registry (ChiCTR2200057805).

2.2. Measurement of Facial Skin Blood Flow

In this study, prototype imaging equipment was used to measure the skin's blood flow. It includes a CCD camera (acA1300-60 gmNIR, Basler AG, Ahrensburg, Germany) and a height-adjustable vertical stand. By starting measurements, a diverging near-infrared laser beam with a wavelength of 830 nm was used to illuminate the imaging area. The reflected light was then collected by the CCD camera with a frame rate of 30 fps and resolution of 640 × 480 (binning 2 × 2). The distance between the laser head and the skin surface was kept at 25 cm [37] and the imaging area was about 30 cm × 30 cm in size.

All the participants, including the healthy subjects and stroke patients, received the facial skin blood flow measurement. The healthy subjects received five minutes of facial blood flow measurement and did not take PMS intervention. Stroke patients sequentially underwent a 5-min pre-intervention blood flow measurement and a 10-min post-intervention blood flow measurement. Figure 1 presents the experimental setup.

Before starting the SkBF measurement, both healthy subjects and stroke patients were asked to rest for 20 min in an air-conditioned room which is maintained at around 22 °C and 40–60% humidity. In addition, the measurements were performed under normal fluorescent lighting conditions. During measurements, the participants were asked to lie down on the examination bed and close their eyes. They were also asked to keep their faces neutral and not to make facial movements. SkBF measurement was performed as soon as the single PMS intervention finished.

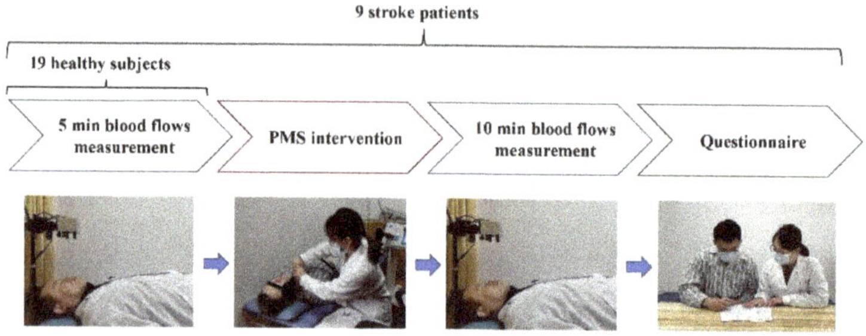

Figure 1. Experimental setup and intervention protocol.

2.3. PMS Intervention

In this study, only stroke patients received PMS intervention. By using a Mag-Pro R30 magnetic device (Tonica Elektronik A/S, Farum, Denmark) and a coil (MMC-140, Tonica Elektronik A/S), PMS intervention was administered. With the special parabola shape, the coil generates focused stimulation. The inner diameter of the coil is 25 mm and the outer diameter is 120 mm. Each stimulation was set as 20 Hz for 1.5 s and the intervals of every two stimulations were set at 3 s. The intensity level of magnetic stimulation was set at 15% of the maximal stimulator output for the device. In total, the entire intervention took about 20 min (1215 s) and produced 270 cycles of stimulation (8100 pulses). During the intervention, the patients maintained the supine position, and they were asked to keep relaxing. The stimulating coil was placed over the affected face of the FP patients and kept perpendicular to the skin to stimulate the outlet of the facial nerve and its branches of the lower part of the face (zygomatic branch, buccal branch, and mandibular branch).

2.4. The Facial Regions of Interest (ROIs)

In this study, the whole face was divided into 14 regions of interest (ROIs) based on previous research [38,39]. The 14 regions can represent the characteristics of different parts of the face in FP patients. There are seven ROIs on each side and are the frontal region (L1/R1), ocular region (L2/R2), infraorbital region and zygomatic region (L3/R3), nasal region (L4/R4), buccal region (L5/R5), lip region (L6/R6) and the chin region (L7/R7). All the ROIs are distributed in pairs on the left and right sides of the face (Figure 2).

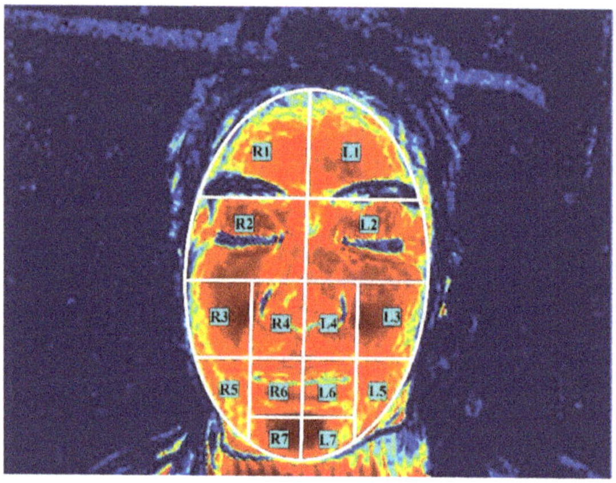

Figure 2. The facial regions of interest. L, left; R, right.

2.5. Safety Section

In order to reflect the patients' treatment experience of PMS, a questionnaire including five subcomponents (tolerance, comfort, preference, pain, and numbness) was designed and applied. A seven-point Likert scale was used, and "1" means "strongly disagree" and "7" means "strongly agree" in the questionnaire. After the post-intervention blood flow measurements, the questionnaire and an open-ended question was answered by the patients. The question is "Use one word to explain your main feelings during intervention" (Question 1). Furthermore, on the next day after the PMS intervention, patients were requested to answer another question "Use one word to explain your intervention-related feelings today" (Question 2).

2.6. Statistics

We used P1 to stand for 0–5 min before the PMS intervention, P2 for 0–5 min after the PMS intervention, P3 for 6–10 min after the PMS intervention, and P4 for 0–10 min after the PMS intervention. Averaged SkBF was calculated for P1, P2, P3, and P4. A *t*-test was conducted to compare the differences in SkBF between the healthy subjects and stroke patients. It is also applied to analyze the skin blood flow in the left and right sides of the faces of healthy subjects and the skin blood flow in the affected and unaffected faces of stroke patients. A paired *t*-test was adopted for the comparison before (P1) and after the PMS intervention (P2, P3, and P4) in stroke patients. Analyses were conducted using SPSS version 23.0 (IBM Inc., Chicago, IL, USA). Data of skin blood flow and scores of five subcomponents of the questionnaire are presented as the mean ± standard deviation. A *p*-value of <0.05 (two-sided) was considered to indicate a significant result.

3. Results

3.1. Left and Right Facial Skin Blood Flow of Healthy and Stroke with FP

Table 2 shows the facial skin blood flow between healthy subjects and stroke patients with facial paralysis. There were no significant differences in the SkBF between the left and right faces of the seven regions and both half faces in the healthy subjects. There were also no significant differences in SkBF between the affected and unaffected face except for a significant difference in Region 7 ($p = 0.046$) between the affected (219.32) and unaffected (231.56) face in the stroke patients with FP. The facial skin blood flow in Region 7 of the affected face was lower than that on the unaffected face.

Table 2. The facial skin blood flow between healthy subjects and stroke patients with facial paralysis.

	Healthy Subjects (n = 19)			Stroke Patients (n = 9) Pre-Intervention		
Region	**Left**	**Right**	***p* Value**	**Affected**	**Unaffected**	***p* Value**
1	151.00	151.36	0.947	145.89	156.43	0.139
2	203.18	201.86	0.659	200.52	206.09	0.378
3	209.23	215.95	0.142	181.84	199.50	0.286
4	233.10	230.75	0.616	235.45	240.20	0.192
5	191.90	191.16	0.931	134.45	166.05	0.181
6	237.20	236.17	0.639	225.00	237.11	0.130
7	232.16	238.53	0.099	219.32	231.56	0.046
half face	197.44	198.14	0.695	193.60	201.30	0.289

Compared to the SkBF of the left (197.44) or right (198.14) face of the healthy subjects ($p = 0.695$), the facial skin blood flow of the stroke patients ($p = 0.289$) on the affected face (193.60) was lower while that of the unaffected face (201.30) was higher. However, no significant differences were found between the two groups.

3.2. *Left and Right Facial Skin Blood Flow before and after PMS in Stroke with FP*

Table 3 shows the facial skin blood flow before and after a single PMS intervention in stroke patients with FP. Before the intervention, the SkBF on the affected face (both on the half face and seven regions) of all patients was lower than that on the healthy side. After the intervention, the SkBF on the affected face (both on the half-face and seven regions) in stroke patients all increased and it even exceeded that of the unaffected side in some areas (half face, Region 2, Region 3, Region 4, Region 5, Region 6, Region 7). There was no statistical difference between the affected and unaffected sides after the PMS intervention, but it shows a trend. For the affected and unaffected half face, the facial skin blood flow changed from 193.60 (P1) to 203.62 (P2) and 205.58 (P3) on the affected face, and from 201.30 (P1) to 200.51 (P2) and 205.13 (P3) on the unaffected face.

Table 3. The facial skin blood flow between the affected and unaffected faces in stroke patients with facial paralysis.

	Pre_0–5 min (P1)			Post_0–5 min (P2)			Post_6–10 min (P3)			Post_0–10 min (P4)		
Region	**Affected**	**Unaffected**	***p* Value**	**Affected**	**Unaffected**	***p* Value**	**Affected**	**Unaffected**	***p* Value**	**Affected**	**Unaffected**	***p* Value**
1	145.89	156.43	0.139	151.87	153.96	0.665	155.63	160.35	0.268	154.01	156.81	0.501
2	200.52	206.10	0.378	209.56	205.15	0.079	208.71	208.44	0.959	209.21	206.54	0.435
3	181.84	199.50	0.286	203.11	198.85	0.581	200.96	205.54	0.783	202.48	201.86	0.958
4	235.45	240.20	0.192	238.36	239.37	0.496	241.08	239.47	0.284	239.71	239.41	0.820
5	134.45	166.05	0.181	181.21	169.77	0.457	182.27	174.71	0.633	182.72	172.68	0.509
6	225.00	237.11	0.130	238.16	228.50	0.054	242.69	236.06	0.124	240.61	232.49	0.064
7	219.32	231.55	0.046	230.06	221.67	0.116	234.33	226.93	0.170	232.53	224.50	0.107
half face	193.60	201.30	0.289	203.62	200.51	0.306	205.58	205.13	0.919	204.81	202.66	0.510

3.3. *The Change of Facial Skin Blood Flow before and after PMS in Stroke with FP*

Table 4 shows the statistical differences between pre-PMS and post-PMS intervention in stroke patients with facial paralysis. On the affected face in stroke patients, the facial skin blood flow increased significantly in Region 5 ($p = 0.014$) and Region 7 ($p = 0.046$) and there was an increasing trend in Region 3 ($p = 0.088$) and Region 6 ($p = 0.069$) before (P1) and after (P2) the PMS intervention. Furthermore, the SkBF on the affected face of patients increased in Region 5 ($p = 0.009$), Region 6 ($p = 0.021$) and Region 7 ($p = 0.023$) significantly, and there was an increasing trend in Region 3 ($p = 0.080$) and left and right face ($p = 0.051$) before (P1) and after (P3) the PMS intervention (Figure 3). However, there was no significant difference in the SkBF on the unaffected face of stroke patients between pre-PMS and post-PMS intervention (Figure 4).

Table 4. The statistical differences of the facial skin blood flow between pre-PMS and post-PMS intervention in stroke patients with facial paralysis. P1, 0–5 min before the PMS intervention; P2, 0–5 min after the PMS intervention; P3, 6–10 min after the PMS intervention; P4, 0–10 min after the PMS intervention.

	Affected Side			Unaffected Side		
Region\Time	**P1-P2**	**P1-P3**	**P1-P4**	**P1-P2**	**P1-P3**	**P1-P4**
1	0.483	0.289	0.362	0.579	0.357	0.929
2	0.150	0.195	0.152	0.823	0.599	0.921
3	0.088	0.080	0.072	0.937	0.538	0.792
4	0.273	0.067	0.115	0.773	0.833	0.800
5	0.014	0.009	0.010	0.778	0.533	0.617
6	0.069	0.021	0.035	0.173	0.832	0.388
7	0.046	0.023	0.023	0.107	0.403	0.197
half face	0.126	0.051	0.077	0.838	0.395	0.744

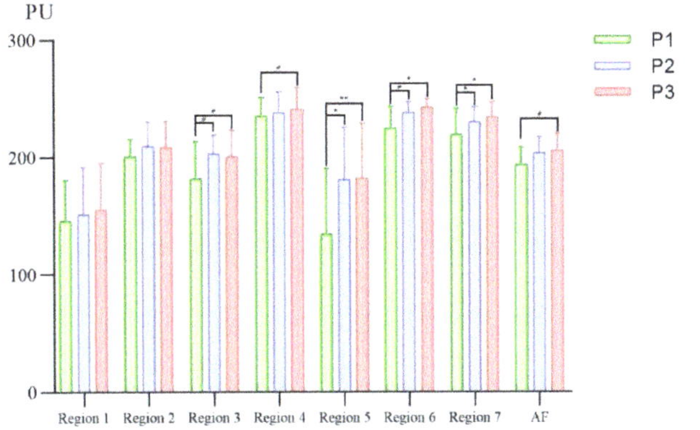

Figure 3. Bar plots of facial skin blood flow of the affected face before and after peripheral magnetic stimulation in stroke patients with facial paralysis. P1, 0–5 min before the PMS intervention; P2, 0–5 min after the PMS intervention; P3, 6–10 min after the PMS intervention; AF, the affected face; PU, perfusion index. #, $0.05 < p < 0.1$; *, $0.01 < p < 0.05$; **, $p < 0.01$.

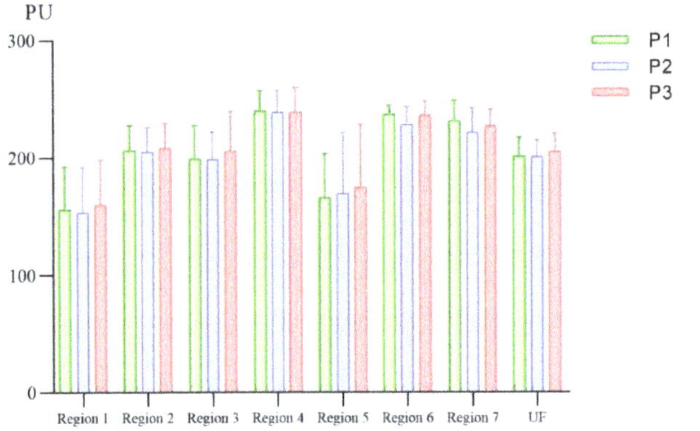

Figure 4. Bar plots of facial skin blood flow of the unaffected face before and after peripheral magnetic stimulation in stroke patients with facial paralysis. P1, 0–5 min before the PMS intervention; P2, 0–5 min after the PMS intervention; P3, 6–10 min after the PMS intervention; UF, the unaffected face; PU, perfusion index.

3.4. Safety Section

Of the nine stroke patients, six felt muscle twitch, one reflexed vibration sensation, one felt uncomfortable with the noise of the equipment, and one reported numbness in Question 1. In Question 2, four patients reported an increase in muscle strength subjectively, two with a feeling of skin tightening, one with a feeling of skin lifting, and two with no special feeling on the next day after PMS intervention. Table 5 shows the results of the questionnaire. The scores of the five subcomponents are tolerance (6.33 ± 0.71), comfort (5.11 ± 1.36), preference (6.56 ± 0.73), pain (1.44 ± 1.33), and numbness (4.11 ± 2.20), respectively. Patients reported high tolerance and almost no pain during and after the PMS intervention.

Table 5. Results of the questionnaire.

Subcomponent (Description)	Scores (Mean ± SD)
Tolerance (I accepted the treatment and stick to finish it until the end easily for me)	6.33 ± 0.71
Comfort (The treatment process is comfortable)	5.11 ± 1.36
Preference (If the treatment effects are the same, I would prefer peripheral magnetic stimulation to other facial treatments)	6.56 ± 0.73
Painful (During the treatment, I felt pain in the treated area)	1.44 ± 1.33
Numbness (During the treatment, I felt numbness)	4.11 ± 2.20

4. Discussion

In this study, we compared the face characteristics of SkBF in 19 healthy subjects and nine stroke patients with FP. The difference in SkBF between healthy subjects and FP patients was analyzed. Furthermore, a single session of PMS was applied to the nine stroke patients with facial paralysis. Through the change of SkBF before and after the PMS intervention, we initially explored the peripheral effects of PMS. The SkBF of 0 to 5 min and 6 to 10 min after the intervention were compared to find the continuous effect of PMS. Moreover, a questionnaire was offered to the patients to test irsafety and to explore their feelings and acceptance of PMS.

4.1. Facial Blood Flow on Both Sides of the Participants

Our results showed no statistical difference between the left side and right side in the facial skin blood flow of healthy subjects. The result was the same as several previous studies [40,41]. As for the stroke patients, some studies suggested that the blood flow of stroke patients on the affected limbs was lower than on the unaffected side. Tiftik et al. [33] showed that the radial and ulnar arteries of the affected side were significantly smaller in volume flow and end-diastolic velocity. Billinger et al. [42] found that the blood flow was also reduced in the femoral artery of the affected body. A major reason for this is likely a lack of physical activity and the disuse of the limbs [32]. Our study firstly explored the facial skin blood flow of both faces in stroke patients and showed similar conclusions, of which the SkBF of the affected side was lower than the unaffected side. However, the differences in SkBF in most of the regions were not statistically significant (R1, R2, R3, R4, R5, R6). This might be related to the anatomy of the face. Unlike the limbs, the face cannot complete facial movement with unilateral muscles, but with the coordinated movement of both sides. It might reduce differences in the blood flow on both sides.

Compared to healthy subjects, the incidence of stroke affects the motor performance of stroke patients. Some studies speculated that it might be related to the hemodynamic changes after the stroke onset [32]. Murphy et al. [43] found that a lower magnitude of muscle perfusion through the femoral artery was observed in the stroke group than in the neurologically intact participants. Zhang et al. [36] demonstrated that superficial perfusion of hands which was measured by laser speckle contrast imaging was lower than healthy volunteers. In our study, compared to healthy volunteers, we also found the affected side face of stroke patients had a lower skin blood flow.

4.2. The Effects of PMS on Facial Skin Blood Flow

Normal muscle function requires a certain amount of SkBF. Decreased perfusion after stroke has been suggested as one of the possible reasons for the impact on muscle performance [36]. Some studies have demonstrated that with the advancement of treatment, motor recovery is accompanied by an increase in blood perfusion [32]. It may suggest the potential of blood perfusion as one of the indicators of exercise improvement. As a pilot study, the outcome measurement was the key to exploring the effectiveness because the common evaluation indicators were hard to reflect the change of a single intervention. A real-time evaluation indicator is thus needed. Unlike the study mentioned above which applied long-term intervention, we chose the facial skin blood flow as the index to monitor the change in muscle status.

In our study, patients presented a higher facial skin blood flow after the PMS intervention. The SkBF in Region 5 and Region 7 both significantly increased in P2 and P3 compared to P1. It is likely that the continuous stimulation of PMS leads to passive facial muscle movement in stroke patients which contributed to the increase in blood flow. Furthermore, the major symptom of central facial paralysis patients is mouth drooping. That is one of the reasons why Region 5 and Region 7 (related regions) have obvious changes compared to other regions [44]. The SkBF in Region 3 maintained an increasing trend in both P2 and P3. Interestingly, as time went on, the SkBF in Region 6 changed from an increasing trend in P2 to a significant increase in P3 compared to P1, which suggested an accumulative effect of the PMS intervention [45]. Besides, there was also an increasing trend in the affected face which covered Region 1 to Region 7. This suggested the activation effect on SkBF from the PMS intervention [28]. Previous studies [46–48] considered that both peripheral magnetic and electrical stimulations can have a modulating and activating effect, which would lead to improvements in sensorimotor function. Additionally, the possible mechanisms that may underlay regional differences in facial SkBF are the autonomic control, and local control of vasomotion in facial skin vessels [49]. That means when facing different physiological or psychological stimulation, human faces present unique responses in facial regions [50].

4.3. *The Acceptance of the Facial PMS Intervention*

According to the questionnaires, patients had a high tolerance and comfort during the PMS intervention. They felt little pain caused by the magnetic stimulation. However, some patients reported a feeling of mild numbness. It might be due to the stimulation affecting the surrounding nerve (trigeminal nerve), which is mainly responsible for facial sensation. Overall, patients had a higher preference for PMS compared to other treatments, which suggested the high acceptance of PMS. In addition, through the open-ended questions, we found that the immediate feeling during treatment and the subsequent feeling the next day after intervention were not the same. During PMS stimulation, most patients felt the twitching of the muscles. On the next day, most patients felt an increase in muscle strength on the affected side. It might be caused by the legacy effects of PMS stimulation on the receptors.

There are some limitations to be noted in this study. First of all, the sample size was small, which consisted of only nine stroke patients and 19 healthy subjects. With a larger sample, it might help to eliminate outliers and present robust data better. Furthermore, although we performed a single PMS intervention, it could not reflect the efficacy of peripheral magnetic stimulation in improving facial function. Indeed, a direct effect would take several weeks to occur [45 s].

5. Conclusions

This study demonstrated that the facial skin blood flow increased on the affected face of stroke patients with facial paralysis after a single session of PMS intervention. The findings of this study extended the possible application of PMS and preliminarily verified the feasibility of applying PMS to stroke patients with facial paralysis.

Author Contributions: Conceptualization, Y.Z., S.C. and J.J.; methodology, Y.Z., S.C. and J.J.; validation, Y.Z., S.C. and J.J.; formal analysis, Y.Z., S.C.; investigation, Y.Z., Y.R. and J.L.; resources, C.L. (Chengdong Li), P.M.; data curation, C.L. (Chengdong Li), P.M.; writing—original draft preparation, Y.Z., S.C.; writing—review and editing, C.L. (Chong Li), S.X., Z.Y. and X.L.; visualization, Y.Z., S.C.; project administration, Y.R., J.L.; funding acquisition, J.J. All authors have read and agreed to the published version of the manuscript.

Funding: This research was funded by the National Key Research and Development Program Project of China (2018YFC2002300), National Natural Integration Project (91948302), National Natural Science Foundation of China (82021002), and the Shanghai Science and Technology Innovation Action Plan (22YF1404200).

Institutional Review Board Statement: The study was conducted in accordance with the Declaration of Helsinki, and approved by the Ethics Committee of Shanghai Jing'an District Central Hospital (KY2022-06).

Informed Consent Statement: Informed consent was obtained from all subjects involved in the study. Written informed consent has been obtained from the patient(s) to publish this paper.

Data Availability Statement: Not applicable.

Acknowledgments: We thank all volunteers for their participation in the study.

Conflicts of Interest: The authors declare no conflict of interest.

References

1. Yew, K.S.; Cheng, E.M. Diagnosis of acute stroke. *Am. Fam. Physician* **2015**, *91*, 528–536. [PubMed]
2. Choi, J.B. Effect of neuromuscular electrical stimulation on facial muscle strength and oral function in stroke patients with facial palsy. *J. Phys. Ther. Sci.* **2016**, *28*, 2541–2543. [CrossRef]
3. Hägg, M.; Tibbling, L. Four-quadrant facial function in dysphagic patients after stroke and in healthy controls. *Neurol. Res. Int.* **2014**, *2014*, 672685. [CrossRef] [PubMed]
4. Pouwels, S.; Sanches, E.E.; Chaiet, S.R.; de Jongh, F.W.; Beurskens, C.; Monstrey, S.J.; Luijmes, R.E.; Siemann, I.; Ramnarain, D.; Marres, H.; et al. Association between duration of peripheral facial palsy, severity, and age of the patient, and psychological distress. *J. Plast. Reconstr. Aesthet. Surg.* **2021**, *74*, 3048–3054. [CrossRef]
5. Coulson, S.E.; O'Dwyer, N.J.; Adams, R.D.; Croxson, G.R. Expression of emotion and quality of life after facial nerve paralysis. *Otol. Neurotol.* **2004**, *25*, 1014–1019. [CrossRef] [PubMed]
6. Teixeira, L.J.; Valbuza, J.S.; Prado, G.F. Physical therapy for Bell's palsy (idiopathic facial paralysis). *Cochrane Database Syst. Rev.* **2011**, CD006283. [CrossRef]
7. Kang, J.; Chun, M.H.; Choi, S.J.; Chang, M.C.; Yi, Y.G. Effects of Mirror Therapy Using a Tablet PC on Central Facial Paresis in Stroke Patients. *Ann. Rehabil. Med.* **2017**, *41*, 347. [CrossRef]
8. Liang, L.; Qiang, F. Observation on the Clinical Effect of Acupuncture and Moxibustion Combined with Repeated Transcranial Magnetic Stimulation on Facial Paralysis. *Comput. Math. Methods Med.* **2021**, *2021*, 9642677. [CrossRef]
9. Yildiz, N.; Yildiz, S.; Ertekin, C.; Aydoğdu, I.; Uludag, B. Changes in the perioral muscle responses to cortical TMS induced by decrease of sensory input and electrical stimulation to lower facial region. *Clin. Neurophysiol.* **2004**, *115*, 2343–2349. [CrossRef] [PubMed]
10. Cao, Z.; Jiao, L.; Wang, H.; Li, J.; Zhong, G.; Zhu, D.; Xu, W.; Jin, M. The efficacy and safety of cupping therapy for treating of intractable peripheral facial paralysis: A protocol for systematic review and meta-analysis. *Medicine* **2021**, *100*, e25388. [CrossRef]
11. Azuma, T.; Nakamura, K.; Takahashi, M.; Ohyama, S.; Toda, N.; Iwasaki, H.; Kalubi, B.; Takeda, N. Mirror biofeedback rehabilitation after administration of single-dose botulinum toxin for treatment of facial synkinesis. *Otolaryngol. Head Neck Surg.* **2012**, *146*, 40–45. [CrossRef]
12. Vanswearingen, J.M.; Brach, J.S. Changes in facial movement and synkinesis with facial neuromuscular reeducation. *Plast Reconstr. Surg.* **2003**, *111*, 2370–2375. [CrossRef] [PubMed]
13. Gobbo, M.; Gaffurini, P.; Vacchi, L.; Lazzarini, S.; Villafane, J.; Orizio, C.; Negrini, S.; Bissolotti, L. Hand Passive Mobilization Performed with Robotic Assistance: Acute Effects on Upper Limb Perfusion and Spasticity in Stroke Survivors. *Biomed Res. Int.* **2017**, *2017*, 2796815. [CrossRef] [PubMed]
14. Obayashi, S.; Takahashi, R. Repetitive peripheral magnetic stimulation improves severe upper limb paresis in early acute phase stroke survivors. *Neurorehabilitation* **2020**, *46*, 569–575. [CrossRef] [PubMed]
15. Grefkes, C.; Fink, G.R. Recovery from stroke: Current concepts and future perspectives. *Neurol. Res. Pract.* **2020**, *2*, 17. [CrossRef]
16. Lee, K.W.; Kim, S.B.; Lee, J.H.; Lee, S.J.; Park, J.G.; Jang, K.W. Effects of Neuromuscular Electrical Stimulation for Masseter Muscle on Oral Dysfunction After Stroke. *Ann. Rehabil. Med.* **2019**, *43*, 11–18. [CrossRef]
17. Oh, D.H.; Park, J.S.; Kim, W.J. Effect of neuromuscular electrical stimulation on lip strength and closure function in patients with dysphagia after stroke. *J. Phys. Ther. Sci.* **2017**, *29*, 1974–1975. [CrossRef]
18. Bampouras, T.M.; Reeves, N.D.; Baltzopoulos, V.; Maganaris, C.N. Muscle activation assessment: Effects of method, stimulus number, and joint angle. *Muscle Nerve* **2006**, *34*, 740–746. [CrossRef]
19. Man, W.D.; Moxham, J.; Polkey, M.I. Magnetic stimulation for the measurement of respiratory and skeletal muscle function. *Eur. Respir. J.* **2004**, *24*, 846–860. [CrossRef]
20. Lampropoulou, S.I.; Nowicky, A.V.; Marston, L. Magnetic versus electrical stimulation in the interpolation twitch technique of elbow flexors. *J. Sports Sci. Med.* **2012**, *11*, 709–718.
21. Krewer, C.; Hartl, S.; Müller, F.; Koenig, E. Effects of Repetitive Peripheral Magnetic Stimulation on Upper-Limb Spasticity and Impairment in Patients with Spastic Hemiparesis: A Randomized, Double-Blind, Sham-Controlled Study. *Arch. Phys. Med. Rehabil.* **2014**, *95*, 1039–1047. [CrossRef] [PubMed]

22. Abe, G.; Oyama, H.; Liao, Z.; Honda, K.; Yashima, K.; Asao, A.; Izumi, S. Difference in Pain and Discomfort of Comparable Wrist Movements Induced by Magnetic or Electrical Stimulation for Peripheral Nerves in the Dorsal Forearm. *Med. Devices* **2020**, *13*, 439–447. [CrossRef] [PubMed]
23. Flamand, V.H.; Schneider, C. Noninvasive and painless magnetic stimulation of nerves improved brain motor function and mobility in a cerebral palsy case. *Arch. Phys. Med. Rehabil.* **2014**, *95*, 1984–1990. [CrossRef]
24. Beaulieu, L.D.; Schneider, C. Effects of repetitive peripheral magnetic stimulation on normal or impaired motor control—A review. *Neurophysiol. Clin.* **2013**, *43*, 251–260. [CrossRef] [PubMed]
25. Flamand, V.H.; Beaulieu, L.D.; Nadeau, L.; Schneider, C. Peripheral magnetic stimulation to decrease spasticity in cerebral palsy. *Pediatr. Neurol.* **2012**, *47*, 345–348. [CrossRef]
26. Gallasch, E.; Christova, M.; Kunz, A.; Rafolt, D.; Golaszewski, S. Modulation of sensorimotor cortex by repetitive peripheral magnetic stimulation. *Front. Hum. Neurosci.* **2015**, *9*, 407. [CrossRef] [PubMed]
27. Struppler, A.; Binkofski, F.; Angerer, B.; Bernhardt, M.; Spiegel, S.; Drzezga, A.; Bartenstein, P. A fronto-parietal network is mediating improvement of motor function related to repetitive peripheral magnetic stimulation: A PET-H2O15 study. *Neuroimage* **2007**, *36*, T174–T186. [CrossRef]
28. Beaulieu, L.D.; Massé-Alarie, H.; Camiré-Bernier, S.; Ribot-Ciscar, É.; Schneider, C. After-effects of peripheral neurostimulation on brain plasticity and ankle function in chronic stroke: The role of afferents recruited. *Neurophysiol. Clin.* **2017**, *47*, 275–291. [CrossRef]
29. Jiang, Y.; Zhang, D.; Zhang, J.; Hai, H.; Zhao, Y.; Ma, Y. A Randomized Controlled Trial of Repetitive Peripheral Magnetic Stimulation applied in Early Subacute Stroke: Effects on Severe Upper-limb Impairment. *Clin. Rehabil.* **2022**, *36*, 693–702. [CrossRef]
30. Miller, T.; Qin, L.; Hung, V.W.Y.; Ying, M.T.C.; Tsang, C.S.L.; Ouyang, H.; Chung, R.C.K.; Pang, M.Y.C. Gait speed and spasticity are independently associated with estimated failure load in the distal tibia after stroke: An HR-pQCT study. *Osteoporosis. Int.* **2022**, *33*, 713–724. [CrossRef]
31. Huang, M.; Miller, T.; Ying, M.; Pang, M.Y.C. Whole-body vibration modulates leg muscle reflex and blood perfusion among people with chronic stroke: A randomized controlled crossover trial. *Sci. Rep.* **2020**, *10*, 1473. [CrossRef] [PubMed]
32. Durand, M.J.; Murphy, S.A.; Schaefer, K.K.; Hunter, S.K.; Schmit, B.D.; Gutterman, D.D.; Hyngstrom, A.S. Impaired Hyperemic Response to Exercise Post Stroke. *PLoS ONE* **2015**, *10*, e0144023. [CrossRef]
33. Tiftik, T.; Kara, M.; özcan, H.N.; Türkkan, C.; Ural, F.G.; Ekiz, T.; Akkuş, S.; özçakar, L. Doppler ultrasonographic evaluation of the radial and ulnar arteries in hemiparetic patients after stroke. *J. Clin. Ultrasound* **2014**, *42*, 277–282. [CrossRef] [PubMed]
34. Wang, S.J.; Lee, C.; Kang, H.G.; Kim, K.W.; Kim, M.; Jeong, H.; Shin, B. Peripheral vasoreactivity in acute ischemic stroke with hemiplegia. *Sci. Rep.* **2021**, *11*, 8531. [CrossRef] [PubMed]
35. Briers, J.D. Laser Doppler, speckle and related techniques for blood perfusion mapping and imaging. *Physiol. Meas.* **2001**, *22*, R35–R66. [CrossRef] [PubMed]
36. Zhang, L.; Ding, L.; Li, M.; Zhang, X.; Su, D.; Jia, J.; Miao, P. Dual-Wavelength Laser Speckle Contrast Imaging (dwLSCI) Improves Chronic Measurement of Superficial Blood Flow in Hands. *Sensors* **2017**, *17*, 2811. [CrossRef]
37. Mahé, G.; Humeau-Heurtier, A.; Durand, S.; Leftheriotis, G.; Abraham, P. Assessment of skin microvascular function and dysfunction with laser speckle contrast imaging. *Circ. Cardiovasc. Imaging* **2012**, *5*, 155–163. [CrossRef]
38. Zhang, Y.; Zhao, L.; Li, J.; Wang, J.; Yu, H. Microcirculation evaluation of facial nerve palsy using laser speckle contrast imaging: A prospective study. *Eur. Arch. Oto-Rhino-Laryngol.* **2019**, *276*, 685–692. [CrossRef]
39. Liu, X.; Wang, Y.; Luan, J. Facial Paralysis Detection in Infrared Thermal Images Using Asymmetry Analysis of Temperature and Texture Features. *Diagnostics* **2021**, *11*, 2309. [CrossRef]
40. Kashima, H.; Ikemura, T.; Hayashi, N. Regional differences in facial skin blood flow responses to the cold pressor and static handgrip tests. *Eur. J. Appl. Physiol.* **2013**, *113*, 1035–1041. [CrossRef]
41. Wang, S.Y.; Qu, X.X.; Song, X.J.; Li, S.Y.; Ma, H.M.; Zhang, D. Blood perfusion in different facial acupoint areas and its changes after acupuncture stimulation of Hegu (LI 4) displayed by laser Doppler imager in healthy volunteers. *Zhen Ci Yan Jiu* **2012**, *37*, 482–487. [PubMed]
42. Billinger, S.A.; Kluding, P.M. Use of Doppler Ultrasound to Assess Femoral Artery Adaptations in the Hemiparetic Limb in People with Stroke. *Cerebrovasc. Dis.* **2009**, *27*, 552–558. [CrossRef] [PubMed]
43. Murphy, S.; Durand, M.; Negro, F.; Farina, D.; Hunter, S.; Schmit, B.; Gutterman, D.; Hyngstrom, A. The Relationship Between Blood Flow and Motor Unit Firing Rates in Response to Fatiguing Exercise Post-stroke. *Front. Physiol.* **2019**, *10*, 545. [CrossRef]
44. Yonezawa, T.; Nomura, K.; Ichimura, S.; Mizoguchi, H.; Takemura, H. Blood Flow-Promoting Effect of Parallel Link Type Human Ankle Rehabilitation Assistive Device—Influence of Difference in Ankle Exercise on Blood Flow in the Lower Limb—. *Trans. Jpn. Soc. Med. Biol. Eng.* **2016**, *54*, 49–57.
45. Khedr, E.M.; Ahmed, M.A.; Alkady, E.A.M.; Mostafa, M.G.; Said, H.G. Therapeutic effects of peripheral magnetic stimulation on traumatic brachial plexopathy: Clinical and neurophysiological study. *Neurophysiol. Clin.* **2012**, *42*, 111–118. [CrossRef]
46. Beaulieu, L.D.; Schneider, C. Repetitive peripheral magnetic stimulation to reduce pain or improve sensorimotor impairments: A literature review on parameters of application and afferents recruitment. *Neurophysiol. Clin.* **2015**, *45*, 223–237. [CrossRef]
47. Chipchase, L.S.; Schabrun, S.M.; Hodges, P.W. Peripheral electrical stimulation to induce cortical plasticity: A systematic review of stimulus parameters. *Clin. Neurophysiol.* **2011**, *122*, 456–463. [CrossRef]

48. Quandt, F.; Hummel, F.C. The influence of functional electrical stimulation on hand motor recovery in stroke patients: A review. *Exp. Transl. Stroke Med.* **2014**, *6*, 9. [CrossRef]
49. Kashima, H.; Hamada, Y.; Hayashi, N. Palatability of Tastes Is Associated with Facial Circulatory Responses. *Chem. Senses* **2014**, *39*, 243–248. [CrossRef]
50. Miyaji, A.; Hayashi, S.; Hayashi, N. Regional differences in facial skin blood flow responses to thermal stimulation. *Eur. J. Appl. Physiol.* **2019**, *119*, 1195–1201. [CrossRef]

brain sciences

MDPI

Article

Effects of Repetitive Transcranial Magnetic Stimulation on Gait and Postural Control Ability of Patients with Executive Dysfunction after Stroke

Huixian Yu [1,2], Sihao Liu [1], Pei Dai [1,2], Zhaoxia Wang [1], Changbin Liu [1] and Hao Zhang [2,*]

[1] Department of Rehabilitation Medicine, Beijing Tiantan Hospital, Capital Medical University, Beijing 100060, China
[2] School of Rehabilitation, China Rehabilitation Research Center, Capital Medical University, Beijing 100068, China
* Correspondence: crrczh2020@163.com; Tel./Fax: +86-010-8756-9345

Abstract: Objective: To assess the effects of repetitive transcranial magnetic stimulation (rTMS) on the gait and postural control ability of patients with executive dysfunction (ED) after stroke. Methods: A total of 18 patients with ED after stroke were randomly assigned into two groups, including an experimental group and a sham group. Patients in both groups received routine rehabilitation therapy, and patients in the experimental group underwent rTMS on the left dorsolateral prefrontal cortex (DLPFC) for 2 weeks (5 HZ, 80%MT, 1200 pulses). In the sham group, patients experienced sham stimulation treatment, in which the coil was placed vertically with the head. Before and after treatment, patients in both groups were subjected to Montreal cognitive assessment (MoCA) scoring, Fugl–Meyer assessment of lower extremity (L-FMA), Stroop color-word test (SCWT), gait analysis, foot plantar pressure test, 10-m walking test (10MWT), Berg balance scale (BBS), and timed up and go test (TUGT). In the SCWT, it was attempted to record the time of each card (SCWT-T), the correct number (SCWT-C), Stroop interference effect-time (SIE-T), and SIE correct count (SIE-C). The TUGT was categorized into four stages: getting up (GT), walking straight (WT), turning around (TT), and sitting down (ST), in which the total time of TUGT was calculated. Results: After two weeks of treatment, the evaluation indexes were improved in the two groups, some of which were statistically significant. In the experimental group, SCWT-T, SIE-T, SIE-C, GT, WT, TT, ST, and TUGT were significantly improved after treatment ($p < 0.05$). SCWT-C, L-FMA score, 10MWT, GT, WT, stride length, step width, foot plantar pressure, pressure center curve, and activities of daily living were not statistically different from those before treatment ($p > 0.05$). After treatment, SCWT-T, SIE-C, SIE-T, BBS score, TT, and ST in the experimental group were significantly shorter than those before treatment, with statistical differences ($p < 0.05$). Compared with the sham group, SCWT-C, L-FMA score, 10MWT, GT, WT, TUGT, stride length, step width, foot plantar pressure, pressure center curve, and motor skills were not significantly improved ($p > 0.05$). Conclusion: It was revealed that post-stroke rTMS treatment of patients with ED could improve executive function, improve postural control function, and reduce the risk of falling. In addition, rTMS of DLPFC could be a therapeutic target for improving postural control ability and reducing the risk of falling.

Keywords: stroke; executive function; postural control; gait; repetitive transcranial stimulation

Citation: Yu, H.; Liu, S.; Dai, P.; Wang, Z.; Liu, C.; Zhang, H. Effects of Repetitive Transcranial Magnetic Stimulation on Gait and Postural Control Ability of Patients with Executive Dysfunction after Stroke. *Brain Sci.* **2022**, *12*, 1185. https://doi.org/10.3390/brainsci12091185

Academic Editors: Maryam Zoghi and Andrea Guerra

Received: 9 August 2022
Accepted: 29 August 2022
Published: 2 September 2022

1. Introduction

The need for post-stroke care due to motor dysfunction and decreased activities of daily living remarkably limits patients' ability to participate in society and poses a great economic burden to their families and society. Decreased postural control after stroke is the main factor affecting patients' daily mobility capability and quality of life. The incidence of post-stroke falling is still noticeable. It has been reported that up to 65% of patients have fallen during hospitalization, and 73% of patients have experienced falling at home or in the community within 6 months after stroke [1].

In our previous study, we found that patients with reduced executive function (EF) had poorer balance and postural control ability and were at a higher risk of falling [2]. EFs reflect a series of cognitive processes that are necessary for the control of cognitive behaviors, including decision-making, planning, cognitive flexibility, attention, working memory, etc. [3]. These important mental abilities can assist people to adapt to complex conditions. When EF is impaired, patients cannot make plans and perform self-adjustment according to rules, remarkably hindering patients' attendance in their families and society. Repetitive transcranial magnetic stimulation (rTMS) is a noninvasive neuromodulation therapeutic technique that uses a series of magnetic stimuli to target brain areas to modulate the excitability of neurons in the cortex at the stimulated site. Which can produce long-term potentiation (LTP) or long-duration long-term depression (LTD) [4]. It is generally believed that low-frequency rTMS are stimuli with frequency < 1 Hz, while high-frequency rTMS have frequency > 5 Hz. Low-frequency rTMS reduces cortical excitability, while high-frequency rTMS upregulate dermal excitability [5]. After a stroke, rTMS can promote functional recovery by inhibiting the unimpaired excitability of the injured motor cortex or increasing the impaired hemispheric cortex.

Studies have shown a consistent improvement in cognitive function with rTMS. It has not been reported that improving post-stroke EF can enhance walking and postural control abilities. However, whether improving executive function can improve motor function and postural control ability, and whether TMS treatment on the dorsolateral prefrontal cortex can improve motor function and postural control after improving executive function has not been reported. In this study, we tried to improve patients' executive function by regulating DLPFC with rTMS and observed whether the patients' motor function, gait, balance, and postural control ability were improved while the patients' executive function was improved. Through this research, we ultimately want to provide a new treatment concept for improving patients' walking and postural control ability.

2. Methods

2.1. Participants

A total of 18 patients with stroke who were admitted to the Department of Rehabilitation Medicine, Beijing Tiantan Hospital Affiliated to Capital Medical University (Beijing, China) from September 2021 to March 2022 were enrolled (like Figure 1). The inclusion criteria were as follows: (1) patients aged 35–65 years old; (2) right-handed patients; (3) patients with a history of the first cerebral hemorrhage or cerebral infarction in basal ganglia; (4) $\leq$3 months post-stroke; (5) patients with educational level of junior high school or above; (6) 15 $\leq$ MOCA score $\leq$ 25; (7) ability to walk more than 10 meters independently. The exclusion criteria were as follows: (1) patients with aggravated/unstable cerebrovascular disease; (2) patients with a history of complications, such as cerebral hemorrhage due to trauma, and other neurological or psychological diseases; (3) with infarction in other brain area or white matter lesions; (4) basal ganglia hemorrhage but no softening foci in the external capsule; (5) patients with serious heart, lung, liver, or renal dysfunction or with malignant tumors; (6) patients with sensory aphasia, abnormal sensory and other cognitive domains, anxiety and depression before or after stroke, and those who were unable to cooperate with assessment and treatment; (7) a history of epilepsy, or a family history of epilepsy; (8) the deterioration of conditions, and the emergence of new infarction or a large area of cerebral infarction. The following criteria were considered for trial suspension: (1) participants with severe adverse reactions or being unable to continue their participation in the study; (2) deterioration of the conditions or serious complications; (3) participants who did not cooperate or did not receive treatment according to regulations; (4) leaving the study by participants and their family members.

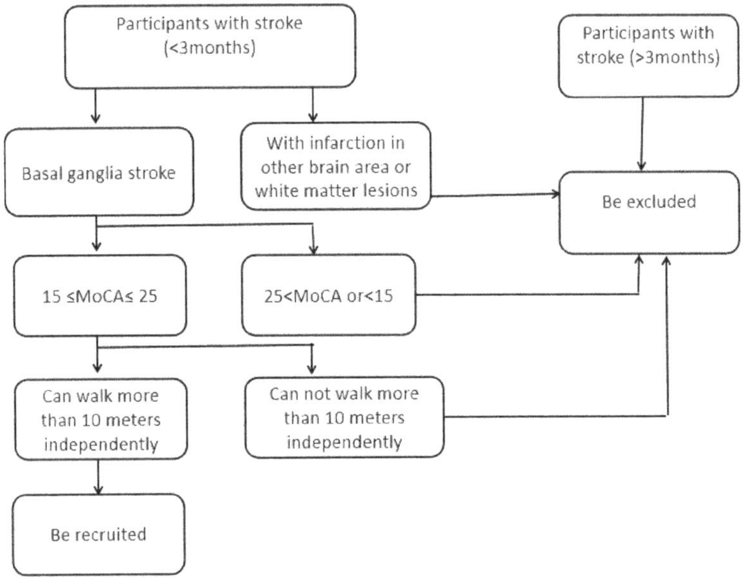

Figure 1. Recruitment flow chart.

A total of 18 patients were finally enrolled in this study. Using the random number table method, patients were assigned into 2 groups ($n = 9$ cases in each group). In the treatment group, there were 7 men and 2 women who were aged (54.6 ± 11.83) years old, including 5 cases of cerebral infarction and 4 cases of cerebral hemorrhage (3 cases of left-sided lesions and 6 cases of right-sided lesions). They had been educated for 9–15 years. In the sham group, there were 8 men and 1 woman who were aged (57.37 ± 12.78) years old, including 5 cases of cerebral infarction and 4 cases of cerebral hemorrhage (5 cases of right-sided lesions and 4 cases of left-sided lesions). There was no statistically significant difference in baseline data between the two groups ($p < 0.05$).

All patients signed informed consent. The study was approved by the Ethics Committee of Beijing Tiantan Hospital Affiliated to Capital Medical University (Approval No. KY2021-040-02).

2.2. Study Design

A randomized, double-blind study was designed. Patients were randomly assigned into two groups, including rTMS group (experimental group) and sham group (control group). All patients were blinded to the treatment. Evaluators were also unaware of patients' grouping. Patients in both groups received routine secondary prevention of cerebrovascular events and routine rehabilitation treatment. Standardized comprehensive rehabilitation treatment program is the use of nerve promotion technology, Bobath therapy, exercise relearning method, and traditional exercise therapy to comprehensively apply to the overall rehabilitation of stroke patients with hemiplegia. Each patient received rehabilitation training for 45 m/day.

The rTMS protocol: in the experimental group, the "8" coil was positioned on the surface of the scalp of the left dorsolateral prefrontal cortex (DLPFC) projection area. The coil was placed vertically in the sham group [6]. Electromyographic electrode was used to record motor evoked potentials (MEPs) at the muscular abdomen of the first dorsal interosseous muscle. According to the guidelines of the International Federation of Clinical Neurophysiology published in 2012, when determining the threshold of resting exercise, subthreshold stimulation should be used to start with the initial detection of 35% maximum output intensity (MOI), and the stimulus intensity gradually increased. Generally, 5% MOI gradually increases, which can continuously lead to MEP with wave amplitude > 50 μV. Then, the stimulus intensity gradually decreases until no more than 5 effective MEPs in 10 stimuli, and an additional 1% increase in the output intensity indicates the resting motor threshold (MT). In the present study, stimulation frequency was 5 Hz, and it was attempted to use a stimulus intensity of 80% MT and 1200 pulses for 5 days/week for 2 weeks. If patients feel uncomfortable, the treatment was immediately stopped, and it was essential to indicate whether there were any uncomfortable symptoms 20 min after the treatment.

At present, the relevant parameters of TMS treatment for motor function, cognitive function, and sensory function after stroke are not unified, and the results are mostly effective, but there is no comparison of the efficacy of two different parameters. According to "Evidence-based guidelines on the therapeutic use of repetitive transcranial magnetic stimulation (rTMS): An update (2014–2018)" [7], Mainly studies choose the stimulation frequency was 5 Hz–20 Hz, stimulus intensity of 80–110% MT and 600–2000 pulses for 5 days/week for 2–4 weeks". Considering that our enrolled patients were all patients in the early stage of stroke, we conservatively chose the prescription of the disclosed dose and frequency, also taking the advice from some experts.

2.3. Assessments

Screening: the scores of MoCA and the Stroop color-word test (SCWT) were utilized as the outcome measures of EF. The lower limb Fugl–Meyer assessment of (L-FMA) was used to assess the lower limb motor function. The 10-m walking test (10MWT), gait analysis, and plantar pressure analysis were employed to assess the gait and postural control ability. Berg balance scale (BBS) and timed up and go test (TUGT) were used to assess the balance and postural control function.

MoCA scoring was developed by Nasreddine et al. [8]. It is a simple screening tool to assess cognitive and attentional/executive functions, and it has also been used in studies on executive function assessment [9]. SCWT was used to measure executive function. It has three cards: card A included 50 color words (yellow, red, blue, and green); card B consisted of dots in four colors (yellow, red, blue, and green); card C covered four color words, which were printed in four different colors (yellow, red, blue, and green). In lieu of thinking about the meaning of each word, subjects were asked to identify color of each word as quickly and accurately as possible. Examiner recorded the time of each card (SCWT-T) and the correct number (SCWT-C). Stroop interference effect (SIE) was calculated as follows: SIE-time (SIE-T) = time of card C − time of card B; SIE correct count (SIE-C) was calculated as follows = correct number of card B − correct number of card C. The greater of the SIE, the worse the interference inhibition function, and the worse the EF.

Analysis of gait and plantar pressure: using the Zebris FDM 1.12 measuring system, subjects were asked to wear tight clothing, and thin socks on test board with their upper limbs swinging in a natural rhythm. "START" was clicked, and data were collected 30 s after adaptation. The following parameters of walking cycle were extracted: step speed, stride length, step width, foot plantar pressure, the peak values of forefoot and rear foot pressure, the length of support line in front and back directions of COP in a single support period, and the difference between the left and right symmetries.

In the TUGT, as described previously [2], the TUGT was categorized into the four stages: getting up (GT), walking straight (WT), turning around (TT), and sitting down (ST), and the total time of TUGT was also recorded.

2.4. Statistical Analysis

Statistical analysis was performed using GraphPad Prism 8.0 software (GraphPad Software, Inc., San Diego, CA, USA). The basic data were presented by frequency, constituent ratio, mean and standard deviation, etc., and the continuous variables were statistically described by mean ± standard error. The measurement data satisfied normal distribution and homogeneity of variance. The paired-sample *t*-test was used for intra-group comparison at different time points, the independent sample *t*-test was employed for inter-group comparison at the same time point, and the chi-square test was utilized for the analysis of count data. A two-sided $p < 0.05$ was considered statistically significant.

3. Results

3.1. Baseline Data

There was no statistically significant difference between the two groups in the baseline data before treatment ($p > 0.05$) (Table 1).

Table 1. The baseline data.

Group	Age (Year)	Sex (*n*)	Hemiplegic Limb (*n*)	Onset Time (Month)	Type (*n*)
Sham group	57.37 ± 12.78	F 1 M 8	L 4 R 5	1.34 ± 0.27	CH 4 CI 5
Experimental group	54.6 ± 11.83	F 2 M 7	L 3 R 6	1.01 ± 0.32	CH 4 CI 5

CH: cerebral hemorrhage; CI: cerebral infarction.

3.2. SCWT before and after Treatment

Before treatment, there was no significant difference in SCWT score between the two groups ($p > 0.05$). After 2 weeks of treatment, SCWT-T, SIE-T, and SIE-C in the experimental group were significantly improved compared with those before treatment ($p < 0.05$). SCWT-C was elevated, while there was no statistical significance ($p > 0.05$). In the sham group, SCWT-T, SCWT-C, SIE-C, and SIE-T were not significantly improved compared with those before treatment ($p > 0.05$). In the experimental group, significant differences were found in SCWT-T, SIE-C, and SIE-T after treatment compared with those in the sham group ($p < 0.05$), while no significant difference was noted in SCWT-C compared with that in the sham group ($p > 0.05$) (Table 2).

Table 2. SCWT and SIE test.

Group	SCWT-T (s)				SCWT-C (*n*)			
	Before	After	T	*p*	Before	After	T	*p*
Sham group	130.36 ± 26.78	118.78 ± 38.34	2.35	0.36	134.90 ± 2.38	140.34 ± 43.25	−2.72	0.23
Experimental group	125.98 ± 31.70	99.26 ± 18.62	5.43	0.006 #	126.47 ± 3.69	146.73 ± 43.25	3.42	0.09
T	1.58	5.69			1.32	−2.79		
p	0.67	0.009 *			0.59	0.25		
Group	**SIE-T (s)**				**SIE-C (*n*)**			
	Before	**After**	**T**	***p***	**Before**	**After**	**T**	***p***
Sham group	35.36 ± 16.78	28.78 ± 11.26	1.98	0.48	11.05 ± 4.27	8.79 ± 2.52	2.47	0.37
Experimental group	41.03 ± 9.37	15.37 ± 8.04	5.79	0.002 †	10.74 ± 3.39	4.28 ± 0.98	5.78	0.002 †
T	2.36	5.21			1.47	6.79		
p	0.35	0.004 ‡			0.49	0.001 ‡		

Before: before treatment; after: after treatment; #: SCWT-T in the experimental group was significantly improved compared with those before treatment ($p < 0.05$); *: In the experimental group, SCWT-T was significant differences compared with those in the sham group after treatment ($p < 0.05$); †: SIE-T and SIE-C in the experimental group were significantly improved compared with those before treatment ($p < 0.05$); ‡: In the experimental group, SIE-T and SIE-C were significantly improved compared with those in the sham group after treatment ($p < 0.05$).

3.3. L-FMA Score before and after Treatment

Before treatment, there was no statistically significant difference in L-FMA score between the two groups ($p > 0.05$). After weeks of treatment, the L-FMA scores in the experimental group were not significantly elevated compared with those before treatment

($p > 0.05$). There was no significant difference in L-FMA score between the two groups before and after treatment ($p > 0.05$) (Table 3).

Table 3. The lower limb Fugl–Meyer assessment.

Group	Before Treatment	After Treatment	T	*p*
Sham group	20.27 ± 7.37	29.82 ± 9.25	−1.98	0.48
Experimental group	24.01 ± 8.27	31.95 ± 10.28	−1.70	0.51
T	−1.99	−1.38		
p	0.43	0.51		

There was no significant difference in L-FMA score between the two groups before and after treatment ($p > 0.05$); there was no significant difference in L-FMA score in each group before and after treatment ($p > 0.05$).

3.4. MWT and BBS Scores before and after Treatment

Before treatment, there was no significant difference in the 10MWT and BBS scores between the two groups ($p > 0.05$). After two weeks of treatment, the BBS score in the experimental group was significantly higher than that before treatment ($p < 0.05$). There was no significant difference in the 10MWT score before and after treatment ($p > 0.05$). After treatment, the BBS score in the experimental group was significantly higher than that in the sham group ($p < 0.05$). There was no significant improvement in the 10MWT score between the two groups, and there was no statistical difference in the 10MWT and BBS scores in the sham group before and after treatment ($p > 0.05$, Table 4).

Table 4. The 10MWT and BBS score.

Group	10MWT (s)				BBS			
	Before	After	T	*p*	Before	After	T	*p*
Sham group	21.57 ± 10.36	16.47 ± 6.36	2.01	0.31	41.73 ± 12.32	46.79 ± 12.51	−2.56	0.39
Experimental group	19.28 ± 7.61	16.28 ± 4.23	1.98	0.42	39.69 ± 13.47	52.37 ± 13.48	−5.12	0.002 #
T	1.27	0.96			2.03	−4.79		
p	0.57	0.64			0.35	0.011 *		

There was no significant difference in 10MWT score between the two groups before and after treatment ($p > 0.05$); there was no significant difference in 10MWT score in each group before and after treatment ($p > 0.05$). #: The score of BBS in the experimental group was significantly improved compared with those before treatment ($p < 0.05$); *: in the experimental group, the score of BBS was significantly higher than those in the sham group after treatment ($p < 0.05$).

3.5. TUGT Score before and after Treatment

Before treatment, there were no significant differences in GT, WT, TT, ST, and TUGT between the two groups ($p > 0.05$). After two weeks of treatment, the total time of GT, WT, and TUGT in the experimental group was not significantly different from that before treatment ($p > 0.05$). In addition, the duration of TT and ST in the experimental group was significantly shortened after treatment compared with that before treatment ($p < 0.05$). There were no significant differences in WT, TT, ST, TT, ST, and TUGT in the sham group compared with those after treatment ($p > 0.05$). After treatment, in the experimental group, the duration of TT and ST significantly decreased compared with that in the sham group ($p < 0.05$). Moreover, GT, WT, and TUGT showed no significant improvement compared with the sham group ($p > 0.05$) (Table 5).

3.6. Gait and Foot Plantar Pressure Parameters before and after Treatment

Stride length, step width, and COP are the line from front to back and bilateral symmetry (the difference between left and right lateral COP trajectories) in a single support period. There was no significant difference between the two groups before and after treatment ($p > 0.05$). After treatment, there were no statistically significant differences in stride length, step width, and COP in the anteroposterior distance and the left and right symmetries between the two groups ($p > 0.05$) (Table 6).

Table 5. TUGT (s).

	Group	Before Treatment	After Treatment	T	p
GT	Sham group	3.27 ± 0.25	2.92 ± 0.56	1.35	0.5
	Experimental group	4.01 ± 0.82	2.95 ± 0.22	1.65	0.51
T		1.90	−0.8		
p		0.63	0.81		
WT	Sham group	12.84 ± 4.3	9.85 ± 2.31	1.78	0.42
	Experimental group	14.01 ± 5.24	10.05 ± 4.26	1.81	0.39
T		−1.61	−1.23		
p		0.48	0.77		
TT	Sham group	4.27 ± 1.34	3.81 ± 0.85	1.75	0.48
	Experimental group	5.01 ± 1.21	1.95 ± 0.68	4.85	0.01 #
T		−1.99	5.38		
p		0.43	0.00 *		
ST	Sham group	3.83 ± 0.31	2.03 ± 0.45	2.18	0.07
	Experimental group	3.90 ± 0.63	1.29 ± 0.08	4.97	0.01 #
T		−1.12	4.63		
p		0.63	0.01 *		
TUGT	Sham group	24.36 ± 7.36	21.36 ± 9.28	2.24	0.28
	Experimental group	26.21 ± 8.39	20.95 ± 8.2	4.29	0.02 #
T		−1.64	1.47		
p		0.33	0.45		

#: Time of the TT, ST, TUGT was significantly shorter compared with those before treatment in the experimental group ($p < 0.05$); *: in the experimental group, the time of ST, TT was significantly higher than those in the sham group after treatment. TUGT: time of stand up and go test; GT: time of getting up; WT: time of walking straight, TT: time of turning around, ST: time of sit down ($p < 0.05$).

Table 6. Gait analysis and plantar pressure parameters.

	Group	Before Treatment	After Treatment	T	p
Stride (cm)	Sham group	35.21 ± 10.24	40.97 ± 16.4	1.37	0.53
	Experimental group	34.01 ± 12.34	42.95 ± 14.52	1.67	0.48
T		1.02	−0.87		
p		0.83	0.76		
Step width (cm)	Sham group	14.85 ± 6.34	11.85 ± 4.31	1.48	0.52
	Experimental group	16.01 ± 5.72	12.05 ± 6.26	1.61	0.39
T		−1.05	−1.03		
p		0.68	0.77		
Front and rear support lines (cm)	Sham group	14.27 ± 1.34	16.81 ± 0.85	−1.25	0.57
	Experimental group	15.01 ± 1.21	18.95 ± 0.68	−1.75	0.41
T		−1.38	−1.49		
p		0.43	0.58		
Bilateral symmetry (cm)	Sham group	4.83 ± 0.31	4.03 ± 0.45	1.68	0.17
	Experimental group	5.42 ± 0.63	3.79 ± 0.08	2.07	0.09
T		−1.18	1.63		
p		0.52	0.31		

There was no significant difference in gait analysis and plantar pressure parameters between the two groups before and after treatment ($p > 0.05$); there was no significant difference in gait analysis and plantar pressure parameters in each group before and after treatment ($p > 0.05$).

4. Discussion

The results of the present study suggested that high-frequency rTMS stimulation of DLPFC could improve the response time and anti-interference ability of patients. Although no significant changes were observed in gait or L-FMA, balance and postural control were significantly improved, and the risk of falling during independent daily activities was significantly reduced.

At present, there is no perfect treatment plan for EF rehabilitation. No controlled study has concentrated on the efficiency of treatment strategies, and no report has guided clinicians in the selection of strategies for individual cases. It has been shown that patients who received rTMS (5~20 Hz at 80%~110% MT) of the left DLPFC could significantly improve ED patients' EF after stroke. rTMS is a non-invasive brain stimulation technique that applies pulsed magnetic field to the brain to cause neuronal excitation or inhibition, thereby affecting brain metabolism and electrical activity. Studies of animal models reported that the beneficial effect of rTMS may be induced by the upregulation of neurotrophic or growth factors [10], and rTMS can improve CI in dementia model rats by changing the activity of N-methyl-d-aspartic acid receptor and brain-derived neurotrophic factor (BDNF) [11]. Studies have shown that cortical plasticity is enhanced after rTMS, which is related to inhibitory cortical circuits and BDNF upregulation in different functional brain regions [12]. The increased concentration of BDNF in the cerebral cortex may complete synaptogenesis and promote the formation and branching of dendritic spines, thus promoting cortical functional remodeling in stroke patients [13].

The cognitive dysfunction after stroke is characterized by impairment of memory, attention, executive ability, and social behavior. In an epidemiological cohort study on chronic brain injury, Jaillard et al. [14] reported that the most common cognitive symptoms were memory impairment (90%), attention impairment (82%), and ED (75%). Different incidence rates of ED have been reported, depending on the cognitive domain tested and the definition of executive function. Post-stroke ED may be ignored under perfect environmental conditions in hospitals with the care of nursing, doctors, therapists, and barrier-free facilities. When they return to their families, communities, or social occupational activities, their disabilities may be revealed. ED was not detected at the early stage and missed treatment time, resulting in more serious consequences [3].

EF plays a critical role in post-stroke recovery and has a high risk of functional dependence. Some patients are unable to perform different tasks and others cannot inhibit erroneous or unrelated behaviors. The majority of patients are only able to complete a single step of a complex problem, while they are unable to present the right solution. In addition, ED patients are mainly unable to return to work and have poor social participation ability [15].

EF in the early stage of a stroke may seriously affect the recovery of motor function [16]. A previous study showed that patients with cognitive dysfunction had a worse motor function recovery one year after stroke. The number of patients with ED who could not recover their motor function was four times higher than that without ED [17]. A cross-sectional study of 20 patients with stroke revealed that patients with ED performed worse on a complex walking test compared with patients with a normal EF [18]. The results of the present study showed that ED had an effect on walking ability with complex postural changes, such as turning and sitting, while it slightly influenced walking straight, which was evidenced by the results of 10MWT, TUGT, and gait analysis.

Disruption of dorsolateral prefrontal subcortical circuitry leads to ED [19]. A previous study [20] showed that the MoCA score decreased after continuous theta-burst stimulation (cTBS) damage to the left DLPFC after temporary virtual injury. However, right DLPFC stimulation did not affect the task performance. The present study suggested that the left DLPFC is associated with EF. Liu-Ambrose et al. [21] confirmed that ED was independently associated with poor balance, mobility, and exercise endurance in patients with chronic stroke. A longitudinal study reported that participants with a poor EF at 3 months and 1 year after a stroke had significantly lower levels of balance and physical activity than participants without these impairments [20]. From a clinical point of view, individuals who exhibit deficits in the management of their thoughts and activities after stroke may have difficulty organizing a family exercise program at discharge [22]. Our previous study also confirmed that patients with a poor ED in the early stage stroke had poor postural control and balance, and balance function and postural control ability were significantly correlated with EF. Horak et al. [23] hypothesized that individuals with cognitive dysfunction may more frequently use existing cognitive processing methods to posture control and falling may be caused by insufficient cognitive processing to posture control, while they are busy with secondary cognitive tasks. The present study showed that patients with improved EF in the TUGT could significantly enhance the indicators of turning around and sitting in the secondary task during walking.

Wagner et al. [24] found that the Stroop task and Wisconsin card sorting test were significantly improved after dorsolateral prefrontal rTMS treatment. Another study reported that [25] the cognitive function index was significantly elevated in patients with mild cognitive impairment who received rTMS (10 Hz at 120% of MT) of the left DLPFC. The results of this study revealed that SCWT-T, SIE-C, and SIE-T of patients significantly improved after 2 weeks of rTMS treatment. In addition, with the improvement of EF, the patient's postural control was significantly enhanced.

According to previous reports, executive dysfunction can hinder the recovery of motor function. People with ED have worse balance and a higher risk of falling. Therefore, in this study, we designed to observe the changes in motor function, gait, balance, and postural control in patients with executive dysfunction before and after treatment. However, the results of this study showed that there was no significant difference between the two groups before and after treatment in gait or L-FMA. This result may suggest that the mechanism of executive function on motor function and gait is different from that of postural control, or that there is little effect of executive function on motor function.

In the present study, it was found that the inhibitory control ability of patients who received high-frequency rTMS of the left DLPFC after stroke was significantly improved, their anti-interference ability was ameliorated, and their postural control ability was raised during walking. With the improvement of EF, patients' abilities to turn around and perform sit-to-stand transfers were significantly improved, BBS was significantly ameliorated, and the risk of falling was significantly reduced. Although it was proven that improved cognition could reduce patients' risk of falling, the gait, and COP were not significantly improved in the present study, which could be related to the sample size or treatment duration. Additionally, in order to avoid the effects of biomechanical factors (abnormal muscle strength, muscle tone, movement pattern) on poor control of posture, patients' L-FMA scores were generally high, and the abnormal movement patterns were not obvious, thus, no significant difference was found in the FMALE score after treatment. Gait and COP may be more influenced by biomechanics, and rhythmic walking requires fewer cognitive resources [2]. Executive function has a greater impact on postural control than motor function and gait. After the left DLPFC rTMS, motor function and gait were not significantly improved with the improvement of executive function, but postural control ability and balance ability were significantly changed.

5. Conclusions

In summary, ED increases the risk of falling. Moreover, post-stroke rTMS treatment of the left DLPFC can improve EF, enhance postural control function, and reduce the risk of falling. It was revealed that rTMS of DLPFC may be a therapeutic target for improving postural control ability and attenuating the risk of falling.

6. Limitations and Prospects

There are some limitations to the study. It is difficult to collect participants in order to ensure the consistency of the affected brain regions, further study is still needed because of the limited cases allotted. In the study, we used the modality to place the coil vertically in the sham group, which does not ensure adequate simulated stimulation—a sham coil would be better. That may also have affected the results. In this study, all patients were in the early stage of stroke, and we conservatively chose the prescription of the disclosed dose and frequency. Further studies are needed to determine whether there is a better treatment option. We will improve them in further research to obtain more meaningful results and guide clinical practice better.

Author Contributions: Conceptualization, H.Z. and H.Y.; methodology, H.Z. and H.Y.; software, C.L.; validation, H.Z., S.L. and H.Y.; formal analysis, Z.W.; investigation, H.Y.; resources, H.Y. and P.D.; data curation, Z.W.; writing—original draft preparation, H.Y.; writing—review and editing, H.Y. and S.L.; visualization, H.Y.; supervision, H.Z.; project administration, H.Z.; funding acquisition, Z.W. All authors have read and agreed to the published version of the manuscript.

Funding: This work was supported by grants from the National Natural Science Foundation of China (Grant Numbers: 82072548, 81974357, and 81772438), and the National Natural Science Foundation of Capital Medical University (grant numbers: XZR2021-114).

Institutional Review Board Statement: The study was approved by the Ethics Committee of Beijing Tiantan Hospital Affiliated with Capital Medical University (approval no. KY2021-040-02).

Data Availability Statement: The data presented in this study are openly available in "Clinical Trial Management Public Platform"(Number: ChiCTR2200055412). Also, the data can be available on request from the corresponding author.

Acknowledgments: Thanks to the experts and colleagues who provided guidance and assistance in this study, and all enrolled patients.

Conflicts of Interest: The authors declare no conflict of interest.

References

1. Guo, Q.; Zhou, T.; Li, W.; Dong, L.; Wang, S.; Zou, L. Single-trial EEG-informed fMRI analysis of emotional decision problems in hot executive function. *Brain Behav.* **2017**, *7*, e00728. [CrossRef] [PubMed]
2. Yu, H.-X.; Wang, Z.-X.; Liu, C.-B.; Dai, P.; Lan, Y.; Xu, G.-Q. Effect of Cognitive Function on Balance and Posture Control after Stroke. *Neural Plast.* **2021**, *2021*, 28. [CrossRef] [PubMed]
3. Sergeev, D.V.; Domashenko, M.A.; Piradov, M.A. Poststroke cognitive impairment and dementia. *Meditsinskiy Sov. Med. Counc.* **2016**, 34–37. [CrossRef]
4. Diekhoff-Krebs, S.; Pool, E.M.; Sarfeld, A.S.; Rehme, A.K.; Eickhoff, S.B.; Fink, G.R.; Grefkes, C. Interindividual differences in motor network connectivity and behavioral response to iTBS in stroke patients. *Neuroimage Clin.* **2017**, *15*, 559–571. [CrossRef] [PubMed]
5. Pacheco-Barrios, K.; Lima, D.; Pimenta, D.; Slawka, E.; Navarro-Flores, A.; Parente, J.; Rebello-Sanchez, I.; Cardenas-Rojas, A.; Gonzalez-Mego, P.; Castelo-Branco, L.; et al. Motor cortex inhibition as a fibromyalgia biomarker: A meta-analysis of transcranial magnetic stimulation studies. *Brain Netw. Modul.* **2022**, *1*, 88–101.
6. Kim, S.H.; Han, H.J.; Ahn, H.M.; Kim, S.A. Effects of five daily high-frequency rTMS on Stroop task performance in aging individuals. *Neurosci. Res.* **2012**, *74*, 256–260. [CrossRef]
7. Lefaucheur, J.P.; Aleman, A.; Baeken, C.; Benninger, D.H.; Brunelin, J.; Di Lazzaro, V.; Filipović, S.R.; Grefkes, C.; Hasan, A.; Hummel, F.C.; et al. Evidence-based guidelines on the therapeutic use of repetitive transcranial magnetic stimulation (rTMS): An update (2014–2018). *Clin. Neurophysiol.* **2020**, *131*, 474–528. [CrossRef]
8. Wonsetler, E.C.; Bowden, M.G. A systematic review of mechanisms of gait speed change post-stroke. Part 2: Exercise capacity, muscle activation, kinetics, and kinematics. *Top Stroke Rehabil.* **2017**, *24*, 394–403. [CrossRef]
9. Xu, B.; Yan, T.; Yang, Y.; Ou, R.; Huang, S. Effect of normal-walking-pattern-based functional electrical stimulation on gait of the lower extremity in subjects with ischemic stroke: A self controlled study. *Neuro Rehabil.* **2016**, *38*, 163–169. [CrossRef]
10. Toledo, R.S.; Stein, D.J.; Sanches, P.R.S.; da Silva, L.S.; Medeiros, H.R.; Fregni, F.; Caumo, W.; Torres, I.L. rTMS induces analgesia and modulates neuroinflammation and neuroplasticity in neuropathic pain model rats. *Brain Res.* **2021**, *1762*, 147427. [CrossRef]
11. Shang, Y.; Wang, X.; Li, F.; Yin, T.; Zhang, J.; Zhang, T. rTMS Ameliorates Prenatal Stress–Induced Cognitive Deficits in Male-Offspring Rats Associated With BDNF/TrkB Signaling Pathway. *Neurorehabilit. Neural Repair* **2019**, *33*, 271–283. [CrossRef] [PubMed]
12. Velioglu, H.A.; Hanoglu, L.; Bayraktaroglu, Z.; Toprak, G.; Guler, E.M.; Bektay, M.Y.; Mutlu-Burnaz, O.; Yulug, B. Left Lateral Parietal rTMS Improves Cognition and Modulates Resting Brain Connectivity in Patients with Alzheimer's Disease: Possible Role of BDNF and Oxidative Stress. *Neurobiol. Learn. Mem.* **2021**, *180*, 107410. [CrossRef] [PubMed]
13. Stanne, T.M.; Åberg, N.D.; Nilsson, S.; Jood, K.; Blomstrand, C.; Andreasson, U.; Blennow, K.; Zetterberg, H.; Isgaard, J.; Svensson, J.; et al. Low Circulating Acute Brain-Derived Neurotrophic Factor Levels Are Associated with Poor Long-Term Functional Outcome After Ischemic Stroke. *Stroke* **2016**, *47*, 1943–1945. [CrossRef]
14. Jaillard, A.; Naegele, B.; Trabucco-Miguel, S.; LeBas, J.F.; Hommel, M. Hidden dysfunctioning in subacute stroke. *Stroke* **2009**, *40*, 2473. [CrossRef] [PubMed]

15. Leśniak, M.; Bak, T.; Czepiel, W.; Seniów, J.; Członkowska, A. Frequency and prognosticvalue of cognitive disorders in stroke patients. *Dement. Geriatr. Cogn. Disord.* **2008**, *26*, 356–363. [CrossRef]
16. Påhlman, U.; Sävborg, M.; Tarkowski, E. Cognitive dysfunction and physical activity after stroke: The Gothenburg Cognitive Stroke Study in the Elderly. *J. Stroke Cerebrovasc. Dis.* **2012**, *21*, 652–658. [CrossRef]
17. Hayes, S.; Donnellan, C.; Stokes, E. Associations between executive function and physical function poststroke: A pilot study. *Physiotherapy* **2013**, *99*, 165–171. [CrossRef]
18. Mega, M.S.; Cummings, J.L. Frontal-subcortical circuits and neuropsychiatric disorders. *J. Neuropsychiatry Clin. Neurosci.* **1994**, *6*, 358–370.
19. Osada, T.; Ohta, S.; Ogawa, A.; Tanaka, M.; Suda, A.; Kamagata, K.; Hori, M.; Aoki, S.; Shimo, Y.; Hattori, N. An Essential Role of the Intraparietal Sulcus in Response Inhibition Predicted by Parcellation-Based Network. *J. Neurosci. Off. J. Soc. Neurosci.* **2019**, *39*, 2509–2521. [CrossRef]
20. Ko, J.; Monchi, O.; Ptito, A.; Bloomfield, P.; Houle, S.; Strafella, A. Theta burst stimulation of dorsolateral prefrontal cortex reveals hemispheric asymmetry in striatal dopamine release during set-shifting task in human. *Technol. Eng.* **2009**, *28*, 2147–2155.
21. Liu-Ambrose, T.; Pang, M.Y.; Eng, J.J. Executive function is independently associated with performances of balance and mobility in community dwelling older adults after mild stroke: Implications for falls prevention. *Cerebrovasc. Dis.* **2007**, *23*, 203–210. [CrossRef] [PubMed]
22. Pahlman, U.; Gutierrez-Perez, C.; Savborg, M.; Knopp, E.; Tarkowski, E. Cognitive function and improvement of balance after stroke in elderly people: The Gothenburg cognitive stroke study in the elderly. *Disabil. Rehabil.* **2011**, *33*, 1952–1962. [CrossRef]
23. Horak, F.B. Postural orientation and equilibrium: What do we need to know about neural control of balance to prevent falls? *Age Ageing* **2006**, *35* (Suppl. S2), ii7–ii11. [CrossRef] [PubMed]
24. Wagner, M.; Rihs, T.A.; Mosimann, U.P.; Fisch, H.U.; Schlaepfer, T.E. Repetitive transcranial magnetic stimulation of the dorsolateral prefrontal cortex affects divided attention immediately after cessation of stimulation. *J. Psychiatr. Res.* **2006**, *40*, 315–321. [CrossRef] [PubMed]
25. Padala, P.; Padala, K.P.; Lensing, S.Y.; Jackson, A.N.; Hunter, C.R.; Parkes, C.M.; Dennis, R.A.; Bopp, M.M.; Caceda, R.; Mennemeier, M.S.; et al. Repetitive transcranial magnetic stimulation for apathy in mild cognitive impairment: A double-blind, randomized, sham-controlled, cross-over pilot study. *Psychiatry Res.* **2018**, *261*, 312–318. [CrossRef] [PubMed]

brain sciences

Case Report

Application of a Brain–Computer Interface System with Visual and Motor Feedback in Limb and Brain Functional Rehabilitation after Stroke: Case Report

Wen Gao [1,†], Zhengzhe Cui [2,†], Yang Yu [1], Jing Mao [1], Jun Xu [1], Leilei Ji [1], Xiuli Kan [1], Xianshan Shen [1], Xueming Li [1], Shiqiang Zhu [2,3,*] and Yongfeng Hong [1,*]

1 Department of Rehabilitation Medicine, The Second Hospital of Anhui Medical University, No. 678 Furong Road, Economic and Technological Development Zone, Hefei 230601, China
2 Zhejiang Laboratory, Department of Intelligent Robot, Keji Avenue, Yuhang Zone, Hangzhou 311100, China
3 Ocean College, Zhejiang University, No. 866 Yuhangtang Road, Xihu Zone, Hangzhou 310030, China
* Correspondence: zhusq@zhejianglab.com (S.Z.); hy_feng@163.com (Y.H.); Tel.: +86-0571-56390588 (S.Z.); +86-0551-65997012 (Y.H.)
† These authors contributed equally to this work.

Abstract: (1) Objective: To investigate the feasibility, safety, and effectiveness of a brain–computer interface (BCI) system with visual and motor feedback in limb and brain function rehabilitation after stroke. (2) Methods: First, we recruited three hemiplegic stroke patients to perform rehabilitation training using a BCI system with visual and motor feedback for two consecutive days (four sessions) to verify the feasibility and safety of the system. Then, we recruited five other hemiplegic stroke patients for rehabilitation training (6 days a week, lasting for 12–14 days) using the same BCI system to verify the effectiveness. The mean and Cohen's w were used to compare the changes in limb motor and brain functions before and after training. (3) Results: In the feasibility verification, the continuous motor state switching time (CMSST) of the three patients was 17.8 ± 21.0s, and the motor state percentages (MSPs) in the upper and lower limb training were 52.6 ± 25.7% and 72.4 ± 24.0%, respectively. The effective training revolutions (ETRs) per minute were 25.8 ± 13.0 for upper limb and 24.8 ± 6.4 for lower limb. There were no adverse events during the training process. Compared with the baseline, the motor function indices of the five patients were improved, including sitting balance ability, upper limb Fugel–Meyer assessment (FMA), lower limb FMA, 6 min walking distance, modified Barthel index, and root mean square (RMS) value of triceps surae, which increased by 0.4, 8.0, 5.4, 11.4, 7.0, and 0.9, respectively, and all had large effect sizes (Cohen's w ≥ 0.5). The brain function indices of the five patients, including the amplitudes of the motor evoked potentials (MEP) on the non-lesion side and lesion side, increased by 3.6 and 3.7, respectively; the latency of MEP on the non-lesion side was shortened by 2.6 ms, and all had large effect sizes (Cohen's w ≥ 0.5). (4) Conclusions: The BCI system with visual and motor feedback is applicable in active rehabilitation training of stroke patients with hemiplegia, and the pilot results show potential multidimensional benefits after a short course of treatment.

Keywords: brain–computer interface; active rehabilitation training; stroke; motor function; brain function

Citation: Gao, W.; Cui, Z.; Yu, Y.; Mao, J.; Xu, J.; Ji, L.; Kan, X.; Shen, X.; Li, X.; Zhu, S.; et al. Application of a Brain–Computer Interface System with Visual and Motor Feedback in Limb and Brain Functional Rehabilitation after Stroke: Case Report. *Brain Sci.* **2022**, *12*, 1083. https://doi.org/10.3390/brainsci12081083

Academic Editors: Jie Jia, Yan Hu, Dingguo Zhang and Konstantin V. Slavin

Received: 27 June 2022
Accepted: 10 August 2022
Published: 16 August 2022

1. Introduction

Stroke is the second leading cause of death worldwide, but is the first leading cause of death in China, the world's most populous country [1–3]. Stroke after interruption of cerebral perfusion causes rapid loss of brain function, often leading to hemiplegia [4], which describes partial or complete paralysis on one side of the body, usually due to extensive cerebral infarction contralateral to the main symptoms [5]. About 60% of stroke survivors experience persistent impairment of motor function and, consequently, need rehabilitation [6]. In addition, stroke survivors often suffer from a range of non-motor disabilities, including visual and cognitive impairment [7], the composite of which has a serious impact on daily activities. Therefore, effective treatment and rehabilitation of stroke patients have been a research focus for many years.

The treatment and rehabilitation of stroke patients entails extensive efforts to help the brain recover damaged neural connections and compensate for broken neuronal pathways. The conventional rehabilitative treatments target motor dysfunctions in the upper and lower limbs, and includes various facilitation techniques [8], functional electrical stimulation (FES) [9], and other interventions, which generally have lesser effects on the functioning of the upper limbs in a patient recovering from a serious stroke. In recent years, some emerging technologies have been applied to the rehabilitation of stroke, such as powered exoskeleton technology [10] and multi-degree-of-freedom stroke rehabilitation robot technology [11], and positive effects have been achieved. These emerging technologies may create new rehabilitation paradigms aimed at accelerating functional recovery in stroke patients [12].

Brain–computer interface (BCI) is a relatively new technology for exchanging information between the brain and external devices. With the help of BCI technology, patients can actively participate in rehabilitation training. BCI has been reported for the rehabilitation of stroke and similar disorders like Parkinson's disease, cerebral palsy, and spinal cord injury, and can significantly promote the recovery of limb function in these patients [13–16]. However, how to get stroke patients to imagine target tasks more effectively and stably; how to monitor the performance of imaginary tasks; how to accurately capture and identify task-related EEG signals; how to convert EEG signals into views, movements, sounds, etc., in order to achieve the enhanced efficacy of BCI training with multiple sensory feedback; and how to solve BCI training fatigue to ensure effective training time are still challenges [17].

Most BCI rehabilitation systems adopt single feedback modality, such as systems based on vision [18–20], kinesthetic sense [21–23], or perception [24,25]. The main purpose is to provide perceptual or sensory feedback, and these feedback modalities can lead to motor function recovery. How these feedback patterns affect clinical outcomes remains elusive. However, a study has shown that sensory feedback of exercise may be a key factor in BCI-based rehabilitation, and single visual feedback is not sufficient to arouse functional gain [26]. In addition, immersive visual feedback may help enhance the effect of feedback [27,28].

In the present report, we introduce a new BCI system, namely the L-B300 Electroencephalogram (EEG) Acquisition and Rehabilitation Training System (Zhejiang Mailian Medical Technology Co., Ltd., Hangzhou, China). Compared with other BCI rehabilitation systems, the BCI rehabilitation system used in this report has the advantage of both visual and motor feedback and high time efficiency: its real-time feedback is only 110 ms, and this parameter is smaller than those of other systems (300 ms [29] and 200 ms [30]); it is so responsive and user-friendly that the user is not easy to feel tired [31]; it is very convenient in clinical use and can guide and timely monitor target task imagination of patients. The purpose of this study was to observe the feasibility and safety of this novel BCI system for rehabilitation of stroke patients with hemiplegia, and the effects of a short course of BCI treatment on patients' limb movement and brain function.

2. Materials and Methods

Eight stroke patients with hemiplegia were recruited in the Department of Rehabilitation Medicine of the Second Hospital of Anhui Medical University to perform BCI rehabilitation training with visual and motor feedback from August 2021 to October 2021.

2.1. Subjects

Inclusion criteria: (1) 18–80 years old, either sex; (2) patients with de novo post-stroke hemiplegia were diagnosed by imaging examination as having had cerebral infarction or cerebral hemorrhage; (3) the strength of all the muscles of the upper and lower limbs on the hemiplegic side was grade 4 or less (manual muscle testing, MMT) [32], while there was no obvious dysfunction on the healthy side; (4) patients could sit without support for 30 min;

(5) stable vital signs; (6) clear awareness and ability to participate in the rehabilitation intervention; (7) patients understood and signed informed consent.

Exclusion criteria: (1) patient's condition continued to deteriorate, vital signs unstable; (2) had severe heart disease, or carried pacemakers that might interfere with the BCI; (3) patients with recurrent ($\geq$2 times) cerebral infarction or cerebral hemorrhage; (4) poor cognitive level, with Mini-mental State Examination (MMSE) score less than 21, and, thus, unable to comply with rehabilitation therapy [33]; (5) patients receiving craniectomy; (6) patients after cranioplasty; (7) patients with motor dysfunction contralateral to the hemiplegic limbs; (8) could not sit alone for 30 min; (9) patients or their families refused to sign informed consent; (10) patients were participating in other clinical experiments.

General information of patients: three patients (48 $\pm$ 15 years old) were recruited for the initial feasibility and safety observation study. After verifying the feasibility and safety of the system, another five patients (48 $\pm$ 9 years old) were recruited for the effectiveness evaluation of the system. The demographic information of all eight patients is shown in Table 1.

Table 1. Information of the eight patients.

Subject	Age	Gender	Sites of Injury	Course of Disease(d)	BCI Treatment Times
1	58	Male	Left basal ganglia cerebral hemorrhage	34	4
2	31	Male	Right basal ganglia cerebral hemorrhage	127	4
3	55	Female	Right basal ganglia cerebral infarction	30	4
1′	34	Male	Left cerebellar hemisphere hemorrhage	41	26
2′	44	Male	Left basal ganglia cerebral hemorrhage	37	26
3′	51	Male	Left basal ganglia cerebral infarction	18	28
4′	52	Female	left basal ganglia cerebral infarction	15	24
5′	58	Male	Left basal ganglia, left paraventricular cerebral infarction	41	26

This study was carried out in the Department of Rehabilitation Medicine of the Second Hospital of Anhui Medical University. The experimental method was approved by the Ethics Committee of the Second Hospital of Anhui Medical University [Approval No. YX2020-103(F1)] and implemented according to the ethical standards of the 1975 Helsinki Declaration (revised in 2008). Written informed consent was obtained from each participant before enrollment.

2.2. L-B300 EEG Acquisition and Rehabilitation Training System

The rehabilitation training system used in this study was the new L-B300 EEG Acquisition and Rehabilitation Training System. In this system, the patient wore an 8-lead EEG cap with electrodes over the left and right prefrontal cortex (FP1, FP2), left and right frontal cortex (F3, F4), left and right central area (C3, C4), frontal midline area (Fz), and central midline area (Cz), respectively. The electrode placement was in line with the 10/20 international standard lead system [34], as shown in Figure 1. The left and right ear clip electrodes (A1 and A2) were, respectively, the reference and bias electrodes. The patients' bilateral upper/lower limbs were fixed on the corresponding left and right rotary shafts of the system for upper/lower limb rehabilitation training. The system provides a training mode, in which the equipment was driven completely by the patient's EEG signals generated through the subject's motor imagery (MI). The display screen in the device established a visual feedback platform between the system and the patient. When the patient intended to perform upper/lower limb exercise training, the researcher needed to set the virtual character on the display screen to the corresponding exercise preparation. Thus, in upper limb training, the virtual character was displayed for swimming preparation, whereas for lower limb training, the display was for cycling preparation. The patient carried out the corresponding motor imagery tasks according to the virtual character training type on the display screen and followed the voice prompt. When the patient's Mscore [35] (the specific

EEG signals) reached a certain threshold, the virtual character on the display screen began to move accordingly. At the same time, the rotary shafts of the system began to rotate to drive the patient's limbs to move accordingly. When the patient's motor intention fell below the set threshold, the virtual character on the display screen stopped its corresponding motion, and the rotary shafts stopped rotating, thus ceasing to drive the patient's limbs.

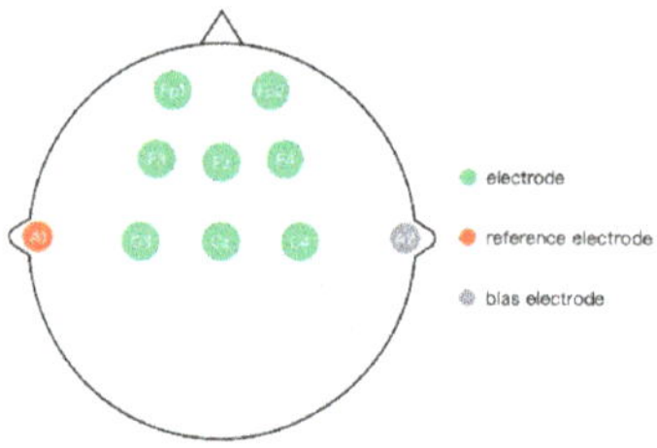

Figure 1. Electrode placement diagram of L-B300 EEG Acquisition and Rehabilitation Training System.

The system gave patients real-time visual and motor perception feedback, that is, during the training, the progress bar on the right side of the display screen showed the intensity of the patient's motor imagery in real time (updates every 110 ms); when the intensity of the patient's motor imagery (i.e., Mscore) reached a certain threshold, the virtual character on the display screen would start corresponding movements (swimming or cycling), and the virtual character's movement would generate visual feedback; meanwhile, the rotary shafts of the system drove the patient's limb movement (update rate > 1 Hz), thus giving the patient motor perception feedback [35,36].

2.3. Training and Evaluation Methods

2.3.1. Feasibility and Safety Verification of the System

First, three stroke patients with hemiplegia were recruited to perform L-B300 system rehabilitation training on a routine basis to verify the feasibility and safety of this system. The training method: with upper and lower limb training twice per day (15 min of upper limb training and 15 min of lower limb training per session, each in the morning and afternoon); thus, a total of 30 min for upper limb training and 30 min for lower limb training per day. The three patients thus completed four training session during two consecutive days. The positioning of a patient during upper and lower limb BCI training is shown in Figure 2.

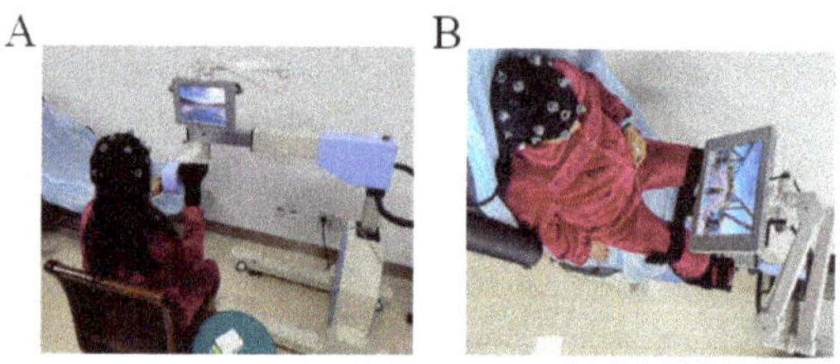

Figure 2. BCI training. (**A**) A patient with right hemiplegia undergoing upper limb BCI training (imagined swimming) (**B**) The same patient undergoing lower limb BCI training (imagined cycling). In the safety evaluation of the system, the three patients were observed and evaluated for any discomfort, seizures, recurrent cerebral hemorrhage, and cerebral infarction during training.

We evaluated the feasibility of the system by first recording the continuous motor state switching time (CMSST) of each patient when using BCI; this refers to the time taken by the patient to switch from a resting state to a concentrated motor intention state that can continuously drive the system [35]. We also recorded the motor state percentage (MSP), which refers to the proportion of time when the patient's motor intention exceeds the selected threshold [35], and the effective training revolution (ETR), which is the number of times that the patient commands the robot to rotate during each training session [35].

2.3.2. Effectiveness Evaluation of the System

Upon finding in the validation study in the three stroke patients with hemiplegia that the L-B300 system was feasible and safe to use for rehabilitation training, we proceeded to study the rehabilitation training of a separate group of five stroke patients with hemiplegia. The rehabilitation training method for these five patients was much as in the feasibility and safety study, but they trained for six days a week to a total of complete 12–14 days; thus, 24–28 sessions of training. We measured limb motor function and brain function indices of these patients at baseline and after rehabilitation treatment.

Detection of limb motor function: (1) to determine sitting balance ability, we used the three-level method to evaluate static sitting balance (level 1), self-dynamic sitting balance (level 2), and other-dynamic sitting balance (level 3). Here, static sitting balance refers to the process of maintaining the stability of sitting posture without the influence of external forces when the participant opens his/her eyes. Self-dynamic sitting balance refers to the process by which the patient can adjust from one posture to another and maintain balance without the influence of external forces. Other-dynamic sitting balance refers to the process whereby the body can quickly adjust its center of mass and posture to maintain balance when the center of gravity of the body changes under an external force [37]. (2) The Fugel–Meyer Assessment (FMA) was used to evaluate the motor function of the upper and lower limbs, where the maximum total score is 100; higher scores indicate better limb motor function [38]. (3) The 10 m walking speed test (m/s) was applied only in those patients who could walk independently. The subjects were asked to walk along a 10 m straight line on a level ground at their fastest speed, which was recorded [39]. (4) A 6 min walking distance (6MWD) is the most widely used clinical submaximal exercise test to evaluate systematic and complete responses during exercise. During the test, subjects were asked to walk back and forth at their fastest speed for six minutes along a 30 m straight and level course, and their total walking distance was recorded [40]. (5) The Modified Barthel Index (MBI) was used to assess their ability to complete activities of daily living, with a total score of 100; higher the score indicated better ability to complete activities of daily living [41]. (6) Surface electromyography (sEMG) signal was acquired by using the Delsys® Trigno wireless EMG acquisition system (Delsys Inc., Natick, MA, USA) and EMGWorks® Acquisition software (version 4.7.6, Delsys Inc., Natick, MA, USA). Test parameters: common mode rejection ratio (CMRR) > 80 dB, noise < 750 nV RMS, analog/digital conversion was 16 bit, sampling frequency was 2000 Hz, each data collection time was 5s, used band-pass filter in the analysis software, bandwidth 20–450 Hz, passband ripple <2%, effective measurement range was ±8000 μV, available channel number was 8. Recorded the sEMG signals of the following muscles: biceps brachialis, triceps brachialis, flexor digitorum, extensor digitorum, abductor pollicis brevis, quadriceps femoris, hamstring muscle, anterior tibial muscle, and triceps surae on the hemiplegic side during maximum isometric contraction (MIVC). From these recordings, we selected the root mean square (RMS) values of the 1s peaks [42]. The values of the 1s peaks referred to the maximum values of the 1s regions containing the strongest signals in the 5s sEMG signals collected. We recorded the sEMG signals sequentially in triplicate, and then calculated the average values.

In the brain function test, the motor evoked potential (MEP) of the M1 region (primary motor cortex) in the cerebral hemisphere both on the lesion side and non-lesion side was collected using a transcranial magnetic stimulator (CR Technology Co., Ltd., Daejeon, Korea) with an 8-wire coil (12.5 cm in diameter, 3.0 T in maximum intensity) [43]. The latent period and amplitude were calculated to detect the conduction of the efferent nerve pathway and the excitability of the underlying cerebral cortex.

2.4. Statistical Analysis

Data were analyzed using the MATLAB 2021a. Quantitative variables were expressed as mean ± standard deviation (mean ± SD). The feasibility and safety evaluation data before and after intervention were statistically compared in terms of numerical size. Cohen's w was used to report the effect size, and thresholds for small, medium, and large effects were 0.10, 0.30, and 0.50, respectively [44].

3. Results

3.1. Feasibility and Safety Verification of the System

All three testing phase patients received four training sessions of the system over two days. The first two sessions and the second two sessions for each patient were counted as stage 1 and stage 2, respectively. In the four training sessions, the CMSST of the three patients was 17.8 ± 21.0 s (range 0.1 to 50.7 s), and the indicator value at stage 2 was lower than that in stage 1, as shown in Figure 3.

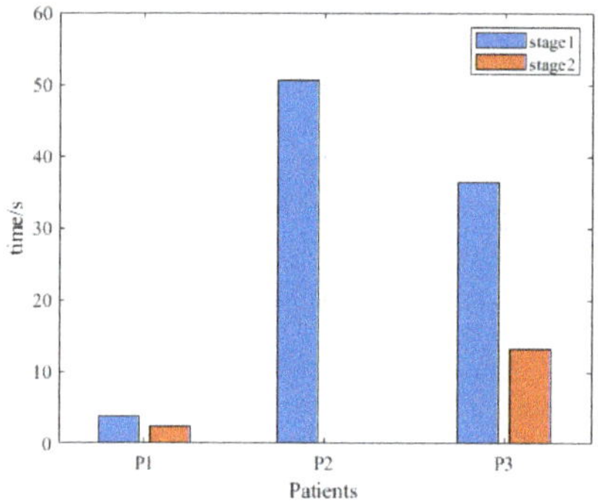

Figure 3. The continuous motor state switching times of the three patients in the feasibility test.

The analysis results of the MSPs and the ETRs per minute of the initial three patients in upper and lower limb training are in Figures 4 and 5. The MSPs in upper and lower limb training were 52.6 ± 25.7% (maximum 86%, minimum 11%) and 72.4 ± 24.0% (maximum 100%, minimum 39.0%), respectively. The ETRs per minute in upper and lower limb training were 25.8 ± 13.0 (maximum 36.3, minimum 3.2) and 24.8 ± 6.4 (maximum 33.3, minimum 18.6), respectively. Comparing stage 2 with stage 1, there were slight declines of these two indicators in the upper limb training of patients P1 and P3. At stage 2, there was a conspicuous improvement in lower limb training of all three patients compared with stage 1.

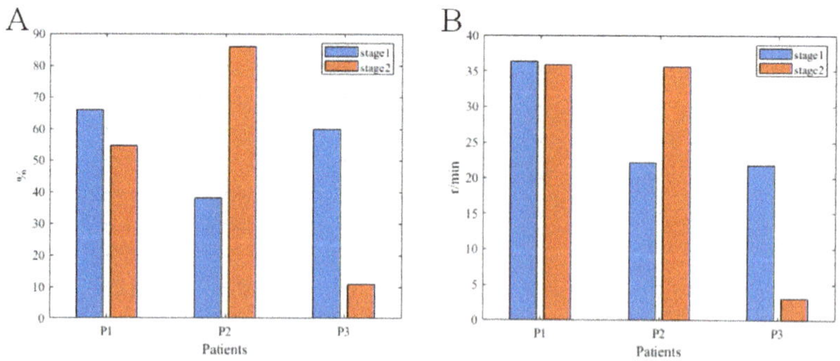

Figure 4. The motor state percentages (**A**) and the effective training revolutions per minute (**B**) of the three test patients in upper limb training at the two stages of training.

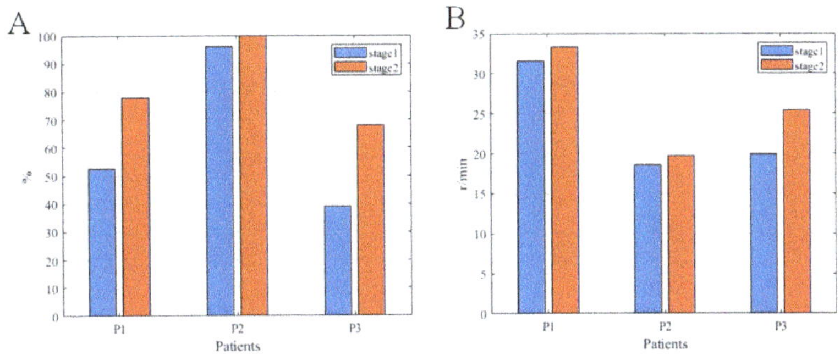

Figure 5. The motor state percentage (**A**) and the effective training revolutions per minute (**B**) of the three pilot patients at the two stages of lower limb training.

During the entire training process, the three pilot patients had no discomfort, recurrence of seizure, or any other adverse events, showing the system to be safe and reliable.

3.2. Rehabilitation Effects of the System

3.2.1. Clinical Indicators in the Limb Motor Function of Patients

We calculated the changes in motor function relative to the baseline condition in the five patients with rehabilitation training. The results indicated conspicuous improvements in the patients' sitting balance ability, upper limb FMA, lower limb FMA, 10 m walking speed, 6MWD, and MBI after treatment. All of the improvements were of large effect size, other than 10 m walking speed (with a small effect size), as shown in Table 2.

Table 2. Clinical efficacy evaluation (mean ± SD) of the five patients.

Assessment Item	Before	After	Difference	Cohen's w
Sitting balance ability	2.4 ± 0.9	2.8 ± 0.5	0.4 ± 0.55	1.22 **
Upper limb FMA	22.2 ± 10.1	30.2 ± 8.9	8.0 ± 5.61	5.18 **
Lower limb FMA	19.6 ± 10.1	25.0 ± 5.7	5.4 ± 5.18	5.44 **
10 m walking speed	0.5 ± 0.2	0.5 ± 0.2	0.04 ± 0.03	0.16
6MWD	155.6 ± 50.0	167.0 ± 48.9	11.4 ± 4.30	2.29 **
MBI	65.0 ± 7.1	72.0 ± 7.6	7.0 ± 2.70	2.06 **

** (Cohen's w ≥ 0.5) indicates a large effect size.

3.2.2. The RMSs of the Limb Muscles on the Hemiplegic Side

The RMS changes showed that, compared with the baseline, the RMSs were numerically increased for the biceps brachii, triceps brachii, extensor digitorum, quadriceps femoris, hamstring muscle, anterior tibial muscle and triceps surae of the five stroke patients. However, the mean RMSs of flexor digitorum and abductor pollicis brevis decreased slightly, as shown in Table 3.

Table 3. Comparison of the RMSs (mean ± SD) before and after treatment in the five patients.

Assessment Item	Examined Position	Before	After	Difference	Cohen's w
RMS (μV)	Biceps brachii	2.9 ± 1.1	3.0 ± 1.1	0.2 ± 0.09	0.25
	Triceps brachii	6.8 ± 7.7	7.0 ± 7.9	0.2 ± 0.25	0.20
	Flexor digitorum	0.6 ± 0.5	0.6 ± 0.4	0.0 ± 0.07	0.11
	Extensor digitorum	0.7 ± 0.8	0.7 ± 0.8	0.0 ± 0.01	0.06
	Abductor pollicis brevis	0.3 ± 0.2	0.3 ± 0.2	0.0 ± 0.03	0.08
	Quadriceps femoris	18.5 ± 12.5	19.0 ± 12.8	0.5 ± 0.68	0.35 *
	Hamstring muscle	15.1 ± 8.0	15.5 ± 8.2	0.4 ± 0.35	0.24
	Anterior tibial muscle	9.0 ± 6.4	9.1 ± 6.5	0.2 ± 0.14	0.14
	Triceps surae	10.0 ± 6.5	10.8 ± 7.6	0.9 ± 1.06	0.71 **

** (Cohen's w ≥ 0.5) indicates a large effect size, * (Cohen's w < 0.5 and ≥0.3) indicates a medium effect size.

3.2.3. Brain Function Test Results of Subjects

The MEP differentials before and after treatment were measured. It was found that the MEP latent periods on the lesion side and non-lesion side were shortened and the amplitudes were enhanced after treatment, All Cohen's w > 0.4, with more than medium effect size, as shown in Table 4.

Table 4. Comparison of the MEPs (mean ± SD) before and after treatment in the five patients.

Assessment Item	Examined Position	Testing Indicator	Before	After	Difference	Cohen's w
MEP	M1 area on the non-lesion side	Latent period (ms)	42.1 ± 8.3	39.5 ± 8.6	−2.6 ± 2.17	1.11 **
		Amplitude (10^{-5})	32.7 ± 10.9	36.2 ± 9.0	3.6 ± 3.78	2.41 **
	M1 area on the lesion side	Latent period (ms)	14.4 ± 5.7	13.8 ± 5.9	−0.6 ± 0.39	0.44 *
		Amplitude (10^{-5})	20.0 ± 7.7	23.9 ± 7.8	3.7 ± 3.89	2.83 **

** (Cohen's w ≥ 0.5) indicates a large effect size, * (Cohen's w < 0.5 and ≥0.3) indicates a medium effect size.

4. Discussion

In this study, we undertook preliminary clinical experiments to investigate the feasibility, safety, and potential rehabilitation efficacy for restoring limb and brain functions of hemiplegic stroke patients using the new BCI system. This system differs from the traditional active/passive rehabilitation training mode with respect to the multichannel feedback, and adopts the active rehabilitation training mode of bidirectional synchronous stimulation of the central and peripheral nervous systems [13,14]. Using this system requires patients to actively participate in the whole process and focus on their training done through motor imagery. Mscore is the specific EEG signals used in this system to timely evaluate the degree of active target task imagination of patients [45,46]. The Mscore was collected through the brain cap, decoded and transmitted to the terminal devices (the rotary shafts and the display screen) via Bluetooth to control the rotary shafts and the virtual character on the display screen. When Mscore meets with certain requirements, the rotary shafts can drive the patient's limb movement and provide motor perception feedback to the patient's body sensation, while simultaneously giving visual feedback to the patient on the display screen [36]. In this study, we first validated the feasibility and safety of the novel system in a pilot test of three stroke patients with hemiplegia. We then proceeded to test the rehabilitative efficacy of the system with 24–28 training sessions in another group of five hemiplegic stroke patients.

In the feasibility verification, we used three indicators (CMSST, MSP, and ETR) to evaluate the usability of the system. Among these indicators, CMSST represents the speed whereby patients enter the active training state. In the pilot study, the mean value of the CMSST was 17.8 s, and this indicator was shortened at stage 2 compared to stage 1, indicating that all three patients could quickly adapt to the rehabilitation training of the system [47]. The factor affecting the MSP is mainly the degree of active participation of the patient. In this study, the mean MSP values of the upper and lower limbs of patients were 52.6 and 72.4%, respectively, which revealed that the three stroke patients with hemiplegia could maintain continuous and high-intensity active rehabilitation training instead of giving up training because of fatigue [47]. The ETRs per minute of the system reflects the amount of exercise of a patient [47]. In this study, the average ETRs per minute in the upper and lower limbs of the patients were 25.8 and 24.8, respectively, suggesting that the upper and lower limbs of the patients were fully trained. As observed in Figures 3 and 4, CMSST, MSPs, and ETRs of the three patients differed greatly, and in MSPs and ETRs, stage 2 of the first and third patients was less than stage 1, while stage 2 of the second patient was larger than stage 1. As can be seen from Figure 5, in MSPs and ETRs, there were not many differences among the three patients, and stage 2 of the three patients was all greater than stage 1. These above results were considered to be related to the fact that cycling is relatively easier to imagine than swimming (since most Chinese people have cycling experience, while many do not have swimming experience) [48]. Therefore, there was no great difference in the performance of the three patients on the task of imagining lower limb cycling, while the imagining upper limb swimming task not only showed greatly different performances among the three patients, but also showed unstable performances in different stages of the same patient [47]. In conclusion, all three patients in the pilot study could effectively complete the training task. More importantly, no discomfort, seizure, or other adverse events occurred in association with the study. Thus, stroke patients with hemiplegia could use the system safely and reliably.

Regarding the efficacy of the system for rehabilitation training, we evaluated motor function at baseline and after 12–14 days of rehabilitation treatment in a group of five patients. Scores numerically improved relative to pretreatment baseline, with respect to sitting balance ability, upper limb FMA, lower limb FMA, 10 m walking speed, 6MWD, and MBI, reflecting an improvement in limb motor function and daily living abilities of patients. The sEMG results showed that the RMSs of all these tested muscles except for flexor digitorum and abductor pollicis brevis rose after treatment, indicating that the intervention boosted the vitality of these muscle groups. The results of MEP differences before and after training displayed that the MEP latent periods on the lesion side and non-lesion side were shortened and the amplitudes were increased, signifying that the functions of bilateral cerebral hemispheres were strengthened after treatment [49,50]. The short-term training using the novel BCI system adopted by these stroke patients with hemiplegia could produce multidimensional effects, which should be related to the system's ability to enhance bidirectional stimulation. Enhancing bidirectional stimulation is the core of the BCI system used in this study. The BCI system selects the characteristic EEG signals related to motor intention during training as the main control index, which is helpful to guide patients to continuously and actively give downward motor control signals. On the one hand, such a design can accurately apply the downward control signals to the peripheral neuromuscular system; on the other hand, repeated high-intensity training of the peripheral neuromuscular system may also improve the function in certain brain areas through visual and motor feedback, thus achieving "bidirectional stimulation" [51]. According to Hebb's theory (Hebb, 1949) [52], such bidirectional stimulation can cause neural reorganization including the reorganization of brain region excitability and brain networks in humans, thereby improving cognitive, language, and motor functions.

5. Limitations

This paper is a case report of 5 BCI rehabilitation training instead of a randomized controlled study. The sample size is relatively small, and the condition of each patient was different, so this report did not conduct paired sample t-tests of pre- and post-intervention data, and only the Cohen's w values were shown. In addition, the CMSST, MSP, and ETR values of each patient were tested only once before and after training without repeated measurements, and this may be one of the reasons for the large variation of these indicators in the three patients during the feasibility verification; moreover, even in discussing rehabilitation effects of the system, the 5 patients only received 12–14 days of rehabilitation treatment, thus 24–28 sessions of training, which means short treatment courses. All of these are the limitations of this paper, which need to be improved in future studies.

6. Conclusions

In summary, the new BCI system including visual and motor feedback is applicable in a program of active rehabilitation training of stroke patients with hemiplegia. It is not only safe, but also enables the patients to enter the active-training state quickly, and attain a sufficient training intensity. In this pilot study, responses after a short course of treatment show promise for therapeutic effects in multiple dimensions, which must be established in a randomized controlled study of a much larger patient population, with follow-up after active training sessions.

Author Contributions: Conceptualization, W.G. and Z.C.; methodology, Y.Y.; software, X.S.; validation, Y.H., X.K. and Z.C.; formal analysis, Z.C.; investigation, J.M.; resources, J.X.; data curation, L.J.; writing—original draft preparation, W.G.; writing—review and editing, Y.H.; visualization, X.L.; supervision, X.S.; project administration, S.Z.; funding acquisition, Y.H. All authors have read and agreed to the published version of the manuscript.

Funding: This study was supported by the Scientific Research Fund Project from Anhui Academy of Translational Medicine (NO. 2021zhyx-C50).

Institutional Review Board Statement: The study was conducted in accordance with the Declaration of Helsinki, and approved by the Ethics Committee of the Second Hospital of Anhui Medical University [Approval No. YX2020-103(F1), 24 February 2021].

Informed Consent Statement: Informed consent was obtained from all subjects involved in the study.

Data Availability Statement: Data are available upon request.

Acknowledgments: We extend our deepest thanks to the nurses and doctors of the hospital for their help with conducting the study. All authors included in this section have consented to the acknowledgement.

Conflicts of Interest: The authors declare no conflict of interest.

References

1. Feigin, V.L.; Forouzanfar, M.H.; Krishnamurthi, R.; Mensah, G.A.; Connor, M.; Bennett, D.A.; Moran, A.E.; Sacco, R.L.; Anderson, L.; Truelsen, T. Global and regional burden of stroke during 1990–2010: Findings from the Global Burden of Disease Study 2010. *Lancet* **2014**, *383*, 245–254. [CrossRef]
2. Zhou, M.; Wang, H.; Zhu, J.; Chen, W.; Wang, L.; Liu, S.; Li, Y.; Wang, L.; Liu, Y.; Yin, P. Cause-specific mortality for 240 causes in China during 1990–2013: A systematic subnational analysis for the Global Burden of Disease Study 2013. *Lancet* **2016**, *387*, 251–272. [CrossRef]
3. Moraga, P.; GBD 2016 Causes of Death Collaborators. Global, regional, and national age-sex specific mortality for 264 causes of death, 1980–2016: A systematic analysis for the Global Burden of Disease Study 2016. *Lancet* **2017**, *390*, 1151–1210.
4. Ono, T.; Shindo, K.; Kawashima, K.; Ota, N.; Ito, M.; Ota, T.; Mukaino, M.; Fujiwara, T.; Kimura, A.; Liu, M.; et al. Brain-Computer Interface with somatosensory feedback improves functional recovery from severe hemiplegia due to chronic stroke. *Front. Neuroeng.* **2014**, *7*, 19. [CrossRef] [PubMed]
5. Al-Qazzaz, N.; Alyasseri, Z.A.A.; Abdulkareem, K.H.; Ali, N.S.; Al-Mhiqani, M.N.; Guger, C. EEG feature fusion for motor imagery: A new robust framework towards stroke patients rehabilitation. *Comput. Biol. Med.* **2021**, *137*, 104799. [CrossRef] [PubMed]
6. Hachinski, V.; Donnan, G.A.; Gorelick, P.B.; Hacke, W.; Cramer, S.C.; Kaste, M.; Fisher, M.; Brainin, M.; Buchan, A.M.; Lo, E.H.; et al. Stroke: Working toward a prioritized world agenda. *Cerebrovasc. Dis.* **2010**, *30*, 127–147. [CrossRef] [PubMed]
7. Al-Qazzaz, N.K.; Ali, S.H.B.; Ahmad, S.A.; Chellappan, K.; Islam, M.; Escudero, J. Role of EEG as biomarker in the early detection and classification of dementia. *Sci. World J.* **2014**, *2014*, 906038. [CrossRef] [PubMed]
8. Junior, V.A.D.S.; Santos, M.D.S.; Ribeiro, N.M.D.S.; Maldonado, I.L. Combining proprioceptive neuromuscular facilitation and virtual reality for improving sensorimotor function in stroke survivors: A randomized clinical trial. *J. Cent. Nerv. Syst. Dis.* **2019**, *11*, 593276910. [CrossRef] [PubMed]
9. Eraifej, J.; Clark, W.; France, B.; Desando, S.; Moore, D. Effectiveness of upper limb functional electrical stimulation after stroke for the improvement of activities of daily living and motor function: A systematic review and meta-analysis. *Syst. Rev.* **2017**, *6*, 40. [CrossRef] [PubMed]
10. Takahashi, K.Z.; Lewek, M.D.; Sawicki, G.S. A neuromechanics-based powered ankle exoskeleton to assist walking post-stroke: A feasibility study. *J. Neuroeng. Rehabil.* **2015**, *12*, 23. [CrossRef]
11. Zhang, Q.; Sun, D.; Qian, W.; Xiao, X.; Guo, Z. Modeling and control of a cable-driven rotary series elastic actuator for an upper limb rehabilitation robot. *Front. Neurorobot.* **2020**, *14*, 13. [CrossRef] [PubMed]
12. Awad, L.N.; Lewek, M.D.; Kesar, T.M.; Franz, J.R.; Bowden, M.G. These legs were made for propulsion: Advancing the diagnosis and treatment of post-stroke propulsion decits. *J. Neuroeng. Rehabil.* **2020**, *17*, 139. [CrossRef] [PubMed]
13. Zulauf-Czaja, A.; Al-Taleb, M.K.H.; Purcell, M.; Petric-Gray, N.; Cloughley, J.; Vuckovic, A. On the way home: A BCI-FES hand therapy self-managed by sub-acute SCI participants and their caregivers: A usability study. *J. Neuroeng. Rehabil.* **2021**, *18*, 44. [CrossRef]
14. Foong, R.; Ang, K.K.; Quek, C.; Guan, C.; Phua, K.S.; Kuah, C.W.K.; Deshmukh, V.A.; Yam, L.H.L.; Rajeswaran, D.K.; Tang, N. Assessment of the efficacy of EEG-based MI-BCI with visual feedback and EEG correlates of mental fatigue for upper-limb stroke rehabilitation. *IEEE. Trans. Biomed. Eng.* **2020**, *67*, 786–795. [CrossRef] [PubMed]
15. Mane, R.; Chouhan, T.; Guan, C. BCI for stroke rehabilitation: Motor and beyond. *J. Neural Eng.* **2020**, *17*, 041001. [CrossRef] [PubMed]

16. Rosenfeld, J.V.; Wong, Y.T. Neurobionics and the brain-computer interface: Current applications and future horizons. *Med. J. Aust.* **2017**, *206*, 363–368. [CrossRef] [PubMed]
17. Mridha, M.F.; Das, S.C.; Kabir, M.M.; Lima, A.A.; Islam, M.R.; Watanobe, Y. Brain-Computer Interface: Advancement and Challenges. *Sensors* **2021**, *21*, 5746. [CrossRef] [PubMed]
18. Chen, X.; Li, K. Robotic arm control system based on augmented reality brain-computer interface and computer vision. *Sheng Wu Yi Xue Gong Cheng Xue Za Zhi* **2021**, *38*, 483–491. [PubMed]
19. Mihara, M.; Hattori, N.; Hatakenaka, M.; Yagura, H.; Kawano, T.; Hino, T.; Miyai, I. Near-infrared spectroscopy-mediated neurofeedback enhances efficacy of motor imagery-based training in poststroke victims: A pilot study. *Stroke* **2013**, *44*, 1091–1098. [CrossRef] [PubMed]
20. Pichiorri, F.; Morone, G.; Petti, M.; Toppi, J.; Pisotta, I.; Molinari, M.; Paolucci, S.; Inghilleri, M.; Astolfi, L.; Cincotti, F.; et al. Brain-computer interface boosts motor imagery practice during stroke recovery. *Ann. Neurol.* **2015**, *77*, 851–865. [CrossRef] [PubMed]
21. Ang, K.K.; Guan, C.; Phua, K.S.; Wang, C.; Zhou, L.; Tang, K.Y.; Ephraim Joseph, G.J.; Kuah, C.W.; Chua, K.S. Brain-computer interface-based robotic end effector system for wrist and hand rehabilitation: Results of a three-armed randomized controlled trial for chronic stroke. *Front. Neuroeng.* **2014**, *7*, 30. [CrossRef]
22. Ang, K.K.; Chua, K.S.; Phua, K.S.; Wang, C.; Chin, Z.Y.; Kuah, C.W.; Low, W.; Guan, C. A Randomized Controlled Trial of EEG-Based Motor Imagery Brain-Computer Interface Robotic Rehabilitation for Stroke. *Clin. EEG Neurosci.* **2015**, *46*, 310–320. [CrossRef]
23. Wang, C.; Phua, K.S.; Ang, K.K.; Guan, C.; Zhang, H.; Lin, R.; Chua, K.S.G.; Ang, B.T.; Kuah, C.W.K. A feasibility study of non-invasive motor-imagery BCI-based robotic rehabilitation for Stroke patients. In Proceedings of the 2009 4th International IEEE/EMBS Conference on Neural Engineering, Antalya, Turkey, 29 April–2 May 2009; pp. 271–274.
24. Vourvopoulos, A.; Jorge, C.; Abreu, R.; Figueiredo, P.; Fernandes, J.C.; Bermúdez, I.; Badia, S. Efficacy and Brain Imaging Correlates of an Immersive Motor Imagery BCI-Driven VR System for Upper Limb Motor Rehabilitation: A Clinical Case Report. *Front. Hum. Neurosci.* **2019**, *13*, 244. [CrossRef] [PubMed]
25. Vourvopoulos, A.; Pardo, O.M.; Lefebvre, S.; Neureither, M.; Saldana, D.; Jahng, E.; Liew, S.L. Effects of a Brain-Computer Interface With Virtual Reality (VR) Neurofeedback: A Pilot Study in Chronic Stroke Patients. *Front. Hum. Neurosci.* **2019**, *13*, 210. [CrossRef] [PubMed]
26. Ono, T.; Mukaino, M.; Ushiba, J. Functional recovery in upper limb function in stroke survivors by using brain-computer interface A single case A-B-A-B design. In Proceedings of the 2013 35th Annual International Conference of the IEEE Engineering in Medicine and Biology Society (EMBC), Osaka, Japan, 3–7 July 2013; pp. 265–268.
27. Montag, M.; Paschall, C.; Ojemann, J.; Rao, R.; Herron, J. A Platform for Virtual Reality Task Design with Intracranial Electrodes. In Proceedings of the 2021 43rd Annual International Conference of the IEEE Engineering in Medicine & Biology Society (EMBC), Virtual Conference, 1–5 November 2021; IEEE: Piscataway, NJ, USA, 2021; pp. 6659–6662.
28. Chmura, J.; Rosing, J.; Collazos, S.; Goodwin, S.J. Classification of Movement and Inhibition Using a Hybrid BCI. *Front. Neurorobot.* **2017**, *11*, 38. [CrossRef] [PubMed]
29. Gomez-Rodriguez, M.; Peters, J.; Hill, J.; Schölkopf, B.; Gharabaghi, A.; Grosse-Wentrup, M. Closing the sensorimotor loop: Haptic feedback facilitates decoding of motor imagery. *J. Neural Eng.* **2011**, *8*, 036005. [CrossRef]
30. Ramos-Murguialday, A.; Broetz, D.; Rea, M.; Läer, L.; Yilmaz, O.; Brasil, F.L.; Liberati, G.; Curado, M.R.; Garcia-Cossio, E.; Vyziotis, A.; et al. Brain-machine interface in chronic stroke rehabilitation: A controlled study. *Ann. Neurol.* **2013**, *74*, 100–108. [CrossRef]
31. Cui, Z.; Fu, X.; Wan, X.; Li, J.; Chen, W.; Zhu, S.; Li, Y. The brain-computer interface based robot gives spinal cord injury patients a full-cycle active rehabilitation. In Proceedings of the 2021 9th International Winter Conference on Brain-Computer Interface (BCI), Gangwon, Korea, 22–24 February 2021; pp. 1–5.
32. Ciesla, N.; Dinglas, V.; Fan, E.; Kho, M.; Kuramoto, J.; Needham, D. Manual muscle testing: A method of measuring extremity muscle strength applied to critically ill patients. *J. Vis. Exp.* **2011**, *50*, 2632. [CrossRef]
33. Coleman, E.R.; Moudgal, R.; Lang, K.; Hyacinth, H.I.; Awosika, O.O.; Kissela, B.M.; Feng, W. Early rehabilitation after stroke: A narrative review. *Curr. Atheroscler. Rep.* **2017**, *19*, 59. [CrossRef]
34. Klem, G.H.; Lüders, H.O.; Jasper, H.H.; Elger, C. The ten-twenty electrode system of the international federation. The internanional federation of clinical nenrophysiology. *Electroencephalogr. Clin. Neurophysiol. Suppl.* **1999**, *52*, 3–6.
35. Cui, Z.; Li, Y.; Huang, S.; Wu, X.; Fu, X.; Liu, F.; Wan, X.; Wang, X.; Zhang, Y.; Qiu, H. BCI system with lower-limb robot improves rehabilitation in spinal cord injury patients through short-term training: A pilot study. *Cogn. Neurodyn.* **2022**, 1–19. [CrossRef]
36. Mousavi, M.; Krol, L.R.; de Sa, V.R. Hybrid brain-computer interface with motor imagery and error-related brain activity. *J. Neural Eng.* **2020**, *17*, 056041. [CrossRef]
37. Cabanas-Valdés, R.; Bagur-Calafat, C.; Girabent-Farrés, M.; Caballero-Gómez, F.M.; Cuchí, G.U. The effect of additional core stability exercises on improving dynamic sitting balance and trunk control for subacute stroke patients: A randomized controlled trial. *Clin. Rehabil.* **2016**, *30*, 1024–1033. [CrossRef]
38. Fugl-Meyer, A.R.; Jääskö, L.; Leyman, I.; Olsson, S.; Steglind, S. A method for evaluation of physical performance. *Scand. J. Rehabil. Med.* **1975**, *7*, 13–31.

39. Thompson, P.; Beath, T.; Bell, J.; Jacobson, G.; Phair, T.; Salbach, N.M.; Wright, F.V. Test–retest reliability of the 10-metre fast walk test and 6-minute walk test in ambulatory school-aged children with cerebral palsy. *Dev. Med. Child. Neurol.* **2008**, *50*, 370–376. [CrossRef]
40. Enright, P.L. The six-minute walk test. *Resp. Care* **2003**, *48*, 783–785.
41. Taghizadeh, G.; Martinez-Martin, P.; Meimandi, M.; Habibi, S.A.H.; Jamali, S.; Dehmiyani, A.; Rostami, S.; Mahmuodi, A.; Mehdizadeh, M.; Fereshtehnejad, S. Barthel index and modified rankin scale: Psychometric properties during medication phases in idiopathic Parkinson disease. *Ann. Phys. Rehabil. Med.* **2020**, *63*, 500–504. [CrossRef]
42. Zhou, Y.; Chen, C.; Cheng, M.; Alshahrani, Y.; Lemos, S. Comparison of machine learning methods in sEMG signal processing for shoulder motion recognition. *Biomed. Signal Process.* **2021**, *68*, 102577. [CrossRef]
43. Kim, W.J.; Min, Y.S.; Yang, E.J.; Paik, N.J. Neuronavigated vs. Conventional Repetitive Transcranial Magnetic Stimulation Method for Virtual Lesioning on the Broca's Area. *Neuromodulation* **2014**, *17*, 16–21. [CrossRef]
44. Parker, R.I.; Hagan-Burke, S. Useful effect size interpretations for single case research. *Behav. Ther.* **2007**, *38*, 95–105. [CrossRef]
45. Sheorajpanday, R.V.; Nagels, G.; Weeren, A.J.; De Surgeloose, D.; De Deyn, P.P. Additional value of quantitative EEG in acute anterior circulation syndrome of presumed ischemic origin. *Clin. Neurophysiol.* **2010**, *121*, 1719–1725. [CrossRef]
46. Sheorajpanday, R.V.; Nagels, G.; Weeren, A.J.; van Putten, M.J.; De Deyn, P.P. Quantitative EEG in ischemic stroke: Correlation with functional status after 6 months. *Clin. Neurophysiol.* **2011**, *122*, 874–883. [CrossRef]
47. Carelli, L.; Solca, F.; Faini, A.; Meriggi, P.; Sangalli, D.; Cipresso, P.; Riva, G.; Ticozzi, N.; Ciammola, A.; Silani, V.; et al. Brain-Computer Interface for Clinical Purposes: Cognitive Assessment and Rehabilitation. *Biomed. Res. Int.* **2017**, *2017*, 1695290. [CrossRef] [PubMed]
48. Feng, W.; Gong, Q.; Liu, K.; Li, H. Analysis of Behavioural Characteristics Related to Unintentional Injury in Southeast Chinese Adolescents: Evidence from a School-Based Survey. *Int. J. Environ. Res. Public Health* **2017**, *14*, 241. [CrossRef]
49. Cakar, E.; Akyuz, G.; Durmus, O.; Bayman, L.; Yagci, I.; Karadag-Saygi, E.; Gunduz, O.H. The relationships of motor-evoked potentials to hand dexterity, motor function, and spasticity in chronic stroke patients: A transcranial magnetic stimulation study. *Acta Neurol. Belg.* **2016**, *116*, 481–487. [CrossRef] [PubMed]
50. Kindred, J.H.; Cash, J.J.; Ergle, J.B.; Charalambous, C.C.; Wonsetler, E.C.; Bowden, M.G. Comparing cortico-motor hotspot identification methods in the lower extremities post-stroke: MEP amplitude vs. latency. *Neurosci. Lett.* **2021**, *754*, 135884. [CrossRef] [PubMed]
51. Hughes, C.; Herrera, A.; Gaunt, R.; Collinger, J. Bidirectional brain-computer interfaces. *Handb. Clin. Neurol.* **2020**, *168*, 163–181.
52. Brown, R.E.; Bligh, T.W.B.; Garden, J.F. The Hebb Synapse Before Hebb: Theories of Synaptic Function in Learning and Memory Before, With a Discussion of the Long-Lost Synaptic Theory of William McDougall. *Front. Behav. Neurosci.* **2021**, *15*, 732195. [CrossRef]

brain sciences

MDPI

Review

A Review of Hand Function Rehabilitation Systems Based on Hand Motion Recognition Devices and Artificial Intelligence

Yuexing Gu [1], Yuanjing Xu [1], Yuling Shen [1,2], Hanyu Huang [3], Tongyou Liu [1], Lei Jin [4], Hang Ren [5] and Jinwu Wang [1,2,*]

1 School of Biomedical Engineering, Shanghai Jiao Tong University, Shanghai 200030, China
2 Shanghai Key Laboratory of Orthopaedic Implants, Department of Orthopaedic Surgery, The Ninth People's Hospital Affiliated to School of Medicine of Shanghai Jiao Tong University, Shanghai 200011, China
3 College of Science, Xi'an Jiaotong-Liverpool University, Suzhou 215028, China
4 Department of Rehabilitation Medicine, The Ninth People's Hospital Affiliated to School of Medicine of Shanghai Jiao Tong University, Shanghai 200011, China
5 School of Health Science and Engineering, University of Shanghai for Science and Technology, Shanghai 200093, China
* Correspondence: wangjw-team@shsmu.edu.cn; Tel.: +86-13301773680

Abstract: The incidence of stroke and the burden on health care and society are expected to increase significantly in the coming years, due to the increasing aging of the population. Various sensory, motor, cognitive and psychological disorders may remain in the patient after survival from a stroke. In hemiplegic patients with movement disorders, the impairment of upper limb function, especially hand function, dramatically limits the ability of patients to perform activities of daily living (ADL). Therefore, one of the essential goals of post-stroke rehabilitation is to restore hand function. The recovery of motor function is achieved chiefly through compensatory strategies, such as hand rehabilitation robots, which have been available since the end of the last century. This paper reviews the current research status of hand function rehabilitation devices based on various types of hand motion recognition technologies and analyzes their advantages and disadvantages, reviews the application of artificial intelligence in hand rehabilitation robots, and summarizes the current research limitations and discusses future research directions.

Keywords: hand function rehabilitation; hand rehabilitation robot; computer vision technology; wearable devices; sensors; artificial intelligence

Citation: Gu, Y.; Xu, Y.; Shen, Y.; Huang, H.; Liu, T.; Jin, L.; Ren, H.; Wang, J. A Review of Hand Function Rehabilitation Systems Based on Hand Motion Recognition Devices and Artificial Intelligence. *Brain Sci.* **2022**, *12*, 1079. https://doi.org/10.3390/brainsci12081079

Academic Editors: Fiorenzo Moscatelli and Konstantin V. Slavin

Received: 10 July 2022
Accepted: 12 August 2022
Published: 15 August 2022

1. Introduction

A stroke is one of the most common causes of adult labor loss. It significantly affects people's quality of life. A patient may endure certain movement disorders after a stroke, such as paralysis of the face, arm, and leg on one side of the body. This is known as hemiplegia [1]. Reduced motor function of the upper limbs, especially the hands, essentially limits the ability of the patients to perform activities of daily living (ADL). The hand, a distal part of the body, is the most challenging part of the upper limb to recover [2]. Accordingly, the degree of rehabilitation of hand function can also be used to measure the rehabilitation of the upper limbs from movement disorders. In recent years, many therapeutic methods for upper limb movement recovery after strokes have been developed, among which rehabilitation robots are considered to be an efficient rehabilitation training method [3], which can not only help patients recover the motor function of their limbs, but also significantly reduce the burden of rehabilitation therapists [4].

Effective hand function rehabilitation training based on rehabilitation systems should, at least, meet the following three principles [5,6]: first, the rehabilitation system can ensure the training motivation of patients and help patients stick with the training. In addition, its training program should be customized according to patients' conditions. Furthermore, the rehabilitation system needs to be able to objectively assess the patient's hand function and training outcomes on a regular basis. Therefore, acquiring and recognizing hand postures is crucial in the rehabilitation and evaluation of hand function. It has the following applications. First, it can be applied to the active training mode of rehabilitation robots. Specifically, the active motion intention of patients can be stimulated, extracted, and utilized through detection technology and modern control technology. This can not only promote the recovery of patients' motor perception, but also help patients reshape the central nervous system circuit. Secondly, gesture recognition can also be applied in the human–computer interaction module of the telerehabilitation system and the evaluation system. The main methods of gesture acquisition can be divided into computer vision technology and sensor-based wearable devices according to the different input devices. The former uses external devices for vision capture and analysis, which poses no interference to patients. The latter requires wearing some sensor devices and recognizes fewer gestures, but is beneficial for portability.

In the development of hand rehabilitation robots, software systems are equally important in the design and production of hardware devices. With the development of artificial intelligence, big data, cloud computing, and 5G technology, the requirements for the software system of hand rehabilitation robots have also increased. It should not only fulfill the basic hardware control function and the human–machine interaction function, but also be more intelligent, diverse, and personalized [7]. Artificial intelligence can be applied to many modules of hand rehabilitation robots, which can not only expand the functions of hand rehabilitation robots, improve the accuracy, effectiveness, and wisdom of the devices, but also reduce the pressure on medical resources and improve the comfort and fun of patients during rehabilitation [8].

The outline of this paper is as follows: Section 2 reviews the developments in the hardware of the hand function rehabilitation systems, which mainly includes the gesture recognition devices applied based on computer vision technology and wearable sensors. Section 3 reviews the developments in the software of the hand function rehabilitation systems, including application of artificial intelligence in the seven modules of the hand function rehabilitation robot, although some of them are still in the research stage and whose actual rehabilitation effects are yet to be verified. Section 4 lists the existing problems and limitations during the current phase and discusses the potential directions for future study.

2. Hand Function Rehabilitation System Based on Gesture Recognition

2.1. Hand Function Rehabilitation System Based on Computer Vision Technology

Hand gesture recognition based on computer vision technology mainly uses external devices to collect image data of gestures, such as cameras, and then processes the images with vision techniques, such as deep convolutional networks, to complete recognition and classification. This method is non-invasive, does not require wearing extra equipment, the user is not easily fatigued, and the calibration procedure is simple and convenient to use. It can be applied to fine hand rehabilitation training and hand function assessment tasks. However, this method also has some shortcomings. First, it has high requirements for the external environment. Second, the recognition speed and accuracy of it are relatively low. Third, sometimes, it needs to affix specific markers. The devices that collect gestures usually include color cameras, depth cameras, etc. These hand gesture recognition techniques based on computer vision have been applied to hand rehabilitation robots and independent hand function rehabilitation game systems.

2.1.1. Hand Function Rehabilitation System Based on the Virtual Environment

First of all, some cameras and computer vision techniques can be used to locate the hand's position and recognize some basic hand gestures, which will provide patients with some more exciting games through augmented reality and virtual reality to enhance their interest in training. Studies have shown that video games are beneficial for improving cognitive dysfunction in patients [9]. Other studies indicated that virtual environment training is significantly more effective than traditional training [10–15]. A virtual environment also provides a safe and customizable training system that can be changed according to users' interests. It can also monitor users' actions to analyze their performance during training [16].

For example, Hondori et al. [17] developed a low-cost augmented reality system for hand rehabilitation training assistance and progress assessment, which provides task instructions through virtual objects projected on the desktop, and uses a web camera to collect and track the color markers of hand recognition to identify patient actions and task completion. This device can allow patients to train in the hospital or at home and can be remotely accessed and controlled by therapists. However, some additional markers need to be worn, which is not very convenient, and the hand positioning recognition ability also needs to be improved.

In addition to webcams, similar hand modeling, tracking, and recognition functions can be accomplished using depth cameras and color cameras without markers. The primary devices currently used are Leap Motion, Microsoft Kinect V1 and V2, etc.

The Leap Motion uses infrared LED and a gray-scale camera, which is cheaper and can handle hand models only. Wang et al. [18] demonstrated that Leap Motion-based virtual reality training could promote cortical reorganization and may aid in the recovery of upper extremity motor function in patients with subacute stroke. However, its effects on severe patients are unknown. Alimanova et al. [19] developed a set of hand rehabilitation games using Leap Motion controllers to help patients relax and train their hand muscles by performing different virtual reality tasks related to daily living activities, such as picking up objects, moving household objects, matching color blocks, throwing garbage, holding objects, etc. These games can also motivate patients by making the rehabilitation process more exciting and effective, and they can help patients relieve muscle tension and restore hand function.

Mukai et al. [20] developed the hand rehabilitation robot "ReRoH". It comprises flexible pneumatic gloves, ERB, an electrical stimulator, Leap Motion non-contact sensor, and game controller. The Leap Motion has an infrared transmitter and receiver that can identify hand coordinates and movements, and the game controller can display an image of the hand on a display in real-time. With rehabilitation games, the ability to grasp and stretch the hand can be trained, and the motor function of the fingers and hands can also be assessed.

The Kinect uses depth cameras, infrared emitters, color sensors, infrared depth sensors, turnover motors, RGB cameras, etc., all of which are needed to generate a full-body or half-body model, resulting in the latter being less efficient and accurate in operation than the former.

For example, Cipresso et al. [21] developed a virtual reality system for rehabilitation by using Kinect V1. It combines rehabilitation technology with virtual environment recognition. It can track patients' hand motions through Kinect's depth images and color space model, and provides real-time feedback. Through the virtual reality of daily life activities with highly realistic visual effects, patients' motivation to participate in treatment is stimulated, and their ADL ability is better trained and evaluated. Likewise, Wang et al. [22] developed a Kinect-based rehabilitation assistance system consisting of the rehabilitation training subsystem, and rehabilitation evaluation subsystem that performed similar functions.

However, these systems lack tactile feedback, game angle, and time-based safety constraints based on the patient's motor ability. Saini et al. [23] solved this problem by designing a "watchdog" to ensure the safety of patients' hand motion angle and time during the game. Additionally, the game framework of the stroke rehabilitation program designed by them only uses Kinect V1 equipment and a single camera to capture human motion, without the need to affix markers.

Avola et al. [24] proposed an interactive and low-cost full-body rehabilitation framework for generating 3D immersive serious games. The hardware part includes Kinect V2 and a head-mounted display (HMD), and acquires depth information in the way of time of flight (TOF), which is different from Kinect V1 using light coding. The software part uses gated recurrent unit recurrent neural networks (GRURNN). The framework's natural user interface (NUIs) can be used for hand modeling, tracking the movement of hand joints and fingers through an infrared stereo camera, and then performing rehabilitation training through a customizable interactive virtual environment. Experiments showed that this system can restore patients' hand function. However, it only has a few hand games to choose from, and HMD may cause vertigo in some patients.

2.1.2. Hand Rehabilitation Robot Based on Computer Vision Technology

In addition to the above applications, computer vision technology can also be used simply for gesture recognition. The hand rehabilitation robot can be controlled by recognized gestures to carry out the corresponding motion. It can also identify the current motion state of the rehabilitation robot and provide feedback to the system for further adjustment of the robot or evaluation of the training situation.

Cordella et al. [25] developed a set of camera-based calibration programs for the bending sensor of the commercial exoskeleton hand rehabilitation robot glove "Gloreha Sininfonia," which uses 8 photoelectric cameras to locate and reconstruct the angles of 18 reflective markers on the glove, and then connects them with the voltage of the glove bending sensor to form closed-loop control, in order to calibrate the angle of the exoskeleton better. The system can also assess a patient's hand function or measure the improvement of hand motion by comparing their range of motion (ROM) before and after treatment.

Farulla et al. [26] proposed a hand exoskeleton system that can be used for master-slave control of telerehabilitation. It uses an RGB-D camera to locate the position of the therapist's hand joint in real-time through the VPE algorithm and remotely transmits the position to the exoskeleton. In this way, the movement of the index finger and thumb of the patient's hand can be controlled. The grip force sensor on the exoskeleton can record the interaction force and feed it back to the therapist for real-time quantitative assessment and adjustment.

Nam et al. [27] developed an exoskeleton that can remotely train the ability of hand grasping and forearm pronation and supination, and also used camera-based computer vision technology to identify the user's intention. However, unlike other systems, this device is equipped with a Microsoft LifeCam Studio camera on the exoskeleton. The patient uses the residual force of the proximal upper limb to move the robot to the target position and identify the target object. Firstly, the recognition algorithm identifies and locates the target through the real-time image collected by the camera. Then, the control system controls the aiming and grasping of the exoskeleton. Finally, the system realizes the motion-vision-sensation closed-loop feedback. To prevent hand injury caused by excessive grasping movements of the robot, the exoskeleton of the hand is placed on the palm side.

There are also many related types of research and achievements in China. For example, Hefei University of technology [28–31] developed a rehabilitation robot system. When the patient completes the specified gesture in front of the camera on the mechanical arm, the processor will display it on the screen after recognition through the internal algorithm. Then, the system can analyze, evaluate, and record the patient's rehabilitation. It can also cooperate with the virtual reality system for more exciting training to improve the patient's cognitive ability and hand function and adjust the training scheme as needed. When the camera cannot capture the complete hand image, the system can automatically identify and locate the position of the patient's hand, adjust the manipulator to the position where the complete gesture can be captured, and use the exoskeleton to compensate for the hand motion.

Nanchang University [32] developed a near-synchronous hand rehabilitation robot. It can collect the motion posture information of the unaffected hand in real-time through Leap Motion, decode and transmit the data through a genetic algorithm and neural network, and then control the exoskeleton to complete the corresponding action and drive the patient's hands for training. The system has a fast response time and high accuracy in gesture recognition and control, but it can only train the thumb, index finger, and middle finger.

Liu Hongmei et al. [33] from Shanghai Normal University developed a flexible hand rehabilitation robot by using the Vicon system, which has eight infrared cameras. They can capture the three-dimensional motion of the hand, obtain the joint angle, and recognize the hand motion to identify the relationship between the extension of the Bowden line and the bending angle of the finger, so as to control the hand rehabilitation robot more accurately.

2.2. Hand Function Rehabilitation System Based on Wearable Devices

Gesture recognition based on wearable devices requires users to wear devices, such as gloves, rings, bracelets, wristbands, armbands, etc., and collect the motion data or physiological signal data of the user's hand movements through the sensors on the devices for recognition. This method can recognize more gestures with small input data and high precision. It can identify hand motion and three-dimensional information in space in real-time. It is not easily disturbed by external interference and has good robustness, but it is usually expensive. Wearing equipment may interfere with the therapist's motion, and the accuracy may be affected when the user is sweating. It is also easy to make the patient tired, and calibration is usually required before each use. According to the types of data collected, wearable devices can be divided into physiological signal sensors, kinematic signal sensors, optical signal sensors, etc. Multiple transmissions are often selected simultaneously as multi-mode fusion data inputs in actual use. Gestures recognized by wearable devices can provide control targets for hand function rehabilitation robots and complete hand function training in the active mode. They can also be used for the evaluation of a patient's rehabilitation.

2.2.1. Physiological Signal Sensor-Based Hand Function Rehabilitation Robot

The bioelectric signals that can be used for hand function rehabilitation robots usually include electroencephalogram (EEG), electro-oculogram (EoG), electromyography (EMG), etc. Generally, the acquisition system collects the required bioelectric signals from the patient's body surface, processes and analyzes the signals to obtain the patient's motion intention, which is equivalent to synchronously identifying the patient's hand action, and then transmits the corresponding motion instructions to the hand rehabilitation robot to drive the patient's hand to make related motions.

Wang Jing et al. [34] from Xi'an Jiaotong University developed the upper limb rehabilitation platform by using the commercialized product Myo gesture control armband to recognize the gesture intention of patients. Gestures are then mapped to a virtual environment, and patients' hand grasping functions are trained through VR glasses and immersive games. The armband is composed of an inertial sensor unit, eight surface electromyography (sEMG) sensors, and a Bluetooth receiver, which is low-cost and portable. Liu Wei et al. [35] from Nanjing University of Aeronautics and Astronautics designed an underactuated hand rehabilitation robot, which also uses MYO gesture control armbands. It can recognize five gestures of the unaffected hand in real-time, and control the exoskeleton to drive the affected hand to complete the corresponding movements for training. Similarly, the low-cost exoskeleton "RobHand" developed by Casnal et al. [36] also completes the bilateral cooperative control of the rehabilitation robot by fixing multiple sEMG sensors. Li et al. [37] designed an exoskeleton that selects 16 muscles in both arms and hands for sEMG acquisition. Combined with the optimized algorithm, it can recognize seven gestures and control the exoskeleton. In addition, it can also estimate the strength of the patient when grasping the object by collecting sEMG signals, and control the rehabilitation robot to provide the required auxiliary force, such as the exoskeleton designed by Leonardis et al. [4]

Soekadar et al. [38] from Germany developed the hand function rehabilitation exoskeleton. This exoskeleton uses an innovative brain/neurocomputer interaction (BNCI) system that integrates EEG and EOG to better compensate for the decline in signal quality and fatigue sensitivity over time. This system can also recognize gestures better and control the exoskeleton. Similarly, Huo Yaopu et al. [39] from Southeast University designed a 3D-printed hand exoskeleton based on the motor imagination brain computer interface (MI-BCI), which also identifies the motion intention of patients by collecting their EEG, and then controls the hand exoskeleton to assist them in completing corresponding actions.

Zhang et al. [40] from Changsha Institute of Mechanical Engineering proposed the multi-mode human–computer interaction flexible rehabilitation robot, which uses three modes, EEG, EOG and EMG. Under the condition of meeting the requirements of classification speed, it improves the accuracy of the classification and dramatically improves the performance and applicability of the system, but also reduces the system's response speed. Similarly, Xi'an Jiaotong University [41] designed the multi-mode human–computer interaction flexible manipulator, which also integrates the instructions of three modes, so that patients can choose their own multi-modal human machine interface (mHMI) mode.

Bioelectrical signals to control hand rehabilitation robots have considerable application prospects. This mode is more in line with the physiological function of the human body; that is, there are physiological signals first, and then muscle activities to produce hand movements. However, the balance and optimization between comfort, diversity, stability, accuracy, timeliness, and timeliness need to be further studied, and the safety of unsupervised training is also worthy of attention.

2.2.2. Kinematics Sensor-Based Hand Function Rehabilitation Robot

The kinematic parameters of hand motion include fingers and joints' coordinates, displacement, angular displacement, motion speed, angular velocity, acceleration, inertia, etc. The kinematic sensors used to measure these parameters in a hand rehabilitation robot mainly include flexible angle sensors, accelerometers, gyroscopes, pressure sensors, etc. Compared with rehabilitation robots based on physiological signals, most rehabilitation robots with integrated kinematic sensors can provide a signal of superior quality and better tolerance with regard to placement of electrodes. They can recognize finer gestures and complete finer-grained training tasks, which is very helpful for the treatment of patients in the later stages of stroke rehabilitation.

Most of the kinematic sensors of hand rehabilitation robots choose the angle sensors, because they can obtain the angle information of each finger joint more directly and then recognize more fine gestures, which can be used for hand function rehabilitation and evaluation. For example, Hong et al. [42] from the National University of Singapore designed a passive flexible mechanical glove. It uses the angle sensor placed on the finger part of the glove to collect the kinematic information of the patient's healthy hand to judge the patient's motion intention, and recognize the gesture. It then uses the pneumatic actuator made of silicone elastic material to generate pressure to drive the affected hand to move. Similarly, Rahman et al. [43] from Sydney University of Technology developed a 15-DOF aluminum hand exoskeleton that also adopts angle sensors and the bilateral cooperative mode.

When the patient has a certain degree of hand function, the tactile sensor and pressure sensor can also be used to identify the motion intention of the affected hand when grasping the object and judge the required force. For example, Nilsson et al. [44] from Sweden developed SEM gloves with tactile sensors on the fingertips and pressure sensors on the palm. After recognizing the patient's motion intention of grasping and judging the vital force, the robot will provide the corresponding auxiliary power to complete the training.

Many devices simultaneously use angle and pressure sensors to obtain more comprehensive kinematic information. For example, Chen et al. [45] proposed a flexible and portable hand fine motor function rehabilitation robot, with ten flexible bending angle sensors at the joints and ten pressure sensors on the palm and fingertips of the unaffected hand's glove. Through these sensors, the joint bending angle and clamping force of each finger can be collected in real-time. Then, 16 gestures and 6 task gestures of a single finger and multiple fingers motion can be recognized, and the affected glove can be controlled to complete the same action-driven training. There are also angle and pressure sensors on the gloves on the affected hand, which can provide feedback on the current parameters for closed-loop control and provide a basis for doctors to evaluate hand function and adjust the training program. Similarly, the rehabilitation robot designed by Rakhtala et al. [46] also uses angle and pressure sensors at the same position of gloves to identify the current hand motion state to achieve a closed-loop control system. The same is true of the pneumatic hand rehabilitation robot designed by Huazhong University of Science and Technology [47].

The angular information during a hand motion is not only the finger joint bending angle mentioned above, but also the opening angle and the degree of overlap between each finger. Sometimes, it is necessary to use an opening angle sensor to measure the degree of the spread between fingers, which can better identify different types of hand gestures and analyze the patient's hand function rehabilitation more comprehensively. For example, Li Nan et al. [48] designed intelligent-assisted rehabilitation gloves, which use bending angle sensors, pressure sensors, and opening angle sensors at the same time.

For the recognition of dynamic hand motions, in addition to static motion information, some dynamic posture information, such as velocity and acceleration, and spatial information, such as relative coordinates, are required. At this time, accelerometers, gyroscopes, and other sensors are needed. These applications are often combined with inertial sensors or posture sensors in practice. For example, Zhengzhou University [49] designed the hand motion rehabilitation training and evaluation system. This system uses bending sensors and posture sensors simultaneously, which can obtain the motion state of the patient's hand and rehabilitation robot in real-time. Then, the software system compares the obtained information with the expected values, and controls the rehabilitation robot to use the appropriate speed and angular speed to complete the required motion. When the system detects that the status exceeds the pre-specified threshold, it will automatically and slowly return to the safe state and inform the medical personnel in a timely manner. The Robot Research Center of Zhejiang University [50] designed a hand function rehabilitation training system that uses bending angle sensors, pressure sensors, and inertial sensors simultaneously. This system can identify the patient's hand actions, spatial motion state, and pressure value of each part during grasping in real-time, and map them to the virtual hand. It is combined with virtual reality to motivate patients' training through more exciting games.

2.2.3. Optical Sensor-Based Hand Function Rehabilitation Robot

Conventional sensors are usually directly mounted on hand rehabilitation robots, which are difficult to integrate with actuators, complex in structures, and challenging to install on flexible actuators. Sensors made of elastomers or conductive liquids will deform when subjected to surface pressure, resulting in non-linear output and compromising accuracy. Optical sensors applied to hand rehabilitation robots mainly include optical fiber sensors and photoelectric sensors. The fiber optic sensor has high sensitivity, a compact structure, and strong anti-interference ability, which means it cannot affect the hand motion when applied to the hand rehabilitation robot. Optical sensors generally work by measuring the deviation of a light beam incident on a photosensitive surface.

He et al. [51] proposed an optical fiber pressure sensor for the hand rehabilitation exoskeleton. This sensor consists of a small piece of optical fiber package attached to a rigid 3D-printed structure. It can capture the interaction force on the exoskeleton in real-time to obtain the current hand motion and grasping situation. The sensor is small, simple, sensitive, safe, and low-cost, and can be easily integrated into the exoskeleton of the hand without affecting actuation. In a later study, the team also proposed a low-cost micro-hand posture sensor based on photoelectric technology that can be integrated into the hand exoskeleton [52], which measures the posture of multi-segment continuous structures in the hand rehabilitation exoskeleton. The sensor has low energy consumption, low noise, high sensitivity, and good real-time performance. It can be used to accurately control the rehabilitation robot, assess patient hand function, and adjust the rehabilitation plan.

Diez et al. [53] proposed a lightweight hand exoskeleton with micro-optical force sensors, which also applies optical principles and can measure human–machine interaction forces to estimate user intentions in rehabilitation scenarios. Due to its miniaturization, the sensor can be inserted between the human interface and the force transmission element. When the patient tries to act, the device can measure the force between the exoskeleton and the patient, identify the patient's intention, and continuously control the exoskeleton to move in the desired direction to achieve the target posture. When the patient has a particular hand motor function and the force measured by the sensor exceeds a pre-calibrated threshold, the exoskeleton will automatically start a complete movement.

Liu Chenglong et al. [54] from Huazhong University of Science and Technology developed a soft actuator for the hand rehabilitation robot. It is embedded with optical fiber curvature sensors. When the finger is bent, the sensor senses different surface pressures and outputs voltage signals in a linear relationship. The software part can convert voltage signals into angle information, and then recognize the gesture. In this way, the rehabilitation robot can be tracked and controlled more accurately to assist in each training mode. At the same time, the system can also display the current gesture with 3D texture animation. The PMMA material is used as the light guiding medium of the sensor, which can effectively eliminate the interference of the extrusion deformation caused by the soft actuator's inflation on the sensor's output and make the output more stable. Table 1 presents a summary of the advantages and disadvantages of these hardware devices for functional hand rehabilitation systems included in the review.

Table 1. This table is a summary of the different input device for the hand function rehabilitation system and indicates the main advantages and disadvantages of these technologies.

Input Device	Specific Device	Reference	Advantage	Disadvantage
Camera	Virtual game	[17–24]	Non-invasive; does not require wearing extra equipment; easy to use	Has high requirements for the external environment; low recognition speed and the accuracy rate; may need markers
	Robot	[25–33]		
Wearable device	Physiological signal sensor	[34–41]	Can recognize more gestures with small input data and high precision in real time; has good robustness	More expensive; require wearing extra equipment; easy to cause fatigue; requires calibration
	Kinematics sensor	[42–50]		
	Optical sensor	[51–54]		

3. Artificial Intelligence Used in Hand Rehabilitation Robots

In addition to the above-mentioned research on hardware devices for hand movement recognition, hand rehabilitation robots also require research in the field of software, combining hardware and software to achieve intelligence and wisdom in the devices. With the development of artificial intelligence technology, many new fields and products have emerged. Artificial intelligence can be applied to various modules of hand rehabilitation robots, such as hand movement recognition, control of hand rehabilitation robots, human-machine intelligent collaboration, interactive game design, training program design and result evaluation, cloud platform, structural design and optimization of hand rehabilitation robots, and so on. However, in practice, the research and application of artificial intelligence in hand rehabilitation robots are still not significant or not deep enough due to technical limitations and insufficient deployment of related medical facilities [7].

3.1. Gesture Recognition Algorithm

In hand rehabilitation robots, gesture recognition mainly requires real-time isolated dynamic gesture recognition, and artificial intelligence algorithms can be used for this recognition. The core idea is mainly to build a matching model from the data training set and then use the model to predict the recognized gestures. The more commonly used methods are mainly linear discriminant analysis (LDA), support vector machines (SVM), convolutional neural networks (CNN), long short-term memory (LSTM) and recurrent neural networks (RNN). For example, Zhang Guangxing [55] from Qingdao University of Science and Technology designed an integrated wrist rehabilitation robot using the LDA method that can recognize five kinds of movements, with an accuracy rate of over 90%. Zhang Fahui [56] from Nanchang University used the SVM model to recognize four kinds of gestures, with an average accuracy rate of 99.3%. Liu Wei [35] from Nanjing University of Aeronautics and Astronautics developed a hand exoskeleton rehabilitation robot using the convolutional neural network, which can recognize four kinds of gestures, with an average accuracy rate of 96.18%. Zhang Jianxi [57] designed a hand rehabilitation robot using a combination of RNN and LSTM algorithms for the recognition of nine gestures, with an average accuracy of 91.44%.

3.2. Control of the Hand Rehabilitation Robot

Safety issues need to be addressed in the control strategy or algorithm of the hand rehabilitation robot. More precise control strategies are needed, as well as balancing the ratio between the degree of control the robot has over the hand and the risk of miscalculation. For example, Jun Wu [58] designed a pneumatic flexible hand rehabilitation robot, used a sliding mode control algorithm based on fuzzy compensation to control the pneumatic muscles, proposed a dynamic surface control based on a nonlinear interference observer to realize the control of the pneumatic muscle system, and used an echo state network (ESN) with recursive least squares (RLS) for PID parallel adaptive control. Yihao Du et al. [59] proposed an adaptive control strategy based on a variable impedance equation model, which can combine the desired trajectory identified by physiological signals to obtain the final trajectory and calculate the required motion of each joint of the rehabilitation robot. Yonghao Yin [60] from Yanshan University also used RBF neural networks to approximate the compensation of errors caused by external perturbations and uncertainties to control the rehabilitation robot to achieve the desired results.

3.3. Human-Robot Intelligence Collaboration

Artificial intelligence can also be applied to the human-robot collaboration of hand rehabilitation robots, mainly in the assisted training mode. For example, Wang Xiangyu [61] from Harbin Institute of Technology designed an impedance control system to carry out motion following the hand rehabilitation robot in the assisted mode, which can identify the bending angle and muscle strength of the patient's fingers when the patient's hand has a certain behavioral ability and apply the appropriate force to help the patient complete the movement, and the system uses a fuzzy neural network.

3.4. Interactive Game Design

In order to increase patients' interest and motivation during rehabilitation training, the hand rehabilitation robot can be equipped with some interactive games, such as interactive control based on voice recognition, virtual reality games based on visual recognition, and games based on brain–computer interface, etc. Artificial intelligence is also applied here. For example, Zhu Xikun [62] from Zhengzhou University designed a finger rehabilitation training system that can interact with active modes through both gesture recognition and voice recognition using algorithms such as neural networks and hidden Markov models. Cao Yali [63] designed a hand function rehabilitation robot software system that uses Unity3D to design different virtual games for different training modalities. Mou Yang et al. [64] designed an Android-based portable virtual reality rehabilitation device that can be applied to a hand rehabilitation robot. Ying Zhang [65] from Beijing University of Posts and Telecommunications designed a monocular vision-based hand grasping interaction training module.

3.5. Training Program Design and Outcome Evaluation

Traditional rehabilitation training programs and assessment of rehabilitation results are mostly conducted by doctors themselves, but this requires a lot of medical resources and sometimes has a certain subjective component. Theoretically, the application of artificial intelligence can improve this problem by digitizing and standardizing the assessment report and training program, which can identify the patient's current hand movement status and physiological data in real time, combine it with the relevant medical program data, assess the patient's current muscle strength level and rehabilitation training effect, and intelligently design the training program based on the assessment results. However, the actual effectiveness of these applications has yet to be clinically validated. For example, Neofect [66] has developed a Rapael Smart Glove, which has an intelligent system that can provide segmented rehabilitation recommendations and evaluation reports, and its unique RAPAEL intelligent rehabilitation algorithm that can build games that meet the patient's rehabilitation plan.

3.6. Cloud Platform

The cloud platform can be used for one-stop implementation of training program design and evaluation of training results, as well as remote rehabilitation and real-time interaction. The cloud platform can monitor equipment parameter data in real time and provide safe and reliable rehabilitation training for patients. It can also apply digital twin technology to break the limitation of time and space and share big data sets of patients' medical records, intelligent rehabilitation assessment reports, and training reports. Through these data, training programs are intelligently designed and pushed to rehabilitation robots, with interactive games, real-time remote training, and full cloud health management. For example, Xinyu Tang [67] from Southeast University designed a rehabilitation training and assessment system that uses cloud platform technology to aggregate, store, analyze, and display patient rehabilitation data. The system uses the DTW algorithm to compare the similarity of patient movement data streams captured by Kinect with standard movement data streams and uses them as indicators to assess the rehabilitation status of patients.

3.7. Hand Rehabilitation Robot Structure Design and Optimization

In addition to the software applications mentioned above, artificial intelligence can be applied to the hardware structure of the rehabilitation robot. For example, AI can optimize the mechanical mechanism based on human body data to make the machinery more ergonomic and better fit the biological curve of the human body to enhance the use experience.

4. Problems and Prospects of the Current Study

The previous context introduces the hardware and software of existing research on hand function rehabilitation robots. However, problems also exist that require further attention in future research. The following list summarizes the existing problems and limitations of the employed techniques in the current studies.

(1) Hand function rehabilitation equipment based on computer vision techniques is sometimes cumbersome, requires affixing markers, and is not convenient or portable enough for the external environment. Some aspects of the equipment will even make users feel dizzy. When using monocular vision, the recognition accuracy is affected by the light and color of the environment, skin color, etc. Although these problems can be improved to some extent when using binocular vision, it requires more complicated calibration and correction, which increases the computational cost and creates other interference factors that affect the image quality. Therefore, it is necessary to continue to improve the equipment and optimize the algorithm.

(2) When using computer vision technology for bare hand gesture recognition and training patients' hand function with games in the virtual environment, the tactile feedback of the affected hand is often not available, ignoring the motion angle and time that

needs to be strictly set according to the patient's motion ability to ensure the safety of the game. The feedback is mandatory during sensorimotor rehabilitation. Therefore, more attention should be paid to the design by adding some threshold limits.

(3) When using computer vision technology only for gesture recognition and rehabilitation training, the type of data is relatively simple. When recognizing complex gestures, it is inevitable to encounter a situation where the acquisition cannot be collected or where the acquisition and recognition are inaccurate. Some other information collection methods, such as physiological signals and so on, can be used to achieve multi-information fusion.

(4) Most hand rehabilitation robots based on wearable device gesture recognition need to wear additional sensors, which increases the cost and at the same time is inconvenient to use and has certain restrictions for patients. The recognition algorithm and the central processor of the wearable device have higher requirements, so there may be some delays. The algorithm also needs to be retrained if the number of sensor positions changes. Therefore, the balance and optimization between comfort, diversity, stability, accuracy, and timeliness in acquisition need to be further studied, and the safety of unsupervised training also deserves attention.

(5) The hand rehabilitation robots based on physiological signal gesture recognition are prone to instability in signal acquisition and transmission, and the amount of data that can be recognized is limited, making it difficult in the application to fine finger motion rehabilitation and the recognition of continuous motion. To address this aspect, multi-mode control strategies can also be used, in conjunction with kinematic signals, optical signals, etc.

(6) Regardless of the techniques used, the rehabilitation robot should be designed with a closed-loop control network, which can, for example, provide force feedback, angular feedback, position feedback, haptic feedback, etc. through sensors to provide timely feedback and adjust parameters according to the real-time status of patients.

(7) Most hand function rehabilitation robots are still in the research stage, and those based on computer vision technologies require far more attention than those found on wearable sensors. Evaluated using the "Technology Readiness Level (TRL) system" by Mankins, most hand function rehabilitation systems based on computer vision technology are still at TRL5 or 6 (technology demonstration). A few of them are at TRL7 or 8 (system/subsystem development), and few reach TRL9 (system test, deployment and ops, the highest level) [68]. On the other hand, those based on wearable devices are at least TRL5 to 7, and many of them reach TRL9.

Besides the above existing problems, the clinical utility of hand function rehabilitation robots has been evaluated in terms of appropriateness, acceptability, and practicability [69]. Most established rehabilitation robots had effective appropriateness, while some robots still in the research stage had relevant appropriateness. Participants' acceptability of rehabilitation robots and computer-vision-based games is mainly related to their effectiveness. Some said that the games could increase their interest in training, and some expressed concerns, such as comfort. Speaking of practicability, most of them perform well in terms of functionality and suitability, but some technical problems hinder the user experience. The variety of functionality and wearing comfort still require further improvements.

In the future, we expect that a hand function rehabilitation robot should first be able to fully simulate a human therapist's approach and achieve complete "human-machine integration". Secondly, it can be upgraded under human guidance to assess the patient's condition, give rehabilitation training plans and evaluate the training effect. Moreover, it can realize a more convenient and intelligent human–machine interaction mode. Finally, it can also assist in optimizing the allocation of medical resources to achieve efficient and interesting telemedicine.

Author Contributions: Conceptualization: Y.G. Data collection, analysis and interpretation: Y.G., L.J. and H.R. Drafting of manuscript: Y.G. Critical revision: Y.S. Visualization: H.H. Project administration: Y.X., T.L. and J.W. All authors have read and agreed to the published version of the manuscript.

Funding: This research was funded by the National Key R&D Program of China (2020YFC2008700) and the Project of Shanghai Science and Technology Commission (19441917500/19441908700).

Institutional Review Board Statement: Not applicable.

Informed Consent Statement: Not applicable.

Acknowledgments: We wish to express our gratitude to the participants and their families in this study.

Conflicts of Interest: The authors declare no conflict of interest.

References

1. Lin, Q.; Li, X.; Cheng, K.; Cheng, A.; Yu, C.; Zhou, Y. Effects of early cognitive rehabilitation training on cognitive function, motor function and activities of daily living in patients with stroke. *Chin. J. Rehabil. Med.* **2015**, *30*, 3.
2. Wang, J. Effects of finger flexion movement combined with comprehensive rehabilitation training on finger range of motion and upper limb function in patients with hemiplegia after stroke. *Chin. Gen. Pract.* **2017**, *20*, 3.
3. Chang, Y.; Meng, Q.; Yu, H. Research progress of hand rehabilitation robot technology. *Beijing Biomed. Eng.* **2018**, *37*, 7.
4. Leonardis, D.; Barsotti, M.; Loconsole, C.; Solazzi, M.; Troncossi, M.; Mazzotti, C.; Castelli, V.P.; Procopio, C.; Lamola, G.; Lamola, C.; et al. An EMG-Controlled robotic hand exoskeleton for bilateral rehabilitation. *IEEE Trans. Haptics* **2015**, *8*, 140–151. [CrossRef]
5. Xiao, X.; Xiao, Y. *Rehabilitation Engineering Technology*; Huazhong University of Science and Technology Press: Wuhan, China, 2019; pp. 367–371.
6. Saa, A.; Aab, A.; Dsk, A. Effectiveness of an intensive, functional, gamified rehabilitation program in improving upper limb motor function in people with stroke: A protocol of the EnteRtain randomized clinical trial. *Contemp. Clin. Trials* **2021**, *105*, 106381.
7. Yu, H. Rehabilitation robots: Ten visionary perspectives for the future. *Chin. J. Rehabil. Med.* **2020**, *35*, 3.
8. Vélez-Guerrero, M.; Callejas-Cuervo, M.; Mazzoleni, S. Artificial Intelligence-Based Wearable Robotic Exoskeletons for Upper Limb Rehabilitation: A Review. *Sensors* **2021**, *21*, 2146. [CrossRef]
9. Harley, L.; Robertson, S.; Gandy, M.; Harbert, S.; Britton, D. The design of an interactive stroke rehabilitation gaming system. In *International Conference on Human-Computer Interaction*; Springer: Berlin/Heidelberg, Germany, 2011.
10. Merians, A.S. Sensorimotor training in a virtual reality environment: Does it improve functional recovery poststroke. *Neurorehabil. Neural Repair* **2006**, *20*, 252–267. [CrossRef]
11. Akn, A.; Atar, E.; Koyiit, H.; Tosun, A.; Kocyi, H. Effects of Kinect-based virtual reality game training on upper extremity motor recovery in chronic stroke. *Somatosens. Mot. Res.* **2018**, *35*, 25–32.
12. Laver, K.E.; Lange, B.; George, S.; Deutsch, E.J.; Saposnik, G. Virtual reality for stroke rehabilitation. *Cochrane Database Syst. Rev.* **2011**, *2*, CD008349.
13. Domínguez-Téllez, P.; Moral-Muñoz, J.; Salazar, A.; Casado-Fernández, E.; Lucena-Antón, D. Game-based virtual reality interventions to improve upper limb motor function and quality of life after stroke: Systematic review and meta-analysis. *Games Health J.* **2019**, *9*, 1–10. [CrossRef]
14. Karamians, R.; Proffitt, R.; Kline, D.; Gauthier, L. Effectiveness of virtual reality- and gaming-based interventions for upper extremity rehabilitation poststroke: A meta-analysis. *Arch. Phys. Med. Rehabil.* **2020**, *101*, 885–896. [CrossRef]
15. Ain, Q.; Khan, S.; Ilyas, S.; Yaseen, A.; Tariq, I.; Liu, T.; Wang, J. Additional effects of Xbox kinect training on upper limb function in chronic stroke patients: A randomized control trial. *Healthcare* **2021**, *9*, 242. [CrossRef]
16. Rizzo, A.; Kim, G. A SWOT Analysis of the field of virtual reality rehabilitation and therapy. *Presence* **2005**, *14*, 119–146. [CrossRef]
17. Mousavi Hondori, H.; Khademi, M.; Dodakian, L.; Cramer, S.C.; Lopes, C.V. A Spatial augmented reality rehab system for post-stroke hand rehabilitation. *Stud. Health Technol. Inform.* **2013**, *184*, 279–285.
18. Wang, Z.; Wang, P.; Xing, L.; Mei, L.; Zhao, J.; Zhang, T. Leap Motion-based virtual reality training for improving motor functional recovery of upper limbs and neural reorganization in subacute stroke patients. *Neural Regen. Res.* **2017**, *12*, 1823–1831.
19. Alimanova, M.; Borambayeva, S.; Kozhamzharova, D.; Kurmangaiyeva, N.; Ospanova, D.; Tyulepberdinova, G.; Gaziz, G.; Kassenkhan, A. Gamification of hand rehabilitation process using virtual reality tools: Using leap motion for hand rehabilitation. In Proceedings of the 2017 First IEEE International Conference on Robotic Computing (IRC), Taichung, Taiwan, 10–12 April 2017.
20. Mukai, H.; Yamabe, K.; Abe, I.; Kikuchi, T.; Ohno, T. Development of Rehabilitation Robot for hand "ReRoH" for hemiplegic patients. In Proceedings of the JSME Annual Conference on Robotics and Mechatronics (Robomec), Tokyo, Japan, 10–13 May 2017; pp. 2063–2068.
21. Cipresso, P.; Serino, S.; Pedroli, E.; Gaggioli, A.; Riva, G. A virtual reality platform for assessment and rehabilitation of neglect using a kinect. *Stud. Health Technol Inform.* **2014**, *196*, 66–68.
22. Wang, L.; Liu, J.; Lan, J. *Feature Evaluation of Upper Limb Exercise Rehabilitation Interactive System Based on Kinect*; IEEE Access: Piscataway, NJ, USA, 2019; p. 1.

23. Saini, S.; Rambli, D.; Sulaiman, S.; Zakaria, M.; Shukri, S. A low-cost game framework for a home-based stroke rehabilitation system. In Proceedings of the 2012 International Conference on Computer & Information Science (ICCIS), Kuala Lumpur, Malaysia, 12–14 June 2012.
24. Avola, D.; Foresti, G.; Cinque, L.; Marini, M. An interactive and low-cost full body rehabilitation framework based on 3d immersive serious games. *J. Biomed. Inform.* **2018**, *89*, 81–100. [CrossRef]
25. Cordella, F.; Scotto Di Luzio, F.; Bravi, M.; Santacaterina, F.; Bressi, F.; Zollo, L. Hand motion analysis during robot-aided rehabilitation in chronic stroke. *J. Biol. Regul. Homeost. Agents* **2020**, *34*, 45–52.
26. Airò Farulla, G.; Russo, L.; Indaco, M.; Pianu, D.; Nerino, R.; Chimienti, A.; Cempini, M.; Cortese, M.; Oddo, C.; Vitiello, N. Vision-Based pose estimation for robot-mediated hand telerehabilitation. *Sensors* **2016**, *16*, 208. [CrossRef]
27. Nam, H.; Hong, N.; Cho, M.; Lee, C.; Seo, H.; Kim, S. Vision-Assisted interactive human-in-the-loop distal upper limb rehabilitation robot and its clinical usability test. *Appl. Sci.* **2019**, *9*, 3106. [CrossRef]
28. Zhao, P.; Chen, Z.; Cheng, K.; Teng, Z.; Yang, T.; Qian, X.; Cai, M. A brain cognitive rehabilitation robot system and training method based on hand recognition. *ASME J. Med. Diagn.* **2020**, *3*, 021108.
29. Zhao, P.; Chen, H.; Zhu, H.; Wang, Y.; Zhao, K. A Mechanical Auxiliary Training Equipment for Cognitive Rehabilitation Training and Its Training Method. CN Patent 109346149A, 12 November 2021.
30. Zhao, P.; Ge, Z.; Zhang, Y.; Deng, X.; Guan, H.; Ge, Q. An Immersive Upper Limb Rehabilitation System. CN Patent 113101612A, 13 July 2021.
31. Zhao, P.; Zhang, Y.; Ge, Z.; Deng, X.; Guan, H.; Ge, Q. An Upper Limb Rehabilitation Robot Based on Motion Mapping and Virtual Reality. CN Patent 13101137A, 13 July 2021.
32. Li, R. Near Synchronous Control System and Method for Finger Symmetry Rehabilitation. Master's Thesis, Jiangxi Nanchang University, Nanchang, China, 2020.
33. Liu, H. Research and Implementation of Control System of Flexible Driven Hand Functional Rehabilitation Robot. Master's Thesis, Shanghai Normal University, Shanghai, China, 2020.
34. Wang, J.; Ren, S.; Le, Z.; Guo, X. VR Upper Limb Rehabilitation Training Platform and Method Based on MYO Armband and Mobile Terminal. CN Patent 108815804A, 16 November 2018.
35. Liu, W. Research on Neural Decoding Control of Hand Exoskeleton Rehabilitation Robot. Master's Thesis, Nanjing University of Aeronautics and Astronautics, Nanjing, China, 2020.
36. Cisnal, A.; Perez-Turiel, J.; Fraile, J.; Sierra, D.; De la Fuente, E. RobHand: A hand exoskeleton with real-time EMG-driven embedded control. In *Quantifying Hand Gesture Recognition Delays for Bilateral Rehabilitation*; IEEE Access: Piscataway, NJ, USA, 2021; pp. 137809–137823.
37. Li, K.; Li, Z.; Zeng, H.; Wei, N. Control of newly-designed wearable robotic hand exoskeleton based on surface Electromyographic signals. *Front. Neurorobot.* **2021**, *15*, 711047. [CrossRef]
38. Soekadar, S.; Witkowski, M.; Vitiello, N.; Birbaumer, N. An EEG/EOG-based hybrid brain-neural computer interaction (BNCI) system to control an exoskeleton for the paralyzed hand. *Biomed. Eng. Biomed. Tech.* **2015**, *60*, 99. [CrossRef]
39. Huo, Y. Research on Finger Rehabilitation System Based on Motor Imagination EEG. Master's Thesis, Southeast University, Nanjing, China, 2019.
40. Zhang, J.; Wang, B.; Zhang, C.; Xiao, Y.; Wang, M. An EEG/EMG/EOG-based multimodal human-machine interface to real-time control of a soft robot hand. *Front. Neurorobot.* **2019**, *13*, 7. [CrossRef] [PubMed]
41. Zhang, R.; Li, Y.; He, S.; Yang, X.; Wang, X.; Li, K.; Huang, Q.; Yu, Z.; Zhang, X.; Tang, D. An EOG-based human–machine interface to control a smart home environment for patients with severe spinal cord injuries. *IEEE Trans. Biomed. Eng.* **2019**, *66*, 89–100. [CrossRef] [PubMed]
42. Yap, H.K.; Lim, J.H.; Yap, H.K.; Low, F.Z.; Goh, J.; Yeow, R. MRC-glove: A fMRI compatible soft robotic glove for hand rehabilitation application. In Proceedings of the 2015 IEEE International Conference on Rehabilitation Robotics (ICORR), Nanyang Ave, Singapore, 11–14 August 2015.
43. Rahman, A.; Al-Jumaily, A. Design and development of a bilateral therapeutic hand device for stroke rehabilitation. *Int. J. Adv. Robot. Syst.* **2013**, *10*, 1. [CrossRef]
44. Nilsson, M.; Ingvast, J.; Wikander, J.; Von Holst, H. The soft extra muscle system for improving the grasping capability in neurological rehabilitation. In Proceedings of the 2012 IEEE-EMBS Conference on Biomedical Engineering and Sciences, Langkawi, Malaysia, 17–19 December 2012.
45. Chen, X.; Gong, L.; Wei, L.; Yeh, S.; Da Xu, L.; Zheng, L.; Zou, Z. A wearable hand rehabilitation system with soft gloves. *IEEE Trans. Ind. Inform.* **2021**, *17*, 943–952. [CrossRef]
46. Rakhtala, S.; Ghayebi, R. Real time control and fabrication of a soft robotic glove by two parallel sensors with MBD approach. *Med. Eng. Phys.* **2022**, *100*, 103743. [CrossRef]
47. Chen, W.; Xiong, C.; Yuan, L.; Li, P.; Zhang, Q. A Flexible Exoskeleton Glove System for Hand Rehabilitation Training. CN Patent 107242958A, 24 September 2019.
48. Li, N.; Yang, G.; Zou, Z.; Zheng, L. An Intelligent Assisted Rehabilitation Glove. CN Patent 106618948A, 10 May 2017.
49. Liu, Y.; Cao, G.; Dou, Y.; Zheng, L.; Zhang, X.; Zhi, Y.; Shi, C.; Xu, Z.; Wang, H.; Xie, H.; et al. A Hand Motion Rehabilitation Training and Evaluation System Based on Soft Robot. CN Patent 109276411A, 29 January 2019.

50. Liu, J.; Xia, Q.; Liu, Y.; Zhu, K. Muscle Weakness Finger Function Rehabilitation Training System Based on Multi-Sensor Data Glove. CN Patent 113126763A, 16 July 2021.
51. He, B.; Li, M.; Chen, J.; Guo, W.; Xu, G.; Xie, J. An intensity-modulated fiber optic pressure sensor for hand-exoskeleton interactive force detection. In Proceedings of the 16th International Conference on Ubiquitous Robots, Jeju, Korea, 24–27 June 2019.
52. He, B.; Li, M.; Liang, R.; Liang, Z.; Yao, W.; Sareh, S.; Xie, J.; Xu, G.; Noh, Y. Optoelectronic-based pose sensing for a hand rehabilitation exoskeleton continuous structure. *IEEE Sens. J.* **2022**, *22*, 5606–5615. [CrossRef]
53. Díez, J.; Blanco, A.; Catalán, J.; Badesa, F.; Lledó, L.; García-Aracil, N. Hand exoskeleton for rehabilitation therapies with integrated optical force sensor. *Adv. Mech. Eng.* **2018**, *10*, 168781401775388. [CrossRef]
54. Liu, C. Design of Bidirectional Soft Actuator for Hand Motor Function Rehabilitation. Master's Thesis, Huazhong University of Science and Technology, Wuhan, China, 2019.
55. Zhang, G. Research on Hand and Wrist Joint Integrated Rehabilitation Robot. Master's Thesis, Qingdao University of Science & Technology, Qingdao, China, 2021.
56. Zhang, F. Design of System on Exoskeleton Finger Rehabilitation Robot. Master's Thesis, Nanchang University, Nanchang, China, 2018.
57. Zhang, J. Design and Research of Finger Rehabilitation Robot Based on MYO Control. Master's Thesis, Nanjing University of Posts and Telecommunications, Nanjing, China, 2020.
58. Wu, J. The Research on Upper Limb Rehabilitation Robot and Related Control Problem. Ph.D. Thesis, Huazhong University of Science and Technology, Wuhan, China, 2012.
59. Du, Y.; Zheng, L.; Bai, X.; Yao, W.; Yu, J.; Wu, X.; Xie, P. Adaptive Control Method and Device for Hand Rehabilitation Robot. CN Patent 109718059A, 7 May 2019.
60. Yin, Y. Design of Hand Rehabilitation Robot Control System Based on sEMG Feedback. Master's Thesis, Yanshan University, Qinhuangdao, China, 2020.
61. Wang, X. Control and Experimental Research of Hand Exoskeleton Based on Active Rehabilitation Strategy. Master's Thesis, Harbin Institute of Technology, Harbin, China, 2015.
62. Zhu, X. Design and Implementation of Finger Rehabilitation Training System. Master's Thesis, Zhengzhou University, Zhengzhou, China, 2020.
63. Cao, Y. Design and Implementation of Software for Hand Function Rehabilitation Training Robot. Master's Thesis, Xidian University, Xi'an, China, 2018.
64. Mou, Y.; Yang, L.; Zhang, F.; Fu, Y.; Mou, Y.; Yang, L.; Zhang, F. Design of an interactive system for hand rehabilitation robot. *Mach. Electron.* **2017**, *35*, 4.
65. Zhang, Y. Research and Implementation of Interactive Body Training System. Master's Thesis, Beijing University of Posts and Telecommunications, Beijing, China, 2021.
66. Weekly AI Application Program Selection: Minimally Invasive Surgical Robot; Artificial Intelligence Exoskeleton Rehabilitation Gloves, etc. Available online: https://baijiahao.baidu.com/s?id=1657577869270444052&wfr=spider&for=pc (accessed on 4 February 2020).
67. Tang, X. Scenario Interactive Rehabilitation Training and Evaluation System Based on Cloud Platform. Master's Thesis, Southeast University, Nanjing, China, 2019.
68. Mankins, J.C. Technology readiness assessments: A retrospective. *Acta Astronaut.* **2009**, *65*, 1216–1223. [CrossRef]
69. Smart, A. A multi-dimensional model of clinical utility. *Int. J. Qual. Health Care* **2006**, *18*, 377–382. [CrossRef]

brain sciences

MDPI

Article

Brain Metabolic Connectivity Patterns in Patients with Prolonged Disorder of Consciousness after Hypoxic-Ischemic Injury: A Preliminary Study

Zhijie He [1,†], Rongrong Lu [1,†], Yihui Guan [2], Yi Wu [1], Jingjie Ge [2], Gang Liu [1], Ying Chen [1], Hongyu Xie [1], Junfa Wu [1,*] and Jie Jia [1,3,4,*]

1 Department of Rehabilitation Medicine, Huashan Hospital, Fudan University, Shanghai 200040, China; hezhijie@fudan.edu.cn (Z.H.); 0356213@fudan.edu.cn (R.L.); wuyi4000@163.com (Y.W.); 16111220062@fudan.edu.cn (G.L.); flyriki@126.com (Y.C.); huangdaitian@hotmail.com (H.X.)

2 PET Center, Huashan Hospital, Fudan University, Shanghai 200235, China; guanyihui@hotmail.com (Y.G.); lovejingjie@fudan.edu.cn (J.G.)

3 National Clinical Research Center for Aging and Medicine, Huashan Hospital, Fudan University, Shanghai 200040, China

4 National Center for Neurological Disorders, Shanghai 200040, China

* Correspondence: junfawu2002@aliyun.com (J.W.); shannonjj@126.com (J.J.); Tel.: +86-13585888698 (J.W.); +86-13617722357 (J.J.)

† These authors contributed equally to this work.

Abstract: Understanding the patterns of brain glucose metabolism and connectivity in hypoxic-ischemic encephalopathy (HIE) patients with prolonged disorders of consciousness (DOC) may be of positive significance to the accurate assessment of consciousness and the optimization of neuromodulation strategy. We retrospectively analyzed the brain glucose metabolism pattern and its correlation with clinical Coma Recovery Scale-Revised (CRS-R) score in six HIE patients with prolonged DOC who had undergone ^{18}F-deoxyglucose brain positron emission tomography scanning (FDG-PET). We also compared the differences in global metabolic connectivity patterns and the characteristics of several brain networks between HIE patients and healthy controls (HC). The metabolism of multiple brain regions decreased significantly in HIE patients, and the degree of local metabolic preservation was correlated with CRS-R score. The internal metabolic connectivity of occipital lobe and limbic system in HIE patients decreased, and their metabolic connectivity with frontal lobe, parietal lobe and temporal lobe also decreased. The metabolic connectivity patterns of default mode network, dorsal attention network, salience network, executive control network and subcortex network of HIE also changed compared with HC. The present study suggested that pattern of cerebral glucose metabolism and network connectivity of HIE patients with prolonged DOC were significantly different from those of healthy people.

Keywords: hypoxic ischemic encephalopathy; disorders of consciousness; metabolic connectivity; positron emission tomography; ^{18}F-fluorodeoxyglucose

Citation: He, Z.; Lu, R.; Guan, Y.; Wu, Y.; Ge, J.; Liu, G.; Chen, Y.; Xie, H.; Wu, J.; Jia, J. Brain Metabolic Connectivity Patterns in Patients with Prolonged Disorder of Consciousness after Hypoxic-Ischemic Injury: A Preliminary Study. *Brain Sci.* **2022**, *12*, 892. https://doi.org/10.3390/brainsci12070892

Academic Editors: Sergio Bagnato and Konstantin V. Slavin

Received: 31 May 2022
Accepted: 5 July 2022
Published: 7 July 2022

1. Introduction

Various causes, such as cardiac arrest and asphyxia, lead to brain injury caused by global cerebral ischemia and hypoxia in adults, which can lead to continuous disorders of consciousness (DOC). Behavioral assessment is the first-line assessment to evaluate the degree of DOC in clinical practice. At present, the most commonly used clinical scale with high sensitivity is the Coma Recovery Scale-Revised (CRS-R) [1], which is possible to distinguish between vegetative state/unresponsive arousal syndrome (VS/UWS; presence of eye opening and reflex behavior), minimally conscious state (MCS; showing repeatable but inconsistent conscious behavior, such as command following or visual tracking) and emerging from MCS (EMCS; patients recover the ability to use objects in a functional manner).

However, neurological deficits caused by hypoxic-ischemic encephalopathy (HIE), such as limb paralysis, spasm and blindness, may affect the results of bedside behavioral evaluation of DOC. In clinical practice, we found that even in VS patients, some still retained emotional response adapted to the external environment, which is not included in the evaluation of CRS-R. Through neuroimaging studies based on specific tasks, Owen AM et al. [2] and Monti MM et al. [3] suggested that even patients with VS may still have a certain degree of cortical activity. Schiff ND et al. [4] defined these DOC patients who were unable to respond to external instructions but still had reactive cortical activity as experiencing "cognitive motor dissociation" (CMD). Thibaut A et al. [5] introduced the concept of "non-behavioral MCS" (MCS star) and diagnosed DOC patients with behavioral evaluation as VS but with brain glucose metabolism preservation, indicated by Positron emission tomography (PET) imaging as MCS star. Compared with VS patients with poor brain glucose metabolism preservation indicated by PET imaging, MCS star patients may have better prognosis.

A number of neuroimaging and electrophysiological studies have shown that the structural and functional connections between bilateral frontal parietal lobe and cingulate cortex in patients with DOC have decreased [6,7], and these brain regions are closely related to arousal and consciousness [8]. The default mode network (DMN) is mainly composed of medial prefrontal cortex, anterior cingulate gyrus, posterior cingulate gyrus, precuneus and bilateral inferior parietal lobules. The functional activity of DMN in patients with DOC is significantly reduced [9]. fMRI studies suggested that the low frequency fluctuations and regional voxel homogeneity of various brain regions in DMN of patients with DOC were reduced [10], while the functional connectivity of DMN is associated with the level of consciousness [11–13]. The connection between medial prefrontal lobe and posterior cingulate gyrus may be related to the prognosis of DOC [14]. In addition, the functional disconnection between cortex and subcortical is also considered to be one of the biological mechanisms of DOC [15]. Patients with DOC have interruption and disorder of the effective connectivity between the left striatum and bilateral precuneus, cingulate gyrus and left middle frontal gyrus [16]. The thalamus is also an important subcortical nucleus for consciousness maintenance. The functional connectivity between medial thalamic nucleus, prefrontal lobe and anterior cingulate gyrus in VS patients decreased significantly [17].

In recent years, various brain stimulation technologies have been explored and applied to enhance the recovery of DOC patients. For example, transcranial pulsed-current stimulation of the prefrontal lobe may enhance local brain functional connection [18]; the treatment of invasive low-intensity focused ultrasound (LIFU) on the thalamus could improve the behavior of patients with DOC, and a functional magnetic resonance imaging (fMRI) study suggested that LIFU can improve the functional connection of the thalamus [19]; meta-analysis showed that deep brain stimulation (DBS) treatment may improve the CRS-R score of DOC patients in some studies, but there was diversity in the targets and parameters of DBS [20]. Therefore, understanding the brain network model of patients with persistent disorders of consciousness after cerebral ischemia and hypoxia may be of positive significance for selecting more appropriate and accurate stimulation targets and neural regulation strategies in the future.

PET imaging is safe, comfortable, and atraumatic and is currently the only imaging technique that can quantitatively evaluate biochemical alterations in vivo, accurately reflecting the biology of the lesion. The present study retrospectively analyzed six DOC patients with hypoxic-ischemic brain injury who underwent brain ^{18}F-deoxyglucose PET scanning in our center, and analyzed the brain glucose metabolism pattern of these HIE patients as well as their correlation with CRS-R score. We also compared the differences in brain metabolic connectivity patterns between HIE patients and healthy subjects, as well as the metabolic connectivity characteristics of major brain networks in HIE patients.

2. Materials and Methods

2.1. Participants

Six patients hospitalized in the Department of Rehabilitation Medicine of Huashan Hospital, affiliated to Fudan University, Shanghai, China, and diagnosed with hypoxic-ischemic encephalopathy (HIE) were included in this study (male/female, 3/3; age, 45.83 ± 16.23 years). The causes of cerebral hypoxia ischemia in these HIE patients were cardiac arrest in 2 cases, anesthesia accident in abdominal surgery in 2 cases, massive bleeding of gastric cancer in 1 case (no evidence of tumor intracranial metastasis) and asphyxia due to food choking in 1 case. All of them had prolonged disorder of consciousness (DOC) after rescue. The average duration of DOC was 20.83 ± 8.93 weeks at the time of PET scanning. The state of consciousness of these HIE patients was assessed according to the Coma Recovery Scale-Revised Version (Chinese version) (CRS-R) [21,22], which was completed by two experienced neurorehabilitation experts according to the standard process of CRS-R [22]. We adopted the highest CRS-R score within 1 week before and after the time of PET scan. Among them, 5 cases were VS and 1 case was MCS. The clinical information and CRS-R assessments of HIE patients are listed in Table 1. In addition, we included 18 gender and age matched healthy people as the healthy control (HC) group. The demographic information is listed in Table 2. All subjects are right-handed. The study was approved by the Ethics Committee of Huashan Hospital and was conducted in accordance with the tenets of the Declaration of Helsinki.

Table 1. Patients with HIE.

Patient No.	Gender	Age (yrs)	Time Since HIE Onset (Weeks)	Cause of HIE	Level of DOC	Total CRS-R Score
1	M	17	29	Cardiac arrest	VS	6
2	F	50	13	Anesthesia accident	VS	5
3	F	39	16	Anesthesia accident	VS	4
4	M	57	27	Massive hemorrhage [a]	VS	7
5	M	63	32	Chocking	VS	5
6	F	49	8	Cardiac arrest	MCS	10

HIE, hypoxic-ischemic encephalopathy. DOC, disorder of consciousness. CRS-R, coma recovery scale-revised version. M, male. F, female. VS, vegetative state. MCS, minimally conscious state. [a] Patient 4 had a history of gastric cancer, but there was no evidence of intracranial metastasis.

Table 2. Demographic data.

	HIE (n = 6)	HC (n = 18)	p Value
Gender (M/F)	3/3	9/9	$p > 0.05$
Age (yrs)	45.83 ± 16.23	52.67 ± 2.28	$p > 0.05$
Handedness (R/L)	6/0	18/0	$p > 0.05$

HIE, hypoxic-ischemic encephalopathy. HC, healthy control. M, male. F, female. L, left. R, right.

2.2. FDG PET Scanning

All subjects were asked to fast for at least 6 h, but had free access to water before PET imaging. PET scans were performed with a United Imaging uMI510 PET/CT (United Imaging, Shanghai, China) in three-dimensional (3D) mode. A CT transmission scan was first performed for attenuation correction. The emission scan was acquired between 60–70 min after intravenous injection of 185 MBq of ^{18}F-fluorodeoxyglucose. The imaging data was digitally registered onto a computer disk to create the sectional images of a patient's brain [23]. As no arterial blood sampling was taken in this clinical imaging protocol, we used radioactivity images to measure changes in relative regional glucose metabolism. All studies in patients and normal individuals were performed in a resting state in a quiet and dimly lit room. All patients and normal individuals were monitored via cameras during the course of uptake and scanning procedure.

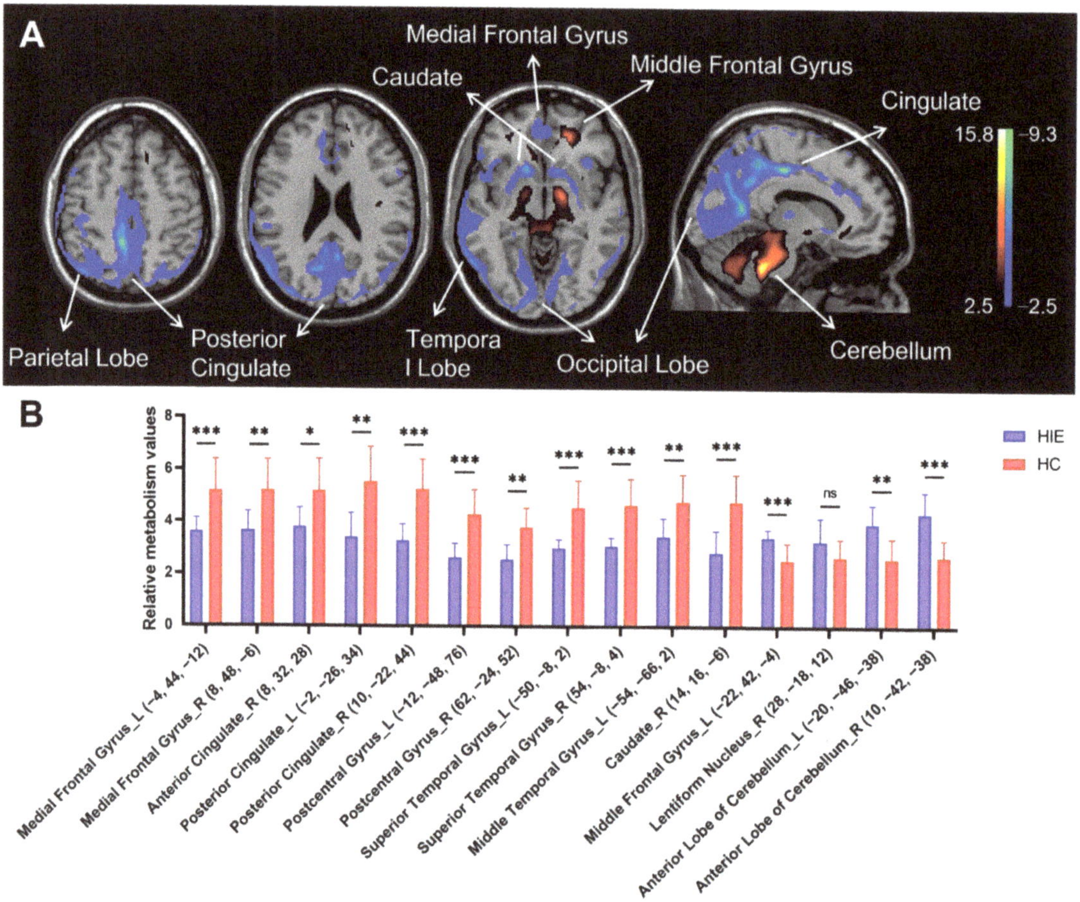

Figure 1. Brain regions with relative abnormal metabolism in patients with hypoxic ischemic encephalopathy (HIE) presenting with disorders of consciousness (DOC). (**A**) Normalized glucose metabolism in the HIE patients decreased (blue) bilaterally in the medial frontal gyrus, posterior cingulate gyrus (extending to parietal-occipital lobe), postcentral gyrus and superior temporal gyrus, and in the right anterior cingulate gyrus and right caudate nucleus, but increased (red) in bilateral anterior cerebellar lobe and left middle frontal gyrus and right lentiform nucleus relative to the healthy controls (HC). The overlays are depicted in neurologic orientation. The gray-scale image is a T1-weighted structural magnetic resonance imaging (MRI) that is representative of Montreal Neurological Institute (MNI) space. The thresholds of the color bars represent T values. (**B**) Differences in regional glucose metabolism in the HIE patients and HC subjects illustrated by post hoc values obtained within a spherical volume of interest (VOI) (3 mm radius) with the center coordinates of each VOI given in the parentheses. The graphs showed the relative metabolic value decreases in the bilateral medial frontal gyrus, posterior cingulate gyrus, postcentral gyrus and superior temporal gyrus, and right anterior cingulate gyrus and right caudate nucleus, while the relative metabolic value increases in bilateral anterior cerebellar lobe and left middle frontal gyrus. The error bars represent standard deviation. ns, no statistical difference. HIE, hypoxic ischemic encephalopathy. HC, healthy control. L, left. R, right. *, $p < 0.05$. **, $p < 0.01$, ***, $p < 0.001$.

Figure 1B shows the differences in relative metabolism values between the HIE and HC groups in the major functional regions (see Figure 1A). The decreased metabolic values in the spherical volume of interests (VOI) centered at the bilateral medial frontal gyrus, posterior cingulate gyrus, postcentral gyrus and superior temporal gyrus, and right anterior cingulate gyrus and right caudate nucleus displayed significant group differences between HIE and healthy individuals ($p < 0.01$, except for the right anterior cingulate gyrus where $p < 0.05$). The increased metabolic value in the VOIs centered at the bilateral anterior cerebellar lobe and left middle frontal gyrus also showed significant group discrimination between patients and controls ($p < 0.01$). There was a trend toward significance in the metabolic value in the VOIs centered at the right lentiform nuclei in the HIE group compared with the HC group ($p = 0.106$).

3.2. Correlation of Consciousness Level with Relative Brain Activity in Patients with HIE

The regression analysis yielded a positive correlation of CRS-R score in HIE patients with metabolic activity bilaterally in the medial frontal gyrus, middle frontal gyrus, anterior cingulate, and caudate, and in the left superior frontal gyrus, left inferior frontal gyrus and right tuber of cerebellum. In contrast, CRS-R correlated negatively with metabolic activity in the left lingual gyrus. (Figure 2A and Table 4). The sample plots for the six major regions from the regression analysis (see Figure 2A) are given in Figure 2B–G. The CRS-R score correlated significantly with relative metabolic values in the right medial frontal gyrus (r = 0.969, $p = 0.002$), left superior frontal gyrus (r = 0.875, $p = 0.023$), right middle frontal gyrus (r = 0.862, $p = 0.027$), left caudate (r = 0.857, $p = 0.029$), right caudate (r = 0.975, $p < 0.001$), and right tuber of cerebellum (r = 0.977, $p < 0.001$).

Table 4. Brain regions correlated with total CRS-R score in patient with HIE.

Structure	Broadmann Area	L/R	MNI Coordinates [a]			Z_{max}	Cluster Size (mm^3)
			x	y	z		
Positive [b]							
Medial Frontal Gyrus [c]	9	L	0	50	26	3.48	104
Anterior Cingulate	32	L	0	40	26	2.79	
Medial Frontal Gyrus	9	R	6	52	2	2.43	5
Anterior Cingulate	32	R	4	32	26	2.44	3
Superior Frontal Gyrus	10	L	−34	60	0	2.84	30
Middle Frontal Gyrus	10	L	−26	52	26	2.7	12
Middle Frontal Gyrus	10	R	40	58	4	2.47	6
Inferior Frontal Gyrus [c]	47	L	−30	32	−20	3.39	82
Caudate	Caudate Head	L	−8	6	−4	2.93	22
Caudate	Caudate Head	R	12	18	−8	2.45	11
Tuber	Cerebellum	R	20	−90	−38	2.83	42
Negative [b]							
Lingual Gyrus	17	L	−14	−86	−6	2.75	113

MNI, Montreal Neurological Institute. L, left. R, right. [a], MNI standard space. [b], Survived at uncorrected $p < 0.01$. [c], Survived at uncorrected $p < 0.001$.

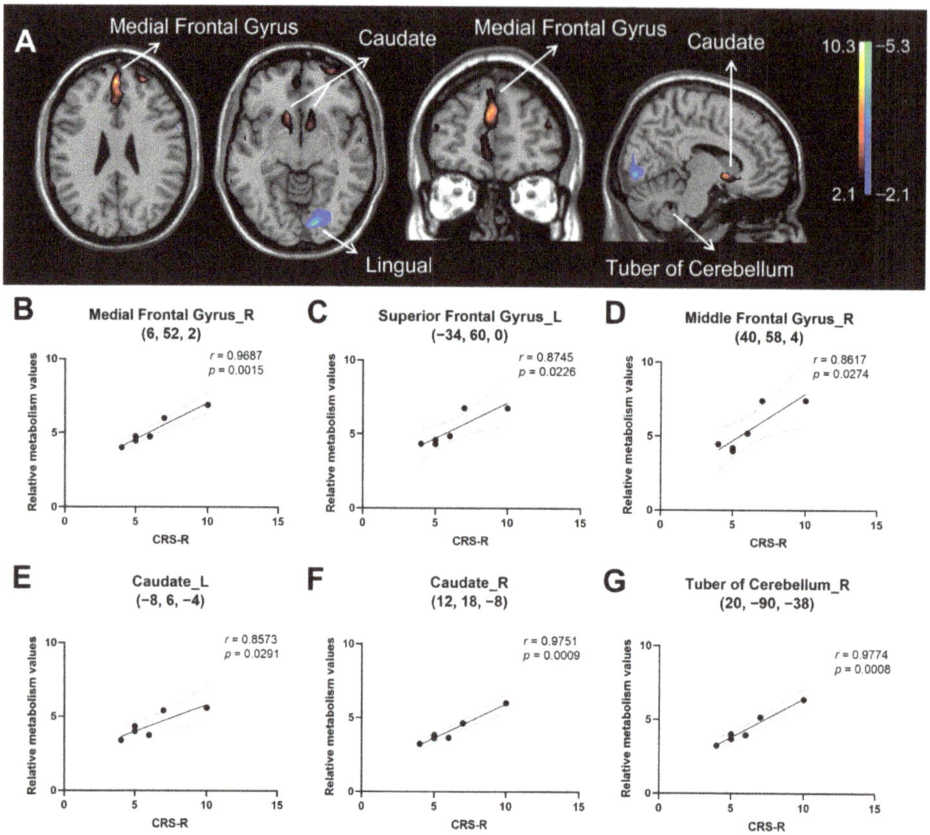

Figure 2. Brain regions correlated with Coma Recovery Scale-Revised (CRS-R) score in hypoxic ischemic encephalopathy (HIE) patients presenting with disorders of consciousness (DOC). (**A**) Regions with positive correlation (red) were observed bilaterally in the medial frontal gyrus, middle frontal gyrus, anterior cingulate and caudate, and in the left superior frontal gyrus, left inferior frontal gyrus and right tuber of cerebellum, whereas those with negative correlation (blue) were found in the left lingual gyrus. The overlays are depicted in neurologic orientation. The gray-scale image is a T1-weighted structural magnetic resonance imaging (MRI) that is representative of Montreal Neurological Institute (MNI) space. The thresholds of the color bars represent T values. (**B–G**) Correlation between relative metabolic values and CRS-R score the right medial frontal gyrus. Dotted lines represent 95% confidence bands of the best-fit line. (**B**), left superior frontal gyrus (**C**), right middle frontal gyrus (**D**), left caudate (**E**), right caudate (**F**), right tuber cerebellum (**G**). The metabolic values were obtained post hoc within a spherical volume of interest (VOI) (3 mm radius) with the center coordinates of each VOI given in the parentheses on each panel. L, left. R, right. CRS-R, coma recovery scale—revised version.

3.3. *Metabolic Connectivity*

The metabolic connectivity matrixes of HIE and HC groups are shown in Figure 3. Compared with the HC group, the global metabolic connectivity decreased in the HIE group. Within each anatomical partition, the internal metabolic connections of frontal, parietal, temporal, and basal ganglia decreased in the HIE group compared with the HC group, but with some degree of preservation remained. In the HIE group, the internal metabolic connections were weakened in the occipital lobe and limbic system, whereas they were enhanced in the cerebellum hemispheres and cerebellum vermis. The metabolic connectivity of the occipital lobe, limbic system, and basal ganglia with other brain regions was reduced in the HIE group compared with the HC group, whereas the cerebellum showed enhanced metabolic connectivity with the frontal, temporal, and occipital lobes.

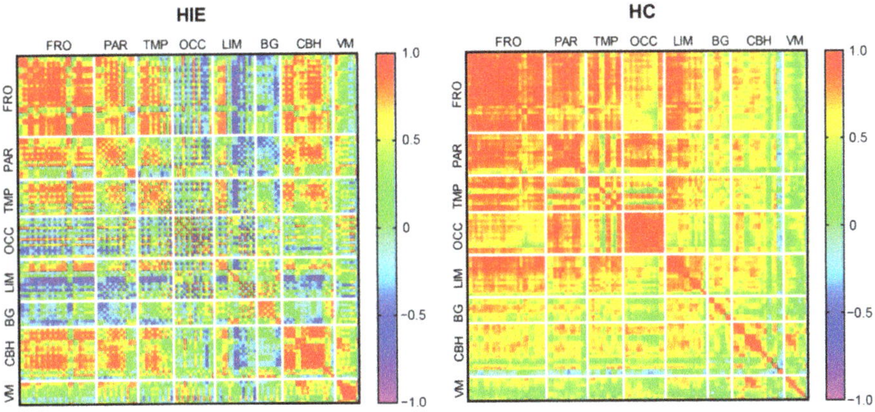

Figure 3. Global metabolic connectivity matrix. Colors in the metabolic connectivity matrix represent the magnitude of the correlation and colors are arranged as a rainbow color from red to purple according to the magnitude of the correlation from positive to negative. HIE, hypoxic ischemic encephalopathy. HC, healthy control. FRO, frontal cortex. PAR, parietal cortex. TMP, temporal cortex. OCC, occipital cortex. LIM, limbic structures. BG, basal ganglia. CBH, cerebellum hemisphere. VM, vermis of cerebellum.

3.4. Brain Network Metabolic Connectivity Patterns

Figure 4A–E demonstrate the metabolic connectivity among the brain regions related to the default mode network (DMN), salience network (SN), dorsal attention network (DAN), executive control network (ECN) and subcortex network in AAL template. In the HIE group, the metabolic connectivity of the bilateral posterior cingulate gyrus with other nodes within the DMN decreased, as did the connectivity of the bilateral precuneus and left angular gyrus with other nodes within the network (Figure 4A). In the SN, the metabolic connectivity of the bilateral insula and left anterior cingulate with other nodes within the network decreased in the HIE group (Figure 4B). In the DAN, the metabolic connectivity between brain regions within both hemispheres were preserved in the HIE group, but the interhemispheric metabolic connections between bilateral superior parietal gyrus, inferior parietal gyrus, supramarginal gyrus, and angular gyrus decreased in the HIE group compared with the HC group (Figure 4C). Similarly, in the ECN, the cross hemispheric metabolic connectivity between the nodes of bilateral parietal lobe in HIE patients decreased, and the metabolic connectivity between the nodes of right frontal lobe and left parietal lobe decreased, but the metabolic connectivity between the nodes of left frontal lobe and right parietal lobe was preserved in the HIE group. Figure 4D). In the subcortex network, the metabolic correlations between the caudate nucleus, putamen, and globus pallidus were enhanced in the HIE group compared with the HC group (Figure 4E). However, there was decreased metabolic correlation between the bilateral hippocampus and amygdala and decreased metabolic connectivity with the contralateral caudate nucleus, putamen, and globus pallidus, respectively, in the HIE group (Figure 4E). Metabolic connectivity between the bilateral thalamus and caudate nucleus was also decreased in HIE patients (Figure 4E).

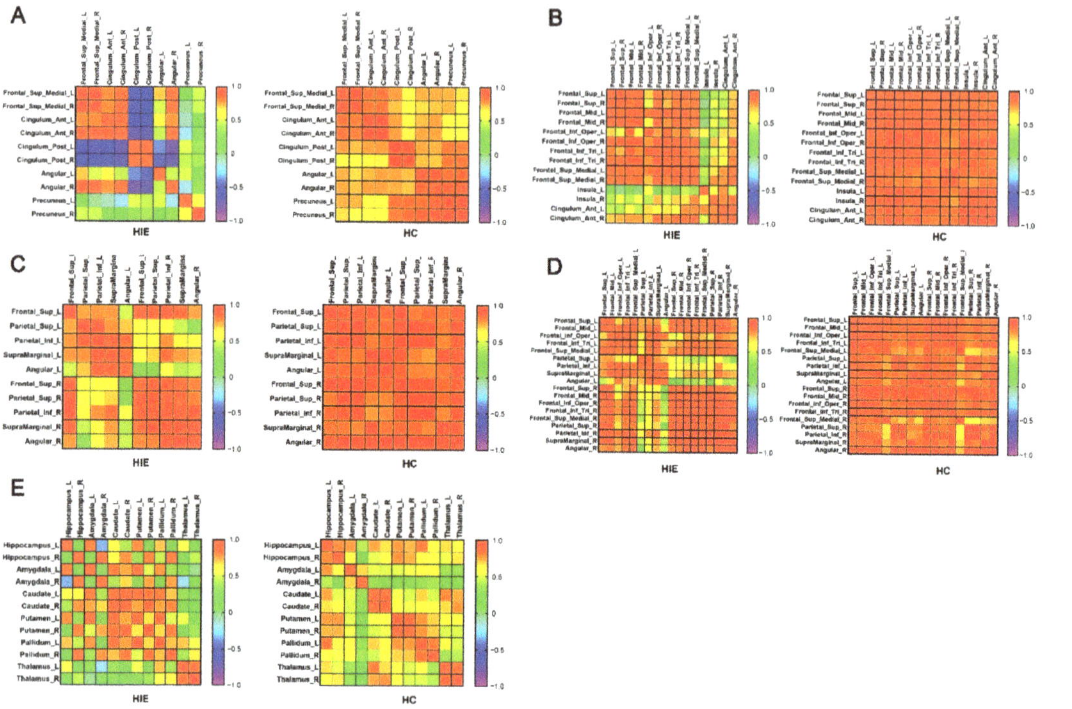

Figure 4. Metabolic connectivity matrix between brain regions associated with different brain networks in the AAL template. (**A**) default mode network (DMN) (**B**) salience network (SN) (**C**) dorsal attention network (DAN) (**D**) executive control network (ECN) (**E**) subcortex network. Colors in the metabolic connectivity matrix represent the magnitude of the correlation and colors are arranged as a rainbow color from red to purple according to the magnitude of the correlation from positive to negative. HIE, hypoxic ischemic encephalopathy. HC, healthy control. L, left. R, right.

4. Discussion

In the present study, we retrospectively analyzed the FDG-PET brain images and clinical information of six patients with hypoxic-ischemic encephalopathy with persistent DOC, and compared and analyzed the characteristics of brain metabolism in HIE patients with healthy people and the correlation between brain metabolism and the evaluation of clinical consciousness level; We also constructed the metabolic connection matrix between HIE patients and healthy people, and compared the brain metabolic connection patterns and characteristics between HIE patients with DOC and healthy people; finally, we analyzed several currently recognized brain networks of HIE patients, and discussed the connectivity mode of key nodes in the brain network of DOC patients.

Our observation of decreased metabolism in the frontal lobe and cingulate gyrus in HIE patients with the presence of DOC and the correlation between the degree of local metabolic preservation and CRS-R scores are similar to the results of previous studies on brain metabolism pattern in DOC patients [34–37]. Through the whole brain functional connectivity analysis by anatomical partition, we found that the internal metabolic connectivity in the frontal, parietal, and temporal lobes of HIE patients, although decreased compared with healthy individuals, were still preserved to some extent compared with other brain regions. However, the more pronounced decrease in metabolic connectivity of the frontal, parietal, and temporal lobes with the occipital and limbic systems in HIE suggests that cognitive processes in these patients may not be in interface with visual input and there might be a dyscoordination of sensory input to motor output from the limbs, but the processing ability of auditory input might be relatively preserved in this subset of patients. This may correspond to the "cognitive motor dissociation" (CMD) [4] or "higher-order cortex motor dissociation" (HMD) [38], as described in previous studies. In clinical practice, we also found that some VS patients had affective reactions that were compatible with the surrounding context, but this partial functional preservation in DOC patients could not be reflected in CRS-R scores. Visual and motor function partial rating items, which corresponded with the behavioral performance of MCS in the CRS-R score, both related to visual perceptual abilities. Therefore, the CRS-R score may not fully describe the level of consciousness in this subset of DOC patients with partially preserved prefrontal cortical function but with a loss of liaison between the frontal and occipital lobes. Clinical evaluation of such patients may also need to incorporate task-related imaging or electrophysiological tests such as fMRI, PET and EEG, etc., and further studies were needed to investigate the prognostic differences between such patients and VS patients without affective reactions.

In terms of several major brain networks of the cortex, we observed a significant loss of connectivity of the bilateral posterior cingulate and precuneus with bilateral medial prefrontal lobes in the DMN of HIE group, which is similar to previous findings of functional connectivity [39–42] and suggests an important role of the precuneus and posterior cingulate in the maintenance of consciousness. We also observed that there were metabolic negative correlations between posterior cingulate and medial prefrontal, suggesting a potential mutual inhibitory interaction between them. We were also able to see a trans-hemispheric loss of contact in the angular gyrus and precuneus, and the same phenomenon with the DAN, especially at various nodes located in the parietal lobe, suggesting a decreased contact between the bilateral parietal lobes in HIE group, which may be related to the decreased higher-order sensory integration in response to environmental stimuli in DOC patients [43]. The connectivity between the frontal and parietal lobes is also closely related to the maintenance of the level of consciousness [44]. In the ECN, we found that the metabolic connectivity between each node of the right frontal lobe and the left parietal lobe decreased in the HIE group, whereas the metabolic connectivity between each node of the left frontal lobe and the right parietal lobe was instead preserved, and the laterality of frontoparietal functions in DOC patients needs further studies for validation and mechanistic exploration. Recent studies have suggested that non-invasive neuromodulation techniques, mainly applied to the prefrontal lobe, may improve local cortical excitability and functional connectivity [18,45], but evidence for their efficacy on the improvement of consciousness levels was insufficient. We speculated whether the optimization of stimulation site and parameters could be performed according to the abnormal metabolic connectivity pattern of frontoparietal network in DOC patients. In addition, we found decreased metabolic connectivity between bilateral insula and various nodes of the prefrontal lobe in the SN of the HIE group. Various sensory stimuli evoke excitation in the insula, an important brain region for overall perception of the forming external environment and intrinsic self-experience [46]. After propofol anesthesia in healthy people, anterior insular function was depressed, which in turn affected the dynamic conversion of the DMN to the DAN [47]. We speculated that the insula might also serve as one of the potential targets of neuromodulation in DOC patients.

Recently, an increasing number of studies have focused on the functional connectivity between subcortical structures, as well as between cortical brain regions, in DOC patients, and a series of clinical investigations with DBS of subcortical structures in DOC patients has been performed. Our results suggested that patients with HIE who present with DOC had hypometabolism in the caudate nucleus and that the degree of hypometabolism in the bilateral caudate nucleus was significantly correlated with the level of consciousness. Metabolic connectivity analysis of subcortex networks suggested enhanced connectivity between various nuclei within the bilateral striatum, while metabolic connectivity between other subcortical structures of the thalamus was decreased. The striatum of DOC patients may have reduced inhibition of the globus pallidus, which may then lead to hyperexcitability of the globus pallidus and, subsequently, increased inhibition of the thalamus [48,49]. In addition, intracranial EEG studies have revealed that the ventral striatum may be involved in the regulation of cortical information flow, which makes it an important part of the experience of conscious perception [50]. It was also believed that the integration of the parietal lobe with striatum and thalamus contributed more than the frontal cortex in the maintenance of consciousness [15], and the metabolic connectivity matrix in our results also showed decreased connectivity between basal ganglia and frontoparietal cortex in the HIE group. Nonhuman primate studies suggested that neurons in the deep layers of the thalamus and cortex were most sensitive to changes in the level of consciousness, stimulation of the thalamus restored wakefulness in anesthetized macaques [51], and DBS to different parts of the thalamus increases both the level of arousal and self-awareness [52], suggesting that the thalamus was one of the important targets for DBS therapy in patients with DOC.

Clearly, the present study still has some limitations. First, although the included patients were all DOC patients after HIE occurrence, the sample size was indeed small. Although there were significant differences in cerebral glucose metabolic and metabolic connectivity in the HIE group compared to the healthy participants, we could no longer perform further subgroup analyses to explore the cerebral metabolic patterns and correlations with clinical scores in the VS and MCS patients. Second, in terms of PET brain imaging processing, we chose the pons as a reference for normalization of whole brain metabolic values, but also lost information on pons metabolism; moreover, there is currently no evidence that pons metabolism is not different in DOC patients compared with healthy individuals. It is possible that in future studies we could choose radioactivity counts at other sites for normalization, such as the soft tissue under the scalp, or perform simultaneous arterial blood collection and radioactivity count measurements with PET scan. Third, the results of the brain metabolic connectivity analysis of the population, which cannot represent the metabolic connectivity of individuals, were not statistically analyzed in intergroup comparisons. We performed the brain metabolic connectivity versus brain network analysis when adopting an anatomical structure based partitioning approach with a relatively small number of nodes. In further studies, we would continue to increase the sample size, as well as conduct long-term follow-up of cases to explore the association of cerebral metabolic patterns and prognosis, and perform subgroup analysis and comparison of VS and MCS; in terms of data correction, we would attempt to acquire subject blood samples for absolute value quantification of radioactivity counts, to reduce data correction bias; we would also apply PET combined with resting-state fMRI and EEG for multimodal measures of brain functional connectivity to compensate for the relative lack of temporal and spatial resolution.

5. Conclusions

Through PET imaging analysis of HIE patients with prolonged DOC, the present study found that patients with HIE had decreased metabolism in the frontal lobe and cingulate gyrus, and that the degree of local metabolic preservation may have a correlation with level of consciousness; the internal metabolic connections in the frontal, parietal, and temporal lobes of HIE patients were to some extent preserved compared to healthy individuals. However, there was a significant decrease in metabolic connectivity of the frontal, parietal, and temporal lobes with the occipital and limbic systems in HIE. There may be abnormal network connectivity patterns in HIE patients in several major brain networks. In the DMN, there was a significant loss of connectivity of the bilateral posterior cingulate and precuneus with bilateral medial prefrontal lobes in patients with HIE, and in the DAN and ECN there was a decline in connectivity between each node in the bilateral parietal lobes in patients with HIE, as well as a decline in metabolic connectivity between each node in the right frontal lobe and the left parietal lobe. Patients with HIE have reduced metabolic connectivity between the bilateral insula and various nodes of the prefrontal lobe in the SN. Patients with HIE may also present with dysconnectivity in subcortex structures, as well as cortico-subcortex dysconnectivity. HIE patients have hypometabolism in the caudate nucleus, and the degree of hypometabolism in the bilateral caudate nucleus correlates significantly with the level of consciousness score. Metabolic connectivity analysis of subcortical networks suggests enhanced functional connectivity between various nuclei within the bilateral striatum, but decreased metabolic connectivity of the thalamus with the other subcortical structures. The HIE group showed decreased connectivity between the basal ganglia and the parietal cortex.

Author Contributions: Conceptualization, Z.H., R.L., J.W. and J.J.; methodology, Z.H., Y.G. and J.G.; validation, Y.G., Y.W., J.W. and J.J.; formal analysis, Z.H., R.L. and J.G.; investigation, Z.H., R.L., J.W., G.L., Y.C. and H.X.; resources, Y.G., J.W., Y.W. and J.J.; data curation, R.L. and J.W.; writing—original draft preparation, Z.H. and R.L.; writing—review and editing, Z.H., R.L., Y.G., Y.W., J.G., J.W. and J.J.; visualization, Z.H., R.L. and J.G.; supervision, Y.G., Y.W. and J.J.; project administration, J.W. and J.J.; funding acquisition, J.J. All authors have read and agreed to the published version of the manuscript.

Funding: This research was funded by the National Key Research & Development Program of China (grant numbers 2018YFC2002300 and 2018YFC2002301) and the National Natural Science Foundation of China (grant numbers 81702229, 81902280 and 81972140).

Institutional Review Board Statement: The study was conducted in accordance with the Declaration of Helsinki, and approved by the ethics committee of Huashan Hospital, Fudan University (protocol code ChiCTR2200060243 and date of approval 18 May 2022).

Informed Consent Statement: Informed consent was obtained from all subjects involved in the study or their legal representatives involved in the study. Written or electronic informed consent has been obtained from all the subjects or their legal representatives to publish this paper.

Data Availability Statement: Not applicable.

Acknowledgments: We wish to express our gratitude to the participants and their families in this study.

Conflicts of Interest: The authors declare no conflict of interest.

References

1. Seel, R.T.; Sherer, M.; Whyte, J.; Katz, D.I.; Giacino, J.T.; Rosenbaum, A.M.; Hammond, F.M.; Kalmar, K.; Pape, T.L.; Zafonte, R.; et al. Assessment scales for disorders of consciousness: Evidence-based recommendations for clinical practice and research. *Arch. Phys. Med. Rehabil.* **2010**, *91*, 1795–1813. [CrossRef] [PubMed]
2. Owen, A.M.; Coleman, M.R.; Boly, M.; Davis, M.H.; Laureys, S.; Pickard, J.D. Detecting awareness in the vegetative state. *Science* **2006**, *313*, 1402. [CrossRef] [PubMed]
3. Monti, M.M.; Vanhaudenhuyse, A.; Coleman, M.R.; Boly, M.; Pickard, J.D.; Tshibanda, L.; Owen, A.M.; Laureys, S. Willful modulation of brain activity in disorders of consciousness. *N. Engl. J. Med.* **2010**, *362*, 579–589. [CrossRef] [PubMed]
4. Schiff, N.D. Cognitive Motor Dissociation Following Severe Brain Injuries. *JAMA Neurol.* **2015**, *72*, 1413–1415. [CrossRef] [PubMed]
5. Thibaut, A.; Panda, R.; Annen, J.; Sanz, L.; Naccache, L.; Martial, C.; Chatelle, C.; Aubinet, C.; Bonin, E.; Barra, A.; et al. Preservation of Brain Activity in Unresponsive Patients Identifies MCS Star. *Ann. Neurol.* **2021**, *90*, 89–100. [CrossRef]
6. Bodart, O.; Gosseries, O.; Wannez, S.; Thibaut, A.; Annen, J.; Boly, M.; Rosanova, M.; Casali, A.G.; Casarotto, S.; Tononi, G.; et al. Measures of metabolism and complexity in the brain of patients with disorders of consciousness. *Neuroimage Clin.* **2017**, *14*, 354–362. [CrossRef]
7. Massimini, M.; Ferrarelli, F.; Sarasso, S.; Tononi, G. Cortical mechanisms of loss of consciousness: Insight from TMS/EEG studies. *Arch. Ital. Biol.* **2012**, *150*, 44–55. [CrossRef]
8. Zeman, A. Consciousness. *Brain* **2001**, *124*, 1263–1289. [CrossRef]
9. Hannawi, Y.; Lindquist, M.A.; Caffo, B.S.; Sair, H.I.; Stevens, R.D. Resting brain activity in disorders of consciousness: A systematic review and meta-analysis. *Neurology* **2015**, *84*, 1272–1280. [CrossRef]
10. Tsai, Y.H.; Yuan, R.; Huang, Y.C.; Yeh, M.Y.; Lin, C.P.; Biswal, B.B. Disruption of brain connectivity in acute stroke patients with early impairment in consciousness. *Front. Psychol.* **2014**, *4*, 956. [CrossRef]
11. Vanhaudenhuyse, A.; Noirhomme, Q.; Tshibanda, L.J.; Bruno, M.A.; Boveroux, P.; Schnakers, C.; Soddu, A.; Perlbarg, V.; Ledoux, D.; Brichant, J.F.; et al. Default network connectivity reflects the level of consciousness in non-communicative brain-damaged patients. *Brain* **2010**, *133*, 161–171. [CrossRef]
12. Norton, L.; Hutchison, R.M.; Young, G.B.; Lee, D.H.; Sharpe, M.D.; Mirsattari, S.M. Disruptions of functional connectivity in the default mode network of comatose patients. *Neurology* **2012**, *78*, 175–181. [CrossRef]

13. Demertzi, A.; Gomez, F.; Crone, J.S.; Vanhaudenhuyse, A.; Tshibanda, L.; Noirhomme, Q.; Thonnard, M.; Charland-Verville, V.; Kirsch, M.; Laureys, S.; et al. Multiple fMRI system-level baseline connectivity is disrupted in patients with consciousness alterations. *Cortex* **2014**, *52*, 35–46. [CrossRef]
14. Silva, S.; de Pasquale, F.; Vuillaume, C.; Riu, B.; Loubinoux, I.; Geeraerts, T.; Seguin, T.; Bounes, V.; Fourcade, O.; Demonet, J.F.; et al. Disruption of posteromedial large-scale neural communication predicts recovery from coma. *Neurology* **2015**, *85*, 2036–2044. [CrossRef]
15. Afrasiabi, M.; Redinbaugh, M.J.; Phillips, J.M.; Kambi, N.A.; Mohanta, S.; Raz, A.; Haun, A.M.; Saalmann, Y.B. Consciousness depends on integration between parietal cortex, striatum, and thalamus. *Cell Syst.* **2021**, *12*, 363–373. [CrossRef]
16. Chen, L.; Rao, B.; Li, S.; Gao, L.; Xie, Y.; Dai, X.; Fu, K.; Peng, X.Z.; Xu, H. Altered Effective Connectivity Measured by Resting-State Functional Magnetic Resonance Imaging in Posterior Parietal-Frontal-Striatum Circuit in Patients with Disorder of Consciousness. *Front. Neurosci.* **2021**, *15*, 766633. [CrossRef]
17. Laureys, S.; Faymonville, M.E.; Luxen, A.; Lamy, M.; Franck, G.; Maquet, P. Restoration of thalamocortical connectivity after recovery from persistent vegetative state. *Lancet* **2000**, *355*, 1790–1791. [CrossRef]
18. Barra, A.; Rosenfelder, M.; Mortaheb, S.; Carriere, M.; Martens, G.; Bodien, Y.G.; Morales-Quezada, L.; Bender, A.; Laureys, S.; Thibaut, A.; et al. Transcranial Pulsed-Current Stimulation versus Transcranial Direct Current Stimulation in Patients with Disorders of Consciousness: A Pilot, Sham-Controlled Cross-Over Double-Blind Study. *Brain Sci.* **2022**, *12*, 429. [CrossRef]
19. Cain, J.A.; Spivak, N.M.; Coetzee, J.P.; Crone, J.S.; Johnson, M.A.; Lutkenhoff, E.S.; Real, C.; Buitrago-Blanco, M.; Vespa, P.M.; Schnakers, C.; et al. Ultrasonic Deep Brain Neuromodulation in Acute Disorders of Consciousness: A Proof-of-Concept. *Brain Sci.* **2022**, *12*, 428. [CrossRef]
20. Rezaei, H.A.; Lythe, V.; Green, A.L. Deep Brain Stimulation for Recovery of Consciousness in Minimally Conscious Patients After Traumatic Brain Injury: A Systematic Review. *Neuromodulation* **2019**, *22*, 373–379. [CrossRef]
21. Zhang, Y.; Wang, J.; Schnakers, C.; He, M.; Luo, H.; Cheng, L.; Wang, F.; Nie, Y.; Huang, W.; Hu, X.; et al. Validation of the Chinese version of the Coma Recovery Scale-Revised (CRS-R). *Brain Inj.* **2019**, *33*, 529–533. [CrossRef] [PubMed]
22. Di, H.; He, M.; Zhang, Y.; Cheng, L.; Wang, F.; Nie, Y.; Huang, W.; Laureys, S.; Schnakers, C. Chinese translation of the Coma Recovery Scale-Revised. *Brain Inj.* **2017**, *31*, 363–365. [CrossRef]
23. Paszkiel, S.; Szpulak, P. Methods of Acquisition, Archiving and Biomedical Data Analysis of Brain Functioning. In *Proceedings of the BCI 2018, Opole, Poland, 13–14 March 2018*; Advances in Intelligent Systems and Computing; Springer: Cham, Switzerland, 2018; Volume 720, pp. 158–171. [CrossRef]
24. Mortensen, K.N.; Gjedde, A.; Thompson, G.J.; Herman, P.; Parent, M.J.; Rothman, D.L.; Kupers, R.; Ptito, M.; Stender, J.; Laureys, S.; et al. Impact of Global Mean Normalization on Regional Glucose Metabolism in the Human Brain. *Neural Plast.* **2018**, *2018*, 6120925. [CrossRef]
25. Laureys, S.; Owen, A.M.; Schiff, N.D. Brain function in coma, vegetative state, and related disorders. *Lancet Neurol.* **2004**, *3*, 537–546. [CrossRef]
26. Fridman, E.A.; Osborne, J.R.; Mozley, P.D.; Victor, J.D.; Schiff, N.D. Presynaptic dopamine deficit in minimally conscious state patients following traumatic brain injury. *Brain* **2019**, *142*, 1887–1893. [CrossRef]
27. Ge, J.; Wu, P.; Peng, S.; Yu, H.; Zhang, H.; Guan, Y.; Eidelberg, D.; Zuo, C.; Ma, Y.; Wang, J. Assessing cerebral glucose metabolism in patients with idiopathic rapid eye movement sleep behavior disorder. *J. Cereb. Blood Flow Metab.* **2015**, *35*, 2062–2069. [CrossRef]
28. Tian, Y.; Margulies, D.S.; Breakspear, M.; Zalesky, A. Topographic organization of the human subcortex unveiled with functional connectivity gradients. *Nat. Neurosci.* **2020**, *23*, 1421–1432. [CrossRef] [PubMed]
29. Uddin, L.Q. Salience processing and insular cortical function and dysfunction. *Nat. Rev. Neurosci.* **2015**, *16*, 55–61. [CrossRef] [PubMed]
30. Vossel, S.; Geng, J.J.; Fink, G.R. Dorsal and ventral attention systems: Distinct neural circuits but collaborative roles. *Neuroscientist* **2014**, *20*, 150–159. [CrossRef] [PubMed]
31. Smith, S.M.; Fox, P.T.; Miller, K.L.; Glahn, D.C.; Fox, P.M.; Mackay, C.E.; Filippini, N.; Watkins, K.E.; Toro, R.; Laird, A.R.; et al. Correspondence of the brain's functional architecture during activation and rest. *Proc. Natl. Acad. Sci. USA* **2009**, *106*, 13040–13045. [CrossRef] [PubMed]
32. Raichle, M.E.; MacLeod, A.M.; Snyder, A.Z.; Powers, W.J.; Gusnard, D.A.; Shulman, G.L. A default mode of brain function. *Proc. Natl. Acad. Sci. USA* **2001**, *98*, 676–682. [CrossRef]
33. Seeley, W.W.; Menon, V.; Schatzberg, A.F.; Keller, J.; Glover, G.H.; Kenna, H.; Reiss, A.L.; Greicius, M.D. Dissociable intrinsic connectivity networks for salience processing and executive control. *J. Neurosci.* **2007**, *27*, 2349–2356. [CrossRef]
34. Hermann, B.; Stender, J.; Habert, M.O.; Kas, A.; Denis-Valente, M.; Raimondo, F.; Perez, P.; Rohaut, B.; Sitt, J.D.; Naccache, L. Multimodal FDG-PET and EEG assessment improves diagnosis and prognostication of disorders of consciousness. *Neuroimage Clin.* **2021**, *30*, 102601. [CrossRef]
35. Zhang, Y.; Lu, J.; Du, J.; Huo, S.; Li, R.; Song, W. Neural correlates of different behavioral response to transcranial direct current stimulation between patients in the unresponsive wakefulness syndrome and minimally conscious state. *Neurol. Sci.* **2020**, *41*, 75–82. [CrossRef]
36. Rosazza, C.; Andronache, A.; Sattin, D.; Bruzzone, M.G.; Marotta, G.; Nigri, A.; Ferraro, S.; Rossi, S.D.; Porcu, L.; Bersano, A.; et al. Multimodal study of default-mode network integrity in disorders of consciousness. *Ann. Neurol.* **2016**, *79*, 841–853. [CrossRef]

37. Stender, J.; Gosseries, O.; Bruno, M.A.; Charland-Verville, V.; Vanhaudenhuyse, A.; Demertzi, A.; Chatelle, C.; Thonnard, M.; Thibaut, A.; Heine, L.; et al. Diagnostic precision of PET imaging and functional MRI in disorders of consciousness: A clinical validation study. *Lancet* **2014**, *384*, 514–522. [CrossRef]
38. Edlow, B.L.; Chatelle, C.; Spencer, C.A.; Chu, C.J.; Bodien, Y.G.; O'Connor, K.L.; Hirschberg, R.E.; Hochberg, L.R.; Giacino, J.T.; Rosenthal, E.S.; et al. Early detection of consciousness in patients with acute severe traumatic brain injury. *Brain* **2017**, *140*, 2399–2414. [CrossRef]
39. Lant, N.D.; Gonzalez-Lara, L.E.; Owen, A.M.; Fernandez-Espejo, D. Relationship between the anterior forebrain mesocircuit and the default mode network in the structural bases of disorders of consciousness. *Neuroimage Clin.* **2016**, *10*, 27–35. [CrossRef]
40. Wu, H.; Qi, Z.; Wu, X.; Zhang, J.; Wu, C.; Huang, Z.; Zang, D.; Fogel, S.; Tanabe, S.; Hudetz, A.G.; et al. Anterior precuneus related to the recovery of consciousness. *Neuroimage Clin.* **2022**, *33*, 102951. [CrossRef]
41. Lemaire, J.J.; Pontier, B.; Chaix, R.; El, O.Y.; Khalil, T.; Sinardet, D.; Achim, V.; Postelnicu, A.; Coste, J.; Germain, V.; et al. Neural correlates of consciousness and related disorders: From phenotypic descriptors of behavioral and relative consciousness to cortico-subcortical circuitry. *Neurochirurgie* **2022**, *68*, 212–222. [CrossRef]
42. Mencarelli, L.; Biagi, M.C.; Salvador, R.; Romanella, S.; Ruffini, G.; Rossi, S.; Santarnecchi, E. Network Mapping of Connectivity Alterations in Disorder of Consciousness: Towards Targeted Neuromodulation. *J. Clin. Med.* **2020**, *9*, 828. [CrossRef]
43. Qin, P.; Wu, X.; Wu, C.; Wu, H.; Zhang, J.; Huang, Z.; Weng, X.; Zang, D.; Qi, Z.; Tang, W.; et al. Higher-order sensorimotor circuit of the brain's global network supports human consciousness. *Neuroimage* **2021**, *231*, 117850. [CrossRef]
44. Ihalainen, R.; Gosseries, O.; de Steen, F.V.; Raimondo, F.; Panda, R.; Bonhomme, V.; Marinazzo, D.; Bowman, H.; Laureys, S.; Chennu, S. How hot is the hot zone? Computational modelling clarifies the role of parietal and frontoparietal connectivity during anaesthetic-induced loss of consciousness. *Neuroimage* **2021**, *231*, 117841. [CrossRef]
45. He, R.H.; Wang, H.J.; Zhou, Z.; Fan, J.Z.; Zhang, S.Q.; Zhong, Y.H. The influence of high-frequency repetitive transcranial magnetic stimulation on endogenous estrogen in patients with disorders of consciousness. *Brain Stimul.* **2021**, *14*, 461–466. [CrossRef]
46. Craig, A.D. How do you feel–now? The anterior insula and human awareness. *Nat. Rev. Neurosci.* **2009**, *10*, 59–70. [CrossRef]
47. Huang, Z.; Tarnal, V.; Vlisides, P.E.; Janke, E.L.; McKinney, A.M.; Picton, P.; Mashour, G.A.; Hudetz, A.G. Anterior insula regulates brain network transitions that gate conscious access. *Cell Rep.* **2021**, *35*, 109081. [CrossRef]
48. Fridman, E.A.; Beattie, B.J.; Broft, A.; Laureys, S.; Schiff, N.D. Regional cerebral metabolic patterns demonstrate the role of anterior forebrain mesocircuit dysfunction in the severely injured brain. *Proc. Natl. Acad. Sci. USA* **2014**, *111*, 6473–6478. [CrossRef]
49. Chen, P.; Xie, Q.; Wu, X.; Huang, H.; Lv, W.; Chen, L.; Guo, Y.; Zhang, S.; Hu, H.; Wang, Y.; et al. Abnormal Effective Connectivity of the Anterior Forebrain Regions in Disorders of Consciousness. *Neurosci. Bull.* **2018**, *34*, 647–658. [CrossRef]
50. Slagter, H.A.; Mazaheri, A.; Reteig, L.C.; Smolders, R.; Figee, M.; Mantione, M.; Schuurman, P.R.; Denys, D. Contributions of the Ventral Striatum to Conscious Perception: An Intracranial EEG Study of the Attentional Blink. *J. Neurosci.* **2017**, *37*, 1081–1089. [CrossRef]
51. Redinbaugh, M.J.; Phillips, J.M.; Kambi, N.A.; Mohanta, S.; Andryk, S.; Dooley, G.L.; Afrasiabi, M.; Raz, A.; Saalmann, Y.B. Thalamus Modulates Consciousness via Layer-Specific Control of Cortex. *Neuron* **2020**, *106*, 66–75. [CrossRef]
52. Tasserie, J.; Uhrig, L.; Sitt, J.D.; Manasova, D.; Dupont, M.; Dehaene, S.; Jarraya, B. Deep brain stimulation of the thalamus restores signatures of consciousness in a nonhuman primate model. *Sci. Adv.* **2022**, *8*, l5547. [CrossRef]

brain sciences

MDPI

Article

Effects of Electromyography Bridge on Upper Limb Motor Functions in Stroke Participants: An Exploratory Randomized Controlled Trial

Qin Zhao [1], Gongwei Jia [1], Lang Jia [1], Yule Wang [1], Wei Jiang [1], Yali Feng [1], Hang Jiang [1], Lehua Yu [1], Jing Yu [2,*] and Botao Tan [1,*]

1 Department of Rehabilitation Medicine, The Second Affiliated Hospital of Chongqing Medical University, Chongqing 400010, China; 2020140156@stu.cqmu.edu.cn (Q.Z.); 302145@cqmu.edu.cn (G.J.); 302116@hospital.cqmu.edu.cn (L.J.); wangyule@hospital.cqmu.edu.cn (Y.W.); 301194@hospital.cqmu.edu.cn (W.J.); 304513@hospital.cqmu.edu.cn (Y.F.); 304772@hospital.cqmu.edu.cn (H.J.); 300895@cqmu.edu.cn (L.Y.)

2 Department of Rehabilitation Medicine, The First Affiliated Hospital of Jinan University, Guangzhou 510630, China

* Correspondence: ave688@hotmail.com (J.Y.); 303518@cqmu.edu.cn (B.T.)

Citation: Zhao, Q.; Jia, G.; Jia, L.; Wang, Y.; Jiang, W.; Feng, Y.; Jiang, H.; Yu, L.; Yu, J.; Tan, B. Effects of Electromyography Bridge on Upper Limb Motor Functions in Stroke Participants: An Exploratory Randomized Controlled Trial. *Brain Sci.* **2022**, *12*, 870. https://doi.org/10.3390/brainsci12070870

Academic Editors: Jie Jia, Yan Hu, Dingguo Zhang, Giovanni Morone and Konstantin V. Slavin

Received: 30 May 2022
Accepted: 28 June 2022
Published: 30 June 2022

Publisher's Note: MDPI stays neutral with regard to jurisdictional claims in published maps and institutional affiliations.

Abstract: The electromyography bridge (EMGB) plays an important role in promoting the recovery of wrist joint function in stroke patients. We investigated the effects of the EMGB on promoting the recovery of upper limb function in hemiplegia. Twenty-four stroke patients with wrist dorsal extension dysfunction were recruited. Participants were randomized to undergo EMGB treatment or neuromuscular electrical stimulation (NMES). Treatments to wrist extensors were conducted for 25 min, twice a day, 5 days per week, for 1 month. Outcome measures: active range of motion (AROM) of wrist dorsal extension; Fugl-Meyer assessment for upper extremity (FMA-UE); Barthel index (BI); and muscle strength of wrist extensors. After interventions, patients in the NMES group had significantly greater improvement in the AROM of wrist dorsal extension at the 4th week and 1st month follow-up ($p < 0.05$). However, patients in the EMGB group had a statistically significant increase in AROM only at the follow-up assessment. No significant differences were observed in the AROM between the EMGB group and the NMES group ($p > 0.05$). For secondary outcomes in the EMGB group, compared to baseline measurements, FMA-UE, BI, extensor carpi radialis and extensor carpi ulnaris muscle strength were significantly different as early as the 4th week ($p < 0.05$). The muscle strength of the extensor digitorum communis muscle showed significant differences at the follow-up ($p < 0.05$). There were no statistically significant differences between patients in the two groups in any of the parameters evaluated ($p > 0.05$). The combination of EMGB or NMES with conventional treatment had similar effects on the improvement of the hemiplegic upper limb as assessed by wrist dorsal extension, FMA-UE, and activities of daily living. The improvement in both groups was maintained until 1 month after the intervention.

Keywords: stroke; hemiplegia; electromyographic bridge; upper limb rehabilitation; randomized controlled trial

1. Introduction

Stroke is the leading cause of adult disability worldwide [1]. More than 50% of stroke survivors exhibit permanent neurological impairments, with motor impairment being the most frequent. Even after standard neurological rehabilitation, approximately 80% of these patients suffer from hand dysfunction [2]. The increased muscle tension of the wrist dorsal extension in stroke patients severely affects the active range of motion (AROM) and the wrist dorsal extension function, and wrist joint dysfunction directly affects the motor control function of the upper limb [3]. The improvement of wrist control improves the quality of life for stroke survivors, reduces comorbidities associated with a loss of independence, and reduces the costs associated with the healthcare system [4–6]. Neuromuscular electrical stimulation (NMES) is one of the most common strategies for improving limb function in the clinical setting. Studies have shown that NMES can improve muscle strength, reduce spasticity, increase joint range of motion by promoting active movement, reorganize the damaged cortico-cerebral circuit, and improve movement control [7–10]. However, during the NMES process, the hemiplegic limb is passively moved, and bilateral limbs exhibit no movement to work together, which greatly reduces the effect of the patient's rehabilitation training. Therefore, the combined modulation of bilateral movement and electrical stimulation potentially play an important role in enhancing patient noncoordinated movement [11,12].

Recently, the State Key Laboratory of Bioelectronics at Southeast University developed a new type of self-controlled NMES system: the electromyography bridge (EMGB) [13,14]. In this instrument, the surface electromyography (sEMG) signals of the nonhemiplegic muscles are converted to control the duration and frequency of the relevant stimulation pulses applied to the muscles of the hemiplegic side. Therefore, the activation state of the control muscles can better simulate the coupling of bimanual exercises and movement responses. EMGB combined with NMES is effective in the short-term for improving upper limb injury in patients with stroke [15]. In a study of eight healthy subjects, EMGB accurately reproduced voluntary muscle forces and was more resistant to fatigue than NMES [13]. Some previous reports have shown that EMGB plays a certain role in promoting the recovery of wrist joint function in stroke patients [16,17], but the results remain controversial. Stroke patients were treated with EMGB for 4 weeks within 6 months of onset. The voluntary surface electromyographic ratio of wrist and finger extensors, Brunnstrom stages for the hand, and FMA-UE were significantly improved compared with the NMES group [16]. However, other articles showed that when thirty-one stroke patients received three weeks of EMGB or NMES treatments, the two treatment modalities showed no significant difference in FMA-UE, self-care FIM, grip strength, or on the modified Ashworth scale [18]. The number of studies of EMGB for stroke patients is limited. The effect of EMGB on wrist function in stroke patients is yet to be elucidated.

Between 1 week and 6 months post-stroke (subacute period of stroke) is a critical time for neural plasticity; most behavioral recovery and rapid changes occur in the first weeks and months post-stroke for the majority of people [19]. Therefore, this study aimed to compare the effects of EMGB and NMES on the recovery of upper limb motor and functional performance in subacute rehabilitation.

2. Materials and Methods

2.1. Study Design

The study was designed as a 2:1, double-blinded, randomized controlled trial. All subjects received 40 treatments twice a day, 5 days per week, for 4 weeks. The assessments were made at baseline, at the 4th week during treatment, and at the 1st month after discharge by a blinded therapist.

2.2. Participants and Setting

Stroke patients who participated in this work suffered from unilateral upper limb hemiparesis, and they could not dorsally extend their wrists. They were hospitalized at the Rehabilitation Medicine and Physical Therapy Department at the Second Affiliated Hospital of Chongqing Medical University between May 2020 and January 2021. The protocol of this study was registered with the Chinese Clinical Trial Registry (registration number: ChiCTR2100051957). The inclusion criteria were as follows: (1) stroke diagnosis that was confirmed by evidence on computed tomography (CT) or magnetic resonance imaging (MRI) scans 3 days to 12 months before the study; (2) a patient of any sex who was aged between 18 and 75 years; (3) poor upper limb function (AROM of the wrist extension was 0°), although the contralateral upper limb functioned well; (4) no progressive stroke and stable vital signs; and (5) the ability to understand and agree to the trial procedures and to sign an informed consent form in accordance with national legislation. Patients with any of the following criteria were excluded: (1) severe cognitive disorders [20] (Mini-Mental State Examination score $\leq$16); (2) severe depression [21] (Hamilton Rating Scale for Depression (HAMD) $\geq$24); (3) a modified Ashworth scale (MAS) score of two or more points for spasticity in carpal extension; (4) carpal contracture; (5) New York Heart Association (NYHA) cardiac function was classified as Level 4; (6) alanine aminotransferase (ALT) and aspartate aminotransferase (AST) were double the upper limit of normal; (7) severe heart, liver, kidney or lung diseases, or cancer; (8) cardiac pacemakers and various implantable electronic devices; (9) pregnant or lactating women; (10) muscles do not respond to functional electrical stimulation (FES); (11) concurrent participation in another similar clinical study during the 3 months before enrollment; and (12) other reasons deemed by the investigators to render the subject unsuitable for this trial.

2.3. Procedure

Out of the 93 patients screened, 24 patients agreed to join the group and were randomized into either the EMGB group (n = 16) or the NMES group (n = 8). The plan accepted by each patient was determined by random allocation. The members of the different groups were recorded in order in a table. The patients' group assignments documented in the table were covered by an opaque coating. Only after scratching off the coating were the patients informed of which group they were assigned to. Two patients in the EMGB group who were discharged and failed to complete follow-up were excluded from the study. Patients in the two groups were well-matched in age, sex, stroke type, hemiplegia side, muscle tone, and HAMD score at baseline. However, the course of stroke onset was unbalanced at baseline ($p < 0.05$). After a detailed analysis of the patients' information, we found that there were 6 patients in the EMGB group who had a relatively long course of stroke (>6 months). Therefore, we removed those patients for further analysis (Table 1). As a result, all remaining patients had similar courses of stroke (ranging from 1–6 months), and other characteristics were also comparable at baseline [22]. The complete data are shown in Supplementary Materials (Tables S1–S3). The Consolidated Standards of Reporting Trials (CONSORT) patient flowchart is shown in Figure 1.

Table 1. Clinical characteristics of the patients in both groups (long course removed).

	EMGB Group (n = 8)	NMES Group (n = 8)	p Value
Age, y	52.75 ± 17.16	53.88 ± 10.70	0.877
Sex, n (%)			
Male	5 (62.5)	5 (62.5)	1
Female	3 (37.5)	3 (37.5)	
Stroke type, n (%)			
Infarction	4 (50.0)	2 (0.25)	0.608
Hemorrhage	4 (50.0)	6 (0.75)	
Hemiplegia side			
Left	6 (0.75)	5 (62.5)	1
Right	2 (0.25)	3 (37.5)	
Muscle tone	0.38 ± 0.52	0.50 ± 0.53	0.642
HAMD	4.75 ± 6.82	5.50 ± 6.72	0.838
Stroke onset, month	1.38 ± 1.06	1.63 ± 1.06	0.645

EMGB: electromyography bridge; NMES: neuromuscular electrical stimulation; HAMD: Hamilton Rating Scale for Depression; y: year. Values are presented as the number of patients (n) or mean ± standard deviation. Significance difference at $p < 0.05$.

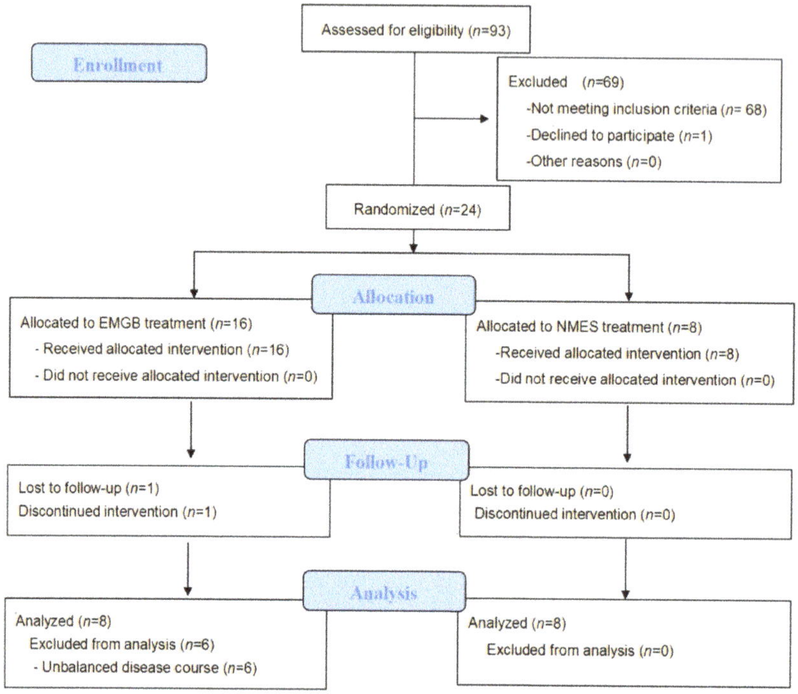

Figure 1. The CONSORT patient flowchart.

2.3.1. EMGB Group

We used the double-channel motor function reconstruction instrument based on the EMGB principle as in previous studies [23]. Similarly, patients were seated in front of a desk with their upper limbs attached to this system. Their elbows were flexed naturally, and their wrists were pronated, fully exposing both forearms. For sEMG detection, the sEMG sensors were placed on the wrist extensors of the nonhemiplegic limb to collect sEMG signals. The stimulation electrode was fixed to the optimal stimulation points for wrist extensors of the hemiplegic limb at a stimulating intensity below the threshold for uncomfortable sensation. A gelled reference electrode was placed over the olecranon. Patients were asked to perform simultaneous bilateral wrist extensions with a cycle comprising 5 s extension and 5 s relaxation periods under the guidance of a rhythmic sound generated by a recorder. The training consisted of two sessions of 10-min EMGB use with a 5-min interval between sessions. Sessions were conducted twice a day (once in the morning and once in the afternoon) for 4 weeks.

2.3.2. NMES Group

The patients were in the same position as the patients undergoing EMGB treatment. The sEMG sensors were placed on the wrist extensors of the hemiplegic limb to collect sEMG signals. A dorsal wrist extension of the hemiplegic side was passively elicited by preprogrammed NMES with the same sound cues.

Licensed therapists with at least 3 years of clinical experience performing manipulative therapies provided all treatments. None of the patients in either group experienced serious adverse effects. In addition to EMGB or NMES treatments, patients were offered conventional therapy (such as manual treatment and acupuncture). Figure 2A,B show the setup for the training tasks completed by patients in the 2 groups.

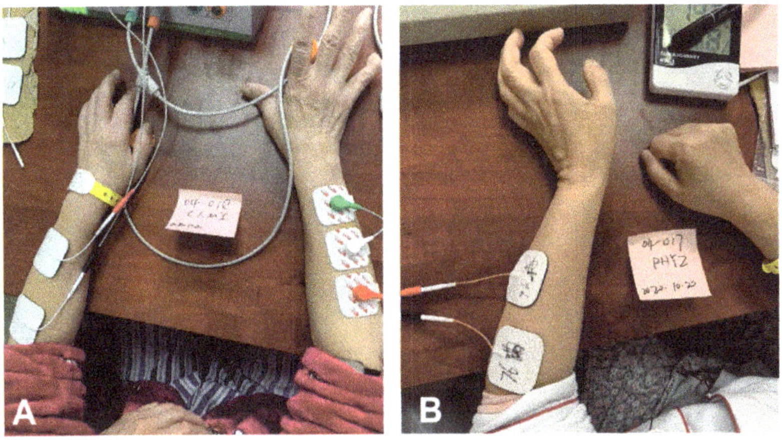

Figure 2. Electromyography bridge(EMGB) group and neuromuscular electrical stimulation(NMES) group. (**A**) Patients undergoing EMGB treatment; (**B**) Patients undergoing NMES treatment.

2.4. Outcome Measurement

Evaluations were performed at baseline, at the 4th week and at the follow-up after the 1st month of the trial by a therapist who had no information about the treatment groups. The primary outcome was an assessment of joint mobility using AROM of wrist dorsal extension. All patients had an AROM of 0° at enrollment. The secondary outcomes were as follows: (1) the Fugl-Meyer Assessment for Upper Extremity (FMA-UE) was used to evaluate motor recovery and motor function of upper limbs; (2) the manual muscle test (MMT) was used to evaluate the muscle strength of the extensor wrist muscles to evaluate muscle function around the wrist; and (3) the Barthel index (BI) was used to assess ADL performance.

2.5. Statistical Analysis

Statistical analyses were performed using SPSS 26.0 (SPSS Inc., Chicago, IL, USA). Data are expressed as the mean ± SD (standard deviation). Before performing the comparisons, we tested the data to determine whether they were normally distributed, and the variances were equal. The Shapiro–Wilk test was used to evaluate the data of the measurable parameters for a normal distribution in each group. To compare the baseline characteristics between the 2 groups, Fisher's exact tests and independent sample t tests were used to analyze variables. Repeated-measures ANOVA was used to compare the AROM of wrist dorsal extension, FMA-UE, MMT, and BI at baseline, at the 4th week, and at the follow-up after the 1st month with 95% confidence intervals. p values < 0.05 were considered statistically significant.

3. Results

3.1. Patient Characteristics

Table 1 shows the baseline characteristics of the studied population. There were no significant differences between groups in most of the demographic data and baseline variables related to stroke and neurological status at the time of admission. The patients in the two groups were well-matched in age, sex, stroke type, hemiplegia side, and HAMD score.

3.2. Primary Outcomes

As shown by the mean changes from baseline (Table 2), AROM of wrist dorsal extension improvements were observed during the trial in both EMGB and NMES groups. AROM improvements in the NMES group were significantly different from baseline at the 4th week and at the follow-up after the 1st month. (The mean change from baseline was equal to 6.92° and 7.70°, $p = 0.009$ and 0.029, respectively.) The significant difference in EMGB was at follow-up after the 1st month. (The mean change from baseline was equal to 7.85°, $p = 0.026$.) Notably, improvement was observed in 8 patients (3/8, 37.50% in the NMES group and 5/8, 62.50% in the EMGB group) at the 4th week and in 10 patients (5/8, 62.50% in both the NMES and EMGB groups) at follow-up. At the follow-up after the 1st month, the AROM increase in the EMGB was slightly higher than that of the NMES (the mean difference between groups was equal to 0.15°, $p = 0.97$), but there was no significant difference between the EMGB and NMES groups.

3.3. Secondary Outcomes

Patients in both groups acquired functional recovery to some extent, as assessed by the FMA-UE, muscle strength of wrist dorsiflexion, and Barthel index.

Briefly, FMA-UE increased after intervention in both groups compared with baseline. Differences in changes from baseline were significant at the 4th week ($p = 0.001$ and 0.004, respectively) and follow-up after the 1st month ($p = 0.001$ and 0.007, respectively). No differences were seen at any time point between groups (Table 2, Figure 3).

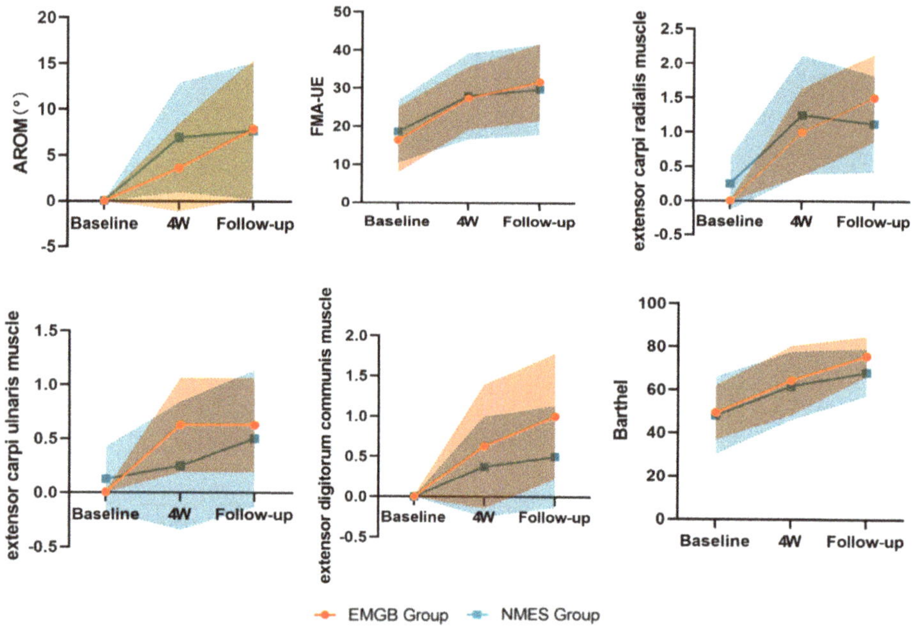

Figure 3. AROM: active range of motion; FMA-UE: Fugl-Meyer Assessment for Upper Extremity. The outcomes changed (mean and 95% CI) across the 3 time points between the EMGB and NMES groups. GraphPad Prism 8 was used to calculate the estimated marginal means: estimated marginal means (y-axis) for the EMGB group (orange); and NMES group (blue) across time points (x-axis).

The muscle strengths of three major wrist dorsiflexion (extensor carpi radialis muscle, extensor carpi ulnaris muscle, extensor digitorum communis muscle) are summarized in Table 2 and Figure 3. Similarly, the strength of the wrist extensor muscles improved in both groups at the 4th week ($p = 0.009$ for carpi radialis, and $p = 0.023$ for carpi ulnaris) and lasted at follow-up ($p = 0.005$ for digitorum communis) (Table 2, Figure 3). No significant differences were seen between the two groups at any time point.

Patients in both groups had improved activities of daily living as early as the 4th week ($p = 0.006$ and $p = 0.01$, respectively). Again, there were no significant differences between the groups at any time point (Table 2, Figure 3).

Table 2. Trial results for the primary and secondary outcomes.

		Baseline		Mean Difference between Groups (95%), p Value	4w		Mean Difference between Groups (95%), p Value	Follow-up		Mean Difference between Groups (95%), p Value
		EMGB	NMES		EMGB	NMES		EMGB	NMES	
	N	8	8		8	8		8	8	
Primary Outcome	AROM	0.00 ± 0.00	0.00 ± 0.00	0.00 (0.00, 0.00)	3.60 ± 5.70	6.92 ± 7.09	−3.32 (−10.22, 3.58), 0.319	7.85 ± 8.98	7.70 ± 8.88	0.15 (−9.42, 9.73), 0.97
	mean change (95% CI) from baseline, *p* value				3.60 (−1.28, 8.47), 0.136	6.92 (2.04, 11.80), 0.009		7.85 (1.08, 14.63), 0.026	7.70 (0.93, 14.47), 0.029	
Secondary Outcomes	FMA-UE	16.38 ± 10.14	18.63 ± 9.74	−2.25 (−12.1, 8.41), 0.66	27.38 ± 9.77	28.00 ± 13.46	−0.63 (−13.24, 11.99), 0.92	31.63 ± 12.03	29.75 ± 14.22	1.875 (−12.25, 16.00), 0.78
	mean change (95% CI) from baseline, *p* value				11.00 (5.10, 16.0), 0.001	9.38 (3.47, 15.28), 0.004		15.25 (7.64, 22.86), 0.001	11.13 (3.51, 18.74), 0.007	
	extensor carpi radialis muscle	0.00 ± 0.00	0.25 ± 0.46	−0.25 (−0.60, 0.10), 0.149	1.00 ± 0.76	1.25 ± 1.04	−0.25 (−1.22, 0.72), 0.590	1.50 ± 0.76	1.13 ± 0.83	0.38 (−0.48, 1.23), 0.362
	mean change (95% CI) from baseline, *p* value				1.00 (0.30, 1.70), 0.009	1.00 (0.30, 1.70), 0.009		1.50 (0.90, 2.10), 0.000	0.88 (0.27, 1.48), 0.008	
	extensor carpi ulnaris muscle	0.00 ± 0.00	0.13 ± 0.35	−0.13 (−0.39, 0.14), 0.334	0.63 ± 0.52	0.25 ± 0.71	0.38 (−0.29, 1.04), 0.246	0.63 ± 0.52	0.50 ± 0.76	0.13 (−0.57, 0.82), 0.705
	mean change (95% CI) from baseline, *p* value				0.63 (0.10–1.15), 0.023	0.13 (−0.40, 0.65), 0.619		0.63 (0.14, 1.11), 0.015	0.38 (−0.11, 0.86), 0.12	
	extensor digitorum communis muscle	0.00 ± 0.00	0.00 ± 0.00	0.00 (0.00, 0.00)	0.63 ± 0.92	0.38 ± 0.74	0.25 (−0.65, 1.15), 0.559	1.00 ± 0.93	0.50 ± 0.76	0.50 (−0.41, 1.41), 0.256
	mean change (95% CI) from baseline, *p* value				0.63 (−0.01, 1.26), 0.053	0.38 (−0.26, 1.01), 0.224		1.00 (0.36, 1.64), 0.005	0.50 (−0.14, 1.14), 0.116	
	BI	49.38 ± 14.74	48.13 ± 21.37	1.25 (−18.44, 20.94), 0.894	64.38 ± 18.79	61.88 ± 18.89	2.50 (−17.70, 22.70), 0.795	75.63 ± 10.84	68.13 ± 13.08	7.50 (−5.38, 20.38), 0.232
	mean change (95% CI) from baseline, *p* value				15.00 (5.10, 24.90), 0.006	13.75 (3.85, 23.65), 0.01		26.25 (17.80, 34.70), 0.000	20.00 (11.55, 28.45), 0.000	

EMGB: electromyography bridge; NMES: neuromuscular electrical stimulation; AROM: active range of motion; FMA-UE: Fugl-Meyer Assessment for Upper Extremity; BI: Barthel Index. Values are presented as the number of patients (*n*) or mean ± standard deviation.

4. Discussion

In this study, we found that EMGB significantly improved the upper limb motor function of patients with subacute stroke. At the 1st-month follow-up, the AROM of wrist dorsal extension and extensor digitorum communis muscle of patients were significantly increased. Moreover, the FMA-UE score, muscle strengths of the extensor carpi radialis muscle and extensor carpi ulnaris muscle, and BI of patients were also significantly improved after 4 weeks of treatment. The results demonstrate that the improvement of wrist and upper limb function led by EMGB can be maintained for at least 1 month.

The instrument used in this research was a two-channel motor function reconstruction instrument for hemiplegic limbs. The instrument combines electromyography and the mean absolute value/number of slope sign changes (MAV/NSS) and co-modulation algorithm (MNDC) to control actions in real time through EMGB technology. Based on the principle of bilateral training, the sEMG of the nonhemiplegic limb was used to detect and collect the real-time motion status data and then generate stimulation pulses by the MNDC algorithm on the corresponding muscles of the hemiplegic limb; this way, the movements of the hemiplegic limb could be guided by the nonparalyzed side [13,24]. Other potential mechanisms of this new instrument for hemiplegia were recently investigated: (1) repeated intentional movement of the nonhemiplegic limb could activate the primary motor cortex of the hemiplegic side, which is helpful for establishing new motor neurofeedback to realize motor relearning and to increase the excitability and recruitment effect of the target muscle contraction on the hemiplegic side [25,26]; (2) EMGB is conducive to promoting the remodeling of the central neural network and triggering the function of movement [27,28]; (3) at the same time, noninvasive stimulation of EMGB increased peripheral blood flow and muscle strength [29,30]. This occurrence is the mechanistic basis for the functional recovery of stroke patients.

Some previous studies demonstrated the effectiveness of EMGB [17,31]. ZHOU [16] administered EMGB treatment to patients for 4 weeks, and the Brunnstrom stages for the FMA-UE, motor status scale, and voluntary sEMG ratio of the wrist and finger extensors of patients' hemiplegic side were improved. The results favor EMGB treatment for augmenting the recovery of volitional wrist motion in stroke patients. Shini et al. [32] investigated the effect of EMG-triggered NMES on functional recovery of the affected hand and related cortical activity in chronic stroke. After the intervention of 10 weeks of EMG-triggered NMES, the hemiplegic hand showed significant improvements in the box and block test (BBT), strength, accuracy index (AI), and on/off set time of muscle contraction. These results suggest that EMG-triggered NMES could improve exercise capacity, exercise accuracy, and effective muscle recruitment in patients with hemiplegia. However, other research articles have different results. By comparing the effectiveness of active and passive neuromuscular electrical stimulation on the upper limbs of hemiplegia, no significant difference was detected in wrist extensor spasticity and upper limb functional between the two stimulation applications [18]. Hemmen and Seelen's [33] study showed that EMG-triggered stimulation did not increase upper limb function recovery relative to NMES in subacute stroke patients. The results of these studies are consistent with our findings. Compared with NMES group, the outcome indicators of the EMGB group showed positive trends toward improved outcomes, but the trends were not statistically significant. Possible explanations for the lack of differential effects between the groups was the small sample size and the fact that only subacute patients were studied. EMGB treatment might accelerate recovery during the subacute stage, but the NMES group might catch up and have similar outcomes 6 months after stroke [22]. In addition, strict inclusion criteria (AROM of wrist dorsal extension was 0° at baseline) limited the number of patients. A total of 24 patients agreed to join our clinical trial, but only 16 patients could be included to balance the patients' course of the disease. Another possible explanation was that conventional therapy was highly effective for the treatment of upper limb dysfunction, and other additional effects on wrist function were too small.

Most patients with stroke have better motor function in the proximal limb than in the distal upper limb. This outcome mainly occurs because patients exert more muscle strength with their shoulders and elbows when required to conduct upper limb movements [34,35]. This motor compensation develops new compensatory muscle activation patterns that differ from those of the unimpaired muscles. However, the flexibility of the hand and wrist has a great impact on the daily life of stroke patients. In some studies related to the rehabilitation of the distal joints, temporary paralysis of the proximal joint muscles was used to reduce the competition between the proximal and distal ends to obtain more distal muscle training [36]. In this research, it was found that EMGB provides a way to improve distal limb AROM. Deanna [37] quantified the ROM required for eight upper-extremity ADLs in healthy participants and found the activities required a total wrist motion of 38° of flexion, 40° of extension, 38° of ulnar deviation, and 28° of radial deviation. Brumfield and Champoux [38] reported that 10° of flexion and 35° of extension were required to accomplish most ADLs. In our study, the AROM of the wrist extension in both groups increased from 0° to approximately 8° at follow-up. They are still not able to complete most functional movements. Future studies should include longer intervention periods to achieve functional recovery.

This study had limitations. Firstly, there were only two groups in the current study, and no control group received conventional rehabilitation treatment alone. This was because patients in the control group would have received 50 min per day less treatment than the other groups, which was a significant medical ethical problem. Secondly, there was a limited number of patients. All participants included in our study were enrolled from a single center, and there was a relatively small sample size. Thirdly, in terms of the selection of evaluation indicators, we selected more indicators of body structure and function, but the level of activity was less-evaluated. As the activity level indicator, the Jebsen hand function test was not analyzed because most patients could not complete it. In addition, the scales used in this paper are ordinal, which means the ability to detect meaningful change may be impaired [39]. Future studies with larger populations, a multicenter clinical trial, and strict, stratified randomization are needed.

5. Conclusions

The findings of the present study suggested that EMGB might be beneficial to upper limb function recovery for patients with subacute stroke. However, our data did not show that EMGB had better effects than traditional NMES treatment in improving hemiplegic wrist extension, FMA-UE, and ADL performance. Further comprehensive studies should include a larger sample size and a longer observation period of stroke patients using balanced enrollment levels.

Supplementary Materials: The following supporting information can be downloaded at: https://www.mdpi.com/article/10.3390/brainsci12070870/s1, Table S1: Demographic and Clinical Information for Patients; Table S2: Demographic and clinical information for Patients (long course Removed); Table S3: Clinical Characteristics of All the Patients in Both Groups.

Author Contributions: Writing—original draft, Q.Z.; Methodology, G.J.; Investigation, L.J., Y.W., W.J. and B.T.; Funding, L.J., L.Y. and B.T.; Data curation, Y.F. and H.J.; Supervision, L.Y.; Project administration, L.Y.; Writing—review and editing, J.Y., Resources, B.T.; Validation, B.T. All authors have read and agreed to the published version of the manuscript.

Funding: Botao Tan, Lang Jia, and Wei Jiang have acquired the rewards of the Kuanren Talents Program of the Second Affiliated Hospital of Chongqing Medical University. This work was partly supported by the Chongqing Health Appropriate Technology Promotion Project (Grant No. 2018jstg046, 2021jstg029). The funders had no role in the study design, data collection and analysis, decision to publish, or preparation of the manuscript.

Institutional Review Board Statement: The study was conducted in accordance with the Declaration of Helsinki and approved by the Ethics Committee of the Second Affiliated Hospital of Chongqing Medical University on 11 June 2019 (Approval No. 2019 (25)).

Informed Consent Statement: Informed consent was obtained from all subjects involved in the study.

Data Availability Statement: The data presented in this study are available on request from the corresponding authors.

Acknowledgments: The authors would like to acknowledge the faculty and staff of the Department of Rehabilitation Medicine and Physical Therapy at the Second Affiliated Hospital of Chongqing Medical University for their assistance in patient recruitment and rehabilitation treatment. The authors thank the medical writers, proofreaders and editors for their helpful comments.

Conflicts of Interest: The double-channel motor function reconstruction instrument was provided by SQ-Med Co., Ltd. in accordance with the Medical Instrument Certification Process. There is no commercial relationship between SQ-Med Co., Ltd. and the Department of Rehabilitation Medicine, Second Affiliated Hospital of Chongqing Medical University.

References

1. Mozaffffarian, D.; Benjamin, E.J.; Go, A.S.; Arnett, D.K.; Blaha, M.J.; Cushman, M.; de Ferranti, S.; Després, J.; Fullerton, H.J.; Howard, V.J.; et al. Heart disease and stroke statistics–2015 update: A report from the American Heart Association. *Circulation* **2015**, *131*, e29–e322.
2. Feigin, V.L.; Lawes, C.M.M.; Bennett, D.A.; Anderson, C.S. Stroke epidemiology: A review of population-based studies of incidence, prevalence, and case-fatality in the late 20th century. *Lancet Neurol.* **2003**, *2*, 43–53. [CrossRef]
3. Park, K.; Chang, P.H.; Kang, S.H. In Vivo Estimation of Human Forearm and Wrist Dynamic Properties. *IEEE Trans. Neural Syst. Rehabil. Eng.* **2017**, *25*, 436–446. [CrossRef] [PubMed]
4. Dawson, J.; Pierce, D.; Dixit, A.; Kimberley, T.J.; Robertson, M.; Tarver, B.; Hilmi, O.; McLean, J.; Forbes, K.; Kilgard, M.P.; et al. Safety, Feasibility, and Efficacy of Vagus Nerve Stimulation Paired with Upper-Limb Rehabilitation after Ischemic Stroke. *Stroke* **2016**, *47*, 143–150. [CrossRef] [PubMed]
5. Cheng, H.Y.; Chair, S.Y.; Chau, J.P.C. Effectiveness of a strength-oriented psychoeducation on caregiving competence, problem-solving abilities, psychosocial outcomes and physical health among family caregiver of stroke survivors: A randomised controlled trial. *Int. J. Nurs. Stud.* **2018**, *87*, 84–93. [CrossRef] [PubMed]
6. Liu, L.; Wang, D.; Wong, K.S.; Wang, Y. Stroke and stroke care in China: Huge burden, significant workload, and a national priority. *Stroke* **2011**, *42*, 3651–3654. [CrossRef] [PubMed]
7. Carson, R.G.; Buick, A.R. Neuromuscular electrical stimulation-promoted plasticity of the human brain. *J. Physiol.* **2021**, *599*, 2375–2399. [CrossRef]
8. Insausti-Delgado, A.; López-Larraz, E.; Omedes, J.; Ramos-Murguialday, A. Intensity and Dose of Neuromuscular Electrical Stimulation Influence Sensorimotor Cortical Excitability. *Front. Neurosci.* **2021**, *15*, 593360. [CrossRef]
9. Yang, J.D.; Liao, C.H.; Huang, S.H.; Tam, K.A.; Liou, T.S.; Lee, Y.U.; Lin, C.H.; Chen, H.U. Effectiveness of electrical stimulation therapy in improving arm function after stroke: A systematic review and a meta-analysis of randomised controlled trials. *Clin. Rehabi.* **2019**, *33*, 1286–1297. [CrossRef]
10. Sentandreu-Mañó, T.; Tomás, J.M.; Ricardo Salom Terrádez, J. A randomised clinical trial comparing 35 Hz versus 50 Hz frequency stimulation effects on hand motor recovery in older adults after stroke. *Sci. Rep.* **2021**, *11*, 9131. [CrossRef]
11. Knutson, J.S.; Harley, M.Y.; Hisel, T.Z.; Makowski, N.S.; Fu, M.J.; Chae, J. Contralaterally controlled functional electrical stimulation for stroke rehabilitation. *Annu. Int. Conf. IEEE. Eng. Med. Biol. Soc.* **2012**, *2012*, 314–317. [PubMed]
12. Knutson, J.S.; Gunzler, D.D.; Wilson, R.D.; Chae, J. Contralaterally Controlled Functional Electrical Stimulation Improves Hand Dexterity in Chronic Hemiparesis: A Randomized Trial. *Stroke* **2016**, *47*, 2596–2602. [CrossRef] [PubMed]
13. Zhou, Y.X.; Wang, H.A.; Bao, X.U.; Lü, X.I.; Wang, Z.H. A frequency and pulse-width co-modulation strategy for transcutaneous neuromuscular electrical stimulation based on sEMG timedomain features. *J. Neural. Eng.* **2016**, *13*, 016004. [CrossRef]
14. Huang, Z.H.; Wang, Z.; Lv, X.; Zhou, Y.; Wang, H.; Zong, S. A novel functional electrical stimulation-control system for restoring motor function of post-stroke hemiplegic patients. *Neural. Regen. Res.* **2014**, *9*, 2102–2110.
15. Monte-Silva, K.; Piscitelli, D.; Norouzi-Gheidari, N.; Batalla, M.A.P.; Archambault, P.; Levin, M.F. Electromyogram-Related Neuromuscular Electrical Stimulation for Restoring Wrist and Hand Movement in Poststroke Hemiplegia: A Systematic Review and Meta-Analysis. *Neurorehabilit. Neural Repair* **2019**, *33*, 96–111. [CrossRef] [PubMed]
16. Zhou, Y.X.; Xia, Y.; Huang, J.; Wang, H.P.; Bao, X.L.; Bi, Z.Y.; Chen, X.B.; Gao, Y.J.; Lü, X.Y.; Wang, Z.G. Electromyographic bridge for promoting the recovery of hand movements in subacute stroke patients: A randomized controlled trial. *J. Rehabil. Med.* **2017**, *49*, 629–636. [CrossRef] [PubMed]
17. Meilink, A.; Hemmen, B.; Seelen, H.A.; Kwakkel, G. Impact of EMG-triggered neuromuscular stimulation of the wrist and finger extensors of the paretic hand after stroke: A systematic review of the literature. *Clin. Rehabil.* **2008**, *22*, 291–305. [CrossRef]
18. Boyaci, A.; Topuz, O.; Alkan, H.; Ozgen, M.; Sarsan, A.; Yildiz, N.; Ardic, F. Comparison of the effectiveness of active and passive neuromuscular electrical stimulation of hemiplegic upper extremities: A randomized, controlled trial. *Int. J. Rehabil. Res.* **2013**, *36*, 315–322. [CrossRef]

19. Bernhardt, J.; Hayward, K.S.; Kwakkel, G.; Ward, N.S.; Wolf, S.L.; Borschmann, K.; Krakauer, J.W.; Boyd, L.A.; Carmichael, S.T.; Corbett, D.; et al. Agreed definitions and a shared vision for new standards in stroke recovery research: The Stroke Recovery and Rehabilitation Roundtable taskforce. *Int. J. Stroke* **2017**, *12*, 444–450. [CrossRef]
20. Folstein, M.F.; Folstein, S.E.; McHugh, P.R. "Mini-mental state". A practical method for grading the cognitive state of patients for the clinician. *J. Psychiatr. Res.* **1975**, *12*, 189–198. [CrossRef]
21. Snaith, R.P. Hamilton rating scale for depression. *Br. J. Psychiatry* **1977**, *131*, 431–432. [CrossRef] [PubMed]
22. Stinear, C.M.; Lang, C.E.; Zeiler, S.; Byblow, W.D. Advances and challenges in stroke rehabilitation. *Lancet Neurol.* **2020**, *19*, 348–360. [CrossRef]
23. Zhou, Y.X.; Wang, H.P.; Cao, X.P.; Bi, Z.Y.; Gao, Y.J.; Chen, X.B.; Lu, X.-Y.; Wang, Z.-G. Electromyographic Bridge-a multi-movement volitional control method for functional electrical stimulation: Prototype system design and experimental validation. *Annu. Int. Conf. IEEE Eng. Med. Biol. Soc.* **2017**, *2017*, 205–208.
24. Wang, Z.G.; Lü, X.Y.; Wang, H.P.; Bao, X.L.; Bi, Z.Y. Electromyographic bridge for motor function rehabilitation of paralyzed limbs. In Proceedings of the 12th National Conference of Chinese Society for Neuroscience, Tianjin, China, 12 October 2017.
25. Stinear, C.M.; Barber, P.A.; Coxon, J.P.; Fleming, M.K.; Byblow, W.D. Priming the motor system enhances the effects of upper limb therapy in chronic stroke. *Brain* **2008**, *131*, 1381–1390. [CrossRef]
26. Stewart, K.C.; Cauraugh, J.H.; Summers, J.J. Bilateral movement training and stroke rehabilitation: A systematic review and meta-analysi. *J. Neurol. Sci.* **2008**, *244*, 89–95. [CrossRef] [PubMed]
27. Khaslavskaia, S.; Sinkjaer, T. Motor cortex excitability following repetitive electrical stimulation of the common peroneal nerve depends on the voluntary drive. *Exp. Brain Res.* **2005**, *162*, 497–502. [CrossRef] [PubMed]
28. Buetefisch, C.; Heger, R.; Schicks, W.; Seitz, R.; Netz, J. Hebbiantype stimulation during robot-assisted training in patients with stroke. *Neurorehabil. Neural. Repair* **2016**, *25*, 645–655. [CrossRef]
29. Ring, H.; Rosenthal, N. Controlled study of neuroprosthetic functional electrical stimulation in sub-acute post-stroke rehabilitation. *J. Rehabil. Med.* **2005**, *37*, 32–36. [CrossRef]
30. Lin, Z.; Yan, T. Long-term effectiveness of neuromuscular electrical stimulation for promoting motor recovery of the upper extremity after stroke. *J. Rehabil. Med.* **2011**, *43*, 506–510.
31. Bolton, D.A.; Cauraugh, J.H.; Hausenblas, H.A. Electromyogram-triggered neuromuscular stimulation and stroke motor recovery of arm/hand functions: A meta-analysis. *J. Neurol. Sci.* **2004**, *223*, 121–127. [CrossRef]
32. Shin, H.K.; Cho, S.H.; Jeon, H.S.; Lee, Y.H.; Song, J.C.; Jang, S.H.; Lee, C.H.; Kwon, Y.H. Cortical effect and functional recovery by the electromyography-triggered neuromuscular stimulation in chronic stroke patients. *Neurosci. Lett.* **2008**, *442*, 174–179. [CrossRef] [PubMed]
33. Hemmen, B.; Seelen, H.A. Effects of movement imagery and electromyography-triggered feedback on arm hand function in stroke patients in the subacute phase. *Clin. Rehabil.* **2007**, *21*, 587–594. [CrossRef] [PubMed]
34. Andrews, A.W.; Bohmmon, R.W. Distribution of muscle strength impairments following stroke. *Clin. Rehabil.* **2000**, *14*, 79–87. [CrossRef] [PubMed]
35. Dewald, J.P.A.; Sheshadri, V.; Dawson, M.L.; Beer, R.F. Upperlimb discoordination in hemiparetic stroke: Implications for neurorehabilitation. *Top. Stroke Rehabil.* **2001**, *8*, 1–12. [CrossRef] [PubMed]
36. Takeuchi, N.; Izumi, S.I. Maladaptive plasticity for motor recovery after stroke: Mechanisms and approaches. *Neural. Plast.* **2012**, *2012*, 359728. [CrossRef]
37. Gates, D.H.; Walters, L.S.; Cowley, J.; Wilken, J.M.; Resnik, L. Range of Motion Requirements for Upper-Limb Activities of Daily Living. *Am. J. Occup. Ther.* **2016**, *70*, 7001350010p1–7001350010p10. [CrossRef]
38. Brumfield, R.H.; Champoux, J.A. A biomechanical study of normal functional wrist motion. *Clin. Orthop.* **1984**, *187*, 23–25. [CrossRef]
39. Piscitelli, D.; Pellicciari, L. Responsiveness: Is it time to move beyond ordinal scores and approach interval measurements? *Clin. Rehabil.* **2018**, *32*, 1426–1427. [CrossRef]

brain sciences

MDPI

Systematic Review

Effects of Non-Invasive Brain Stimulation on Post-Stroke Spasticity: A Systematic Review and Meta-Analysis of Randomized Controlled Trials

Xiaohan Wang [1,†], Le Ge [2,†], Huijing Hu [1], Li Yan [1,*] and Le Li [1,*]

1 Institute of Medical Research, Northwestern Polytechnical University, Xi'an 710072, China; xhwang616@mail.nwpu.edu.cn (X.W.); huhuijing@nwpu.edu.cn (H.H.)
2 Department of Rehabilitation Medicine, The First Affiliated Hospital, Sun Yat-sen University, Guangzhou 510080, China; gele3@mail.sysu.edu.cn
* Correspondence: yanli1130@nwpu.edu.cn (L.Y.); lile5@nwpu.edu.cn (L.L.); Tel.: +86-186-2939-5063 (L.Y.); +86-135-6041-5367 (L.L.)
† These authors contributed equally to this work.

Abstract: In recent years, the potential of non-invasive brain stimulation (NIBS) for the therapeutic effect of post-stroke spasticity has been explored. There are various NIBS methods depending on the stimulation modality, site and parameters. The purpose of this study is to evaluate the efficacy of NIBS on spasticity in patients after stroke. This systematic review and meta-analysis was conducted according to Preferred Reporting Items for Systematic reviews and Meta-Analyses (PRISMA) guidelines. PUBMED (MEDLINE), Web of Science, Cochrane Library and Excerpta Medica Database (EMBASE) were searched for all randomized controlled trials (RCTs) published before December 2021. Two independent researchers screened relevant articles and extracted data. This meta-analysis included 14 articles, and all included articles included 18 RCT datasets. The results showed that repetitive transcranial magnetic stimulation (rTMS) (MD = −0.40, [95% CI]: −0.56 to −0.25, $p < 0.01$) had a significant effect on improving spasticity, in which low-frequency rTMS (LF-rTMS) (MD = −0.51, [95% CI]: −0.78 to −0.24, $p < 0.01$) and stimulation of the unaffected hemisphere (MD = −0.58, [95% CI]: −0.80 to −0.36, $p < 0.01$) were beneficial on Modified Ashworth Scale (MAS) in patients with post-stroke spasticity. Transcranial direct current stimulation (tDCS) (MD = −0.65, [95% CI]: −1.07 to −0.22, $p < 0.01$) also had a significant impact on post-stroke rehabilitation, with anodal stimulation (MD = −0.74, [95% CI]: −1.35 to −0.13, $p < 0.05$) being more effective in improving spasticity in patients. This meta-analysis revealed moderate evidence that NIBS reduces spasticity after stroke and may promote recovery in stroke survivors. Future studies investigating the mechanisms of NIBS in addressing spasticity are warranted to further support the clinical application of NIBS in post-stroke spasticity.

Keywords: non-invasive brain stimulation; stroke; spasticity; meta-analysis

Citation: Wang, X.; Ge, L.; Hu, H.; Yan, L.; Li, L. Effects of Non-Invasive Brain Stimulation on Post-Stroke Spasticity: A Systematic Review and Meta-Analysis of Randomized Controlled Trials. *Brain Sci.* **2022**, *12*, 836. https://doi.org/10.3390/brainsci12070836

Academic Editors: Jie Jia, Yan Hu, Dingguo Zhang and Konstantin V. Slavin

Received: 13 May 2022
Accepted: 24 June 2022
Published: 27 June 2022

1. Introduction

Post-stroke spasticity, as a neurological manifestation with a typical syndrome of increased muscle tone, was reported to have a prevalence rate of up to 25% in stroke survivors [1]. Spasticity leads to complications such as pain, muscle spasticity, abnormal joint positions and anchylosis, which further decrease the motor function of patients after stroke and bring great challenges to their daily activities [2]. Therefore, effective interventions for post-stroke spasticity are very important. Current management regimens for post-stroke spasticity include electrical stimulation of muscles, botulinum toxin injections, oral anti-spasticity drugs and wearable exoskeletons devices, etc. [3,4]. However, common side effects of drugs and the invasiveness of local treatment are undesirable, which limits their effectiveness.

In recent years, non-invasive brain stimulation (NIBS) has been actively explored in various diseases of the nervous system. Among various NIBS techniques, transcranial magnetic stimulation (TMS) and transcranial direct current stimulation (tDCS) are most often used to treat patients with post-stroke spasticity [5,6]. Spasticity usually occurs within one to six weeks after stroke and is caused by abnormal or hyperexcitable spinal reflexes [7,8]. NIBS induces excitatory changes in the underlying cerebral cortex in a non-invasive manner and lasting changes in neuroplasticity [9]. NIBS works by altering the excitability of the cerebral motor cortex and indirectly reducing the excitability of motor neurons in the spinal cord through the H-reflex [10].

Currently, the effects of NIBS on post-stroke spasticity are contradictory. Although some studies have reported a beneficial effect of NIBS in the treatment of post-stroke spasticity [11–13], other studies have shown no significant benefit of NIBS in reducing muscle spasticity. A meta-analysis published in 2020 showed no significant effect of rTMS in spasticity management. However, it included only five RCTs [14]. Results from two published meta-analyses of tDCS for post-stroke spasticity also showed some variability without uniform criteria [15,16]. Therefore, the aim of this study is to conduct a systematic review and meta-analysis of the effectiveness of NIBS in the management of spasticity in patients after stroke.

2. Methods

2.1. Literature Search Strategy

This meta-analysis was performed in accordance with the PRISMA guidelines for systematic reviews and meta-analysis [17]. The PICO principles consist of four parts: population, interventions, control and outcome and all articles included in systematic reviews and meta-analyses are retrieved according to the PICO principles [18]. The inclusion criteria for articles are (1) Population: patients who have been diagnosed as stroke patients by clinical examinations and have post-stroke spasticity; (2) Interventions: NIBS; (3) Control: sham stimulation; (4) Outcome: MAS; and (5) Research type: RCT. The research language is limited to English. Two authors independently searched electronic databases, including PUBMED (MEDLINE), Web of Science, Cochrane Library and EMBASE. We searched the database for related articles published as of December 2021 by using MeSH terms including "Stroke", "Non-invasive Brain Stimulation" and "spasticity". If there is a disagreement in the article inclusion process, it will be discussed with the third author to determine the eligibility for inclusion.

2.2. Study Selection

The article search strategy is shown in Figure 1. We retrieved a total of 2482 publications in our first search. The two authors screened titles and abstracts to determine relevant research articles and then further reviewed the full text to finally determine the research articles included in the meta-analysis. Any disagreements during the inclusion process were discussed and resolved by the third author.

2.3. Quality Assessment

All included RCTs were independently evaluated by two authors using the Cochrane risk of bias assessment tool [19]. It included six items: selection bias: random sequence generation and allocation concealment; performance bias: blinding of participants and personnel; detection bias: blinding of outcome assessment; attrition bias: incomplete outcome data; reporting bias: selective reporting; and other biases [20]. If there was a disagreement in the evaluation, it would be resolved through a discussion with the third author.

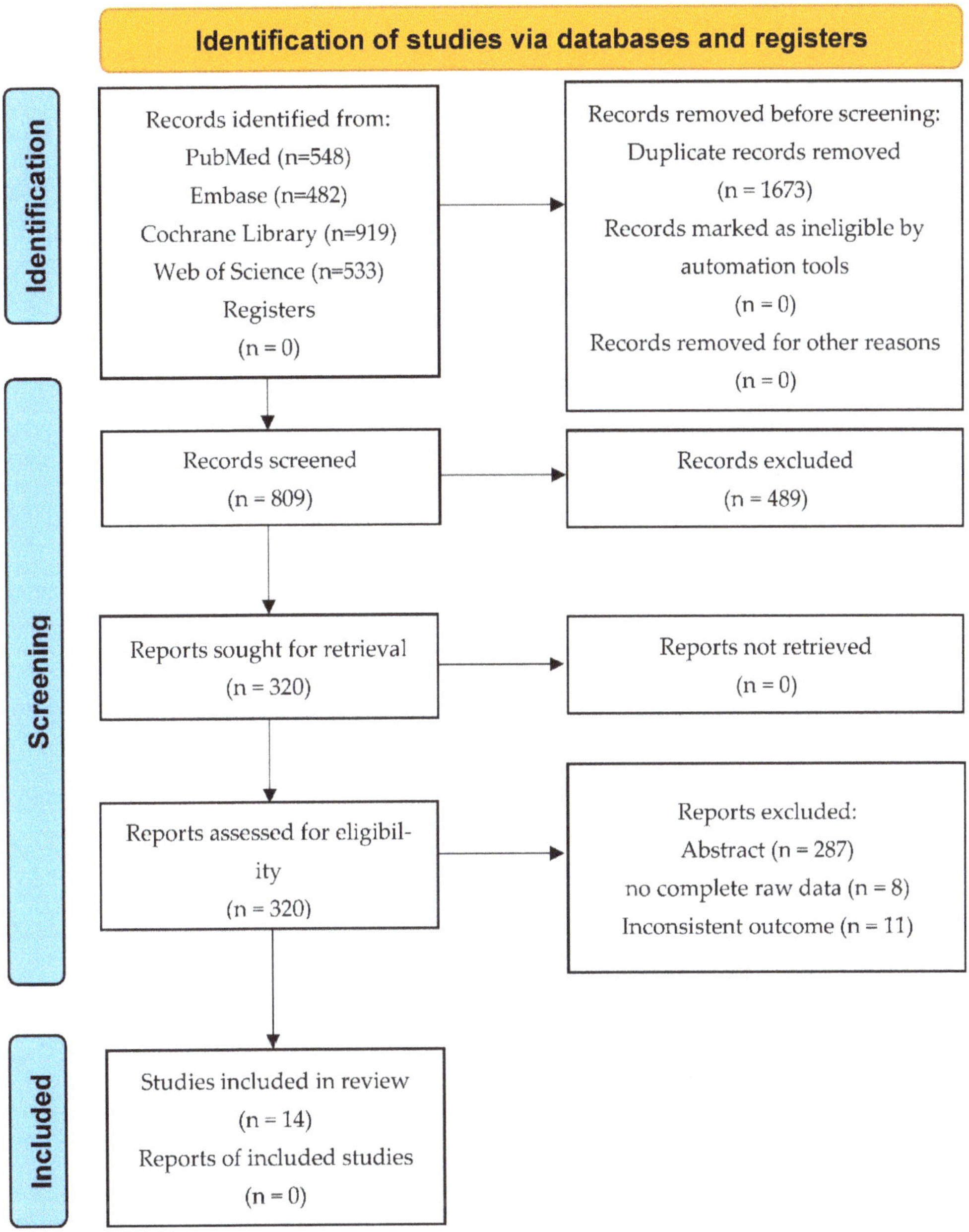

Figure 1. PRISMA flow diagram for search strategy and study selection.

2.4. Data Extraction

For each study that met the inclusion criteria, relevant information about experimental design and result analysis was extracted. All extracted information included research characteristics (author, publication year and sample size), treatment parameters (stimulation method, stimulation parameters, stimulation time and control group) and main measurement results (MAS).

2.5. Statistical Analysis

A meta-analysis of the extracted studies was performed. Meta-analyses are useful for assessing the strength of evidence for treatment from multiple studies. The aim is to determine whether there is an effect, either positive or negative, and to obtain a single pooled estimate of effect rather than a single estimate of individual studies. In this meta-analysis, for each outcome related to continuous data, we calculated a pooled estimate and 95% confidence interval (CI) of the mean difference (MD) between the experimental and control groups after the intervention.

This meta-analysis used RevMan 5.4 (The Nordic Cochrane Centre, The Cochrane Collaboration, Copenhagen, Denmark) for statistical analysis. This was performed by entering the mean and standard deviation of all continuous data in each study into the software and calculating the mean difference (MD) of the 95% confidence interval (CI) to analyze the results. Cochran's Q test and the I^2 index were used to assess the heterogeneity of all studies included in the meta-analysis. Statistical heterogeneity between these studies was calculated using Cochran's Q test and the I^2 index. An I^2 index > 50% and $p < 0.10$ of the Cochran's Q test indicated high heterogeneity, and the random-effects model was used; otherwise, the fixed-effects model was used. The results of all data analyses in this meta-analysis were shown by forest plots.

Funnel plots and Egger's test to assess potential publication bias were applied. Still, because the number of studies included in each meta-analysis was less than 10, the funnel plot and Egger's test could produce misleading results in this case [21]. Therefore, the funnel plot and Egger's test were not used in this meta-analysis to assess publication bias.

3. Results

3.1. Study Identification and Selection

A total of 2482 publications were retrieved from two authors independently by searching the database. The search results are shown in Figure 1. Of these, 1673 duplicate publications were firstly deleted, then 489 publications were screened based on titles, and then 287 publications were based on abstracts, and finally, 33 full-text articles were retrieved. Through the final full-text review, 14 articles were ultimately included for this review. This study included eight research articles [22–29] on rTMS, one of which included three data sets, one article included two data sets and the other articles each had one data set. A total of 128 patients received rTMS in all studies, and 104 patients served as the control group. At the same time, this study included six research articles [13,30–34] on tDCS. One article included two data sets, and the other articles had one data set. A total of 199 patients in all studies received tDCS, and 146 patients served as the control group. The information extracted from all research related to rTMS is shown in Table 1, and the information extracted from all studies related to tDCS is shown in Table 2.

Details of each study are provided in Tables 1 and 2. In rTMS, the pooled sample size was 135 individuals receiving rTMS, with sample sizes ranging from 7 to 22 participants per group. In terms of study design, all articles in this review were RCTs. In tDCS, the pooled sample size was 196 individuals receiving tDCS, with sample sizes ranging from 10 to 45 participants per group. In terms of study design, all articles in this review were RCTs.

Table 1. Research Characteristics of rTMS.

Study	Participant				Mean Severity (SD)		Intervention	Control	Outcomes	Muscle
	Intervention		Control		Intervention	Control				
	Mean Age (SD)	N (Male/Female)	Mean Age (SD)	N (Male/Female)	MAS					
Askı et al. (2017)	56.75 (11.46)	20 (14/6)	58.80 (12.02)	20 (15/5)	3.2 (0.75)	2.8 (0.75)	LF-rTMS + PT 1200 pulses, 1 Hz, 90% RMT	Sham rTMS + PT	MAS	upper limb
Barros Galvao et al. (2014)	57.4 (12.0)	10 (6/4)	64.6 (6.8)	10 (7/3)	2.5 (0.5)	2.4 (0.5)	LF-rTMS + PT 1500 pulses, 1 Hz; 90% RMT	Sham rTMS +PT	MAS	wrist
Chen et al. (2019)	52.9 (11.1)	11 (7/4)	52.6 (8.3)	11 (7/4)	3.90 (2.10)	4.05 (1.56)	iTBS 50 Hz 80% AMT	Sham iTBS	MAS	upper limb
Chen et al. (2021)	54.36 (10.56)	12 (8/4)	48.95 (9.63)	11 (10/1)	0.87 (0.54)	0.94 (0.69)	iTBS + VCT 50 Hz 80% AMT	Sham iTBS + VCT	MAS	upper limb
Chervyakov et al. (2018a)	54.2 (11.1)	11 (5/6)	61.4 (11.4)	10 (5/5)	1.2 (0.9)	1.4 (1.0)	LF-rTMS 1200 pulses, 1 Hz, 100% RMT	Sham rTMS	MAS	arm
Chervyakov et al. (2018b)	58.6 (10.4)	13 (10/3)	61.4 (11.4)	10 (5/5)	1.84 (0.8)	1.4 (1.0)	HF-rTMS 200 pulses, 10-Hz, 80% RMT	Sham rTMS	MAS	arm
Chervyakov et al. (2018c)	60.7 (9.6)	8 (6/2)	61.4 (11.4)	10 (5/5)	1.5 (0.9)	1.4 (1.0)	LF-rTMS 1 Hz 100% RMT HF-rTMS 10 Hz 80% RMT	Sham rTMS	MAS	arm
Gottlieb et al. (2021)]	63.93 (10.91)	14 (9/5)	62.43 (11.46)	14 (3/11)	1.86 (1.35)	1.71 (1.27)	LF-rTMS 1200 pulses, 1 Hz	Sham-rTMS	MAS	upper limb
Kuzu et al. (2021a)	56.3 (11.5)	7 (4/3)	65.0 (4.6)	6 (2/4)	1.8 (0.4)	2.3 (0.6)	LF-rTMS 1200 pulses, 1 Hz	Sham rTMS	MAS	upper limb
Kuzu et al. (2021b)	61.3 (9.8)	7 (6/1)	65.0 (4.6)	6 (2/4)	2.1 (0.6)	2.3 (0.6)	cTBS 50 Hz	Sham cTBS	MAS	upper limb
Xu et al. (2021)	79.50 (1.49)	22 (17/5)	68.86 (3.09)	22 (15/7)	2.32 (0.48)	2.41 (0.50)	LF-rTMS + CRT 550 pulses, 1 Hz 90% RMT	Sham rTMS + CRT	MAS	upper limb

HF-rTMS: high-frequency repetitive transcranial magnetic stimulation; LF-rTMS: low-frequency repetitive transcranial magnetic stimulation; cTBS: continuous theta-burst repetitive transcranial magnetic stimulation; iTBS: intermittent theta-burst repetitive transcranial magnetic stimulation; AMT: active motor threshold; RMT: resting motor threshold; MAS: modified Ashworth scale; PT: physical therapy; VCT: virtual reality-based cycling training; CRT: conventional rehabilitation treatment.

Table 2. Research Characteristics of tDCS.

Study	Participant				Mean Severity (SD)		Intervention	Control	Outcomes	Muscle
	Intervention		Control		MAS					
	Mean Age (SD)	N (Male/Female)	Mean Age (SD)	N (Male/Female)	Intervention	Control				
Andrade et al. (2017)	54.08 (3.72)	40 (22/18)	54.76 (4.28)	20 (12/8)	3.3 (0.36)	3.6 (0.5)	tDCS (Anodal) + CIMT 0.7 mA, 10 sessions	Sham-tDCS + CIMT	MAS	upper limb
Hesse et al. (2012a)	63.9 (10.5)	32 (20/12)	65.6 (10.3)	32 (21/11)	1.6 (2.9)	1.4 (2.7)	tDCS (Anodal) 2.0 mA, 30 sessions	Sham-tDCS	MAS	upper limb
Hesse et al. (2012b)	65.4 (8.6)	32 (18/14)	65.6 (10.3)	32 (21/11)	1.0 (1.8)	1.4 (2.7)	tDCS (Cathodal) 2.0 mA, 30 sessions	Sham-tDCS	MAS	upper limb
Lee and Chun (2014)	63.1 (10.3)	20 (12/8)	60.6 (14.1)	20 (9/11)	0.4 (0.5)	0.5 (0.4)	tDCS (Cathodal) + VRT 2.0 mA, 15 sessions	Sham-tDCS + VRT	MAS	upper limb
Mazzoleni et al. (2019)	67.50 (16.30)	20 (8/12)	68.74 (15.83)	19 (7/12)	1.1 (1.86)	1.58 (2.34)	tDCS (Anodal) + wrist robot-assisted rehabilitation 2.0 mA, 30 sessions	Sham-tDCS + wrist robot-assisted rehabilitation	MAS	wrist
Viana et al. (2014)	56.0 (10.2)	10 (9/1)	55.0 (12.2)	10 (7/3)	1.5 (0.7)	1.5 (0.52)	tDCS (Anodal) + VRT 2.0 mA, 15 sessions	Sham-tDCS + VRT	MAS	upper limb
Wu et al. (2013)	45.9 (11.2)	45 (34/11)	49.3 (12.6)	45 (35/10)	2.0 (0.75)	2.0 (0.5)	tDCS (Cathodal) + PT 1.2 mA, 20 sessions	Sham-tDCS + PT	MAS	elbow, wrist

tDCS: transcranial direct current stimulation; MAS: modified Ashworth scale; CIMT: constraint-induced movement therapy; VRT: virtual reality therapy; PT: physical therapy.

3.2. Effects of rTMS

A total of 11 RCTs on the effect of rTMS on post-stroke spasticity were included in the study, and the outcome measure of all the studies was MAS. The meta-analysis showed that compared with the control group, rTMS had significant benefits for patients with post-stroke spasticity, and the MAS was significantly reduced (MD: −0.40, 95% CI: −0.56 to −0.25, $p < 0.01$). The meta-analysis showed that there was no significant heterogeneity between the various studies ($p = 0.42$, $I^2 = 3\%$) (Figure 2A).

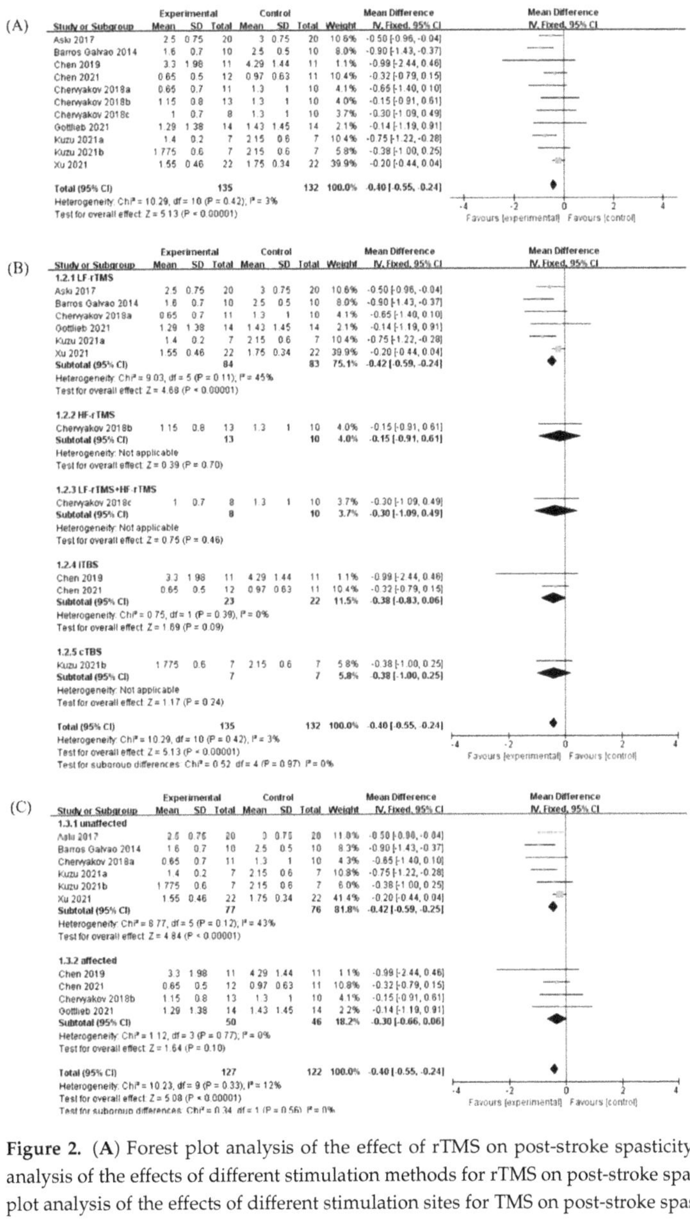

Figure 2. (**A**) Forest plot analysis of the effect of rTMS on post-stroke spasticity. (**B**) Forest plot analysis of the effects of different stimulation methods for rTMS on post-stroke spasticity. (**C**) Forest plot analysis of the effects of different stimulation sites for TMS on post-stroke spasticity.

The different stimulation methods of rTMS were divided into different subgroups. Six of all studies used LF-rTMS, two studies used intermittent theta-burst rTMS (iTBS), and high-frequency rTMS (HF-rTMS), LF-rTMS combined with HF-rTMS and continuous theta-burst rTMS (cTBS) each had one study. The meta-analysis showed that compared with the control group, LF-rTMS had significant benefits for post-stroke spasticity, and the MAS was significantly reduced (MD: −0.51, 95% CI: −0.78 to −0.24, $p < 0.01$). However, although other studies had shown certain benefits, they did not reach statistical differences (Figure 2B).

The different stimulation sites of rTMS were divided into different subgroups. Six of the studies included the unaffected hemispheres of patients with post-stroke spasticity, and the other four studies included the affected hemispheres of patients. The meta-analysis showed that compared with the control group, rTMS applied to stimulate the unaffected hemispheres of patients with post-stroke spasticity had significant benefits, and the MAS was significantly reduced (MD: −0.58, 95% CI: −0.80 to −0.36, $p < 0.01$). However, stimulation of the affected hemispheres also had certain benefits but did not reach statistical differences (Figure 2C).

3.3. *Effects of tDCS*

A total of seven RCTs on the effects of tDCS on post-stroke spasticity were included in the study, and the measurement outcome for all studies was the MAS. The meta-analysis showed that compared with the control group, tDCS had significant benefits for patients with post-stroke spasticity, and the MAS was significantly reduced (MD: −0.65, 95% CI: −1.07 to −0.22, $p < 0.01$). This meta-analysis showed that there was heterogeneity between different studies ($p < 0.01$, $I^2 = 78\%$) (Figure 3A).

The stimulation types of tDCS were divided into different subgroups. Four studies used anodal stimulation, and three studies used cathodal stimulation. The meta-analysis showed that compared with the control group, anodal stimulation had significant benefits for patients with post-stroke spasticity (MD: −0.74, 95% CI: −1.35 to −0.13, $p < 0.05$); however, although cathode stimulation also had certain benefits, it did not reach a statistical difference (MD: −0.51, 95% CI: −1.31 to 0.29, $p = 0.22$) (Figure 3B).

The stimulation intensities of tDCS were divided into different subgroups. There were five studies with a stimulation intensity of 2.0 mA and the other two studies with a stimulation intensity of 0.7 mA and 1.2 mA, respectively. The meta-analysis showed that compared with the control group, the stimulation intensity of tDCS of 0.7 mA (MD: −1.20, 95% CI: −1.40 to −1.00, $p < 0.01$) and 1.2 mA (MD: −1.00, 95% CI: −1.26 to −0.74, $p < 0.01$) had significant effect on patients with post-stroke spasticity. However, the measurement results of other studies had changed but did not reach statistical differences (Figure 3C).

3.4. *Risk of Bias and Sensitivity Analysis*

In this meta-analysis, three of the included articles [26,28,31] designed different experimental groups based on the stimulation method. There was no mutual interference between the different experimental groups, so each study was treated as an RCT. Finally, a total of 18 studies were obtained from 14 articles in the meta-analysis. Two authors independently assessed the risk of bias assessment of 18 included studies. The results of the risk of bias for all studies are shown in Figure 4. The risk of bias was assessed using the Cochrane Collaboration recommendations, and the sensitivity results indicated that the results of our meta-analysis appeared to be stable [20].

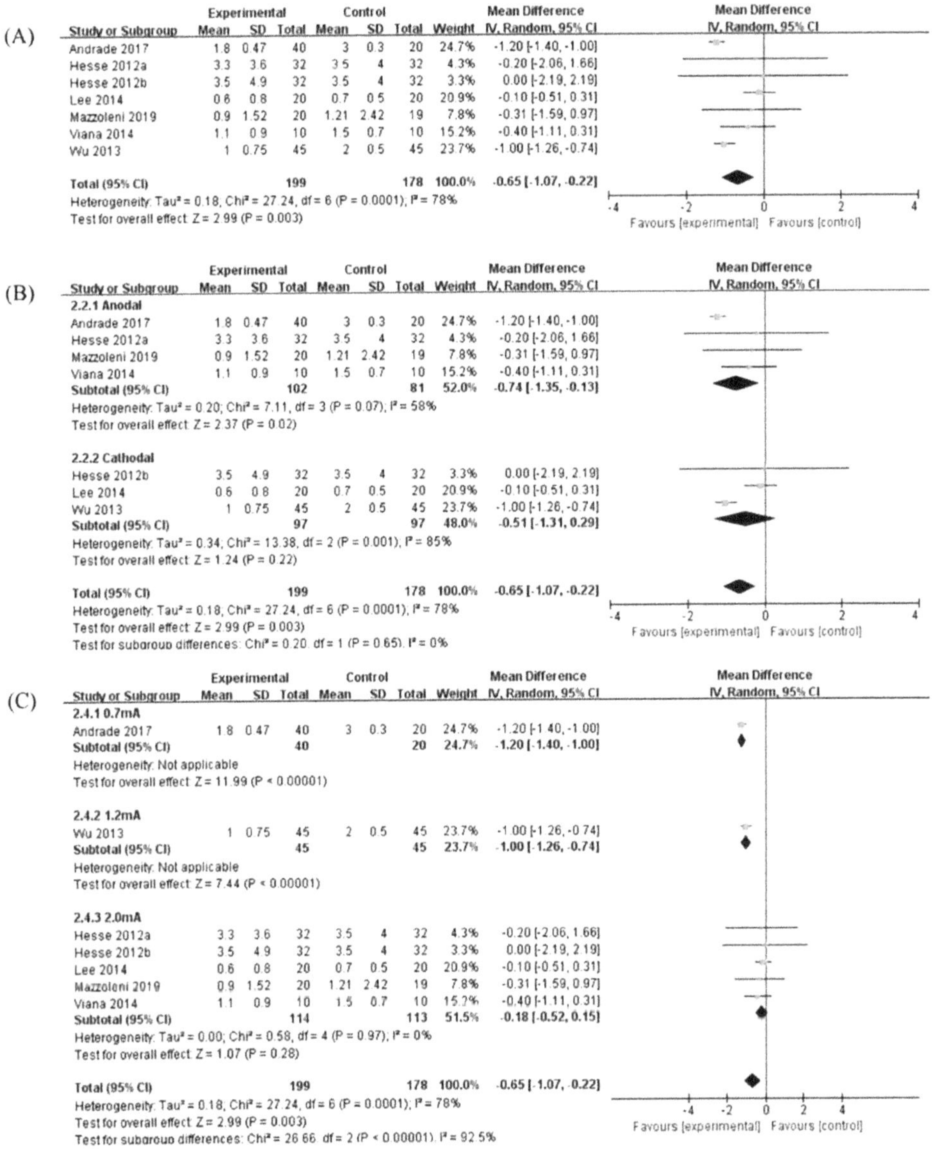

Figure 3. (**A**) Forest plot analysis of the effect of tDCS on post-stroke spasticity. (**B**) Forest plot analysis of the effects of different stimulation types for tDCS on post-stroke spasticity. (**C**) Forest plot analysis of the effects of different stimulation intensities for tDCS on post-stroke spasticity.

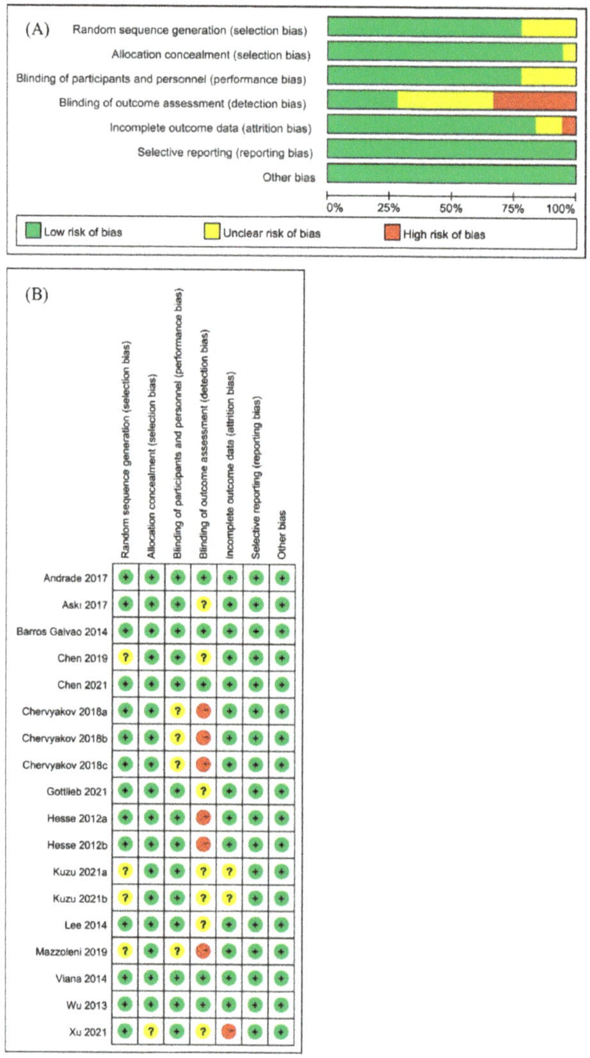

Figure 4. Risk of bias in the systematic review. (**A**) Risk of bias graph: review of the authors' judgments about each risk of bias item, presented as percentages across all included studies. (**B**) Risk of bias summary: review of authors' judgments about each risk of bias item for each included study.

4. Discussion

In this current study, a meta-analysis of the effect of NIBS on spasticity for post-stroke populations was performed. It included 18 RCTs, with the most relevant RCTs to date based on stringent inclusion and exclusion criteria. The results of the meta-analysis proved that NIBS has a positive effect on post-stroke spasticity. In addition, the sub-group analysis of NIBS (i.e., tDCS and TMS) on post-stroke spasticity was also conducted.

In terms of rTMS, the results of different subgroup analyses showed that LF-rTMS had a significant benefit in the unaffected hemispheres of patients with post-stroke spasticity (Figure 2B,C). This finding is in line with clinical evidence-based guidelines, which have shown that LF-rTMS acts on the unaffected hemisphere to promote post-stroke motor function recovery [35]. rTMS uses magnetic signals of different frequencies to stimulate the central nervous system in the corresponding parts and relieve limb spasticity in patients after stroke, and induce brain plasticity and brain network reorganization, promote the rehabilitation of the primary and secondary motor cortex [36]. Studies have shown that joint application of LF-rTMS acting on the unaffected hemisphere and HF-rTMS acting on the affected hemisphere can achieve better therapeutic effects by regulating the excitability of bilateral hemispheres [37]. However, there is no consistent standard for different stimulation methods. The possible mechanism of LF-rTMS for addressing spasticity may be related to the changes in the excitability of the cerebral motor cortex, thereby reducing the excitability of spinal motor neurons [13].

For the stimulation types of tDCS, anodal stimulation has significant benefits for spasticity treatment in post-stroke patients (Figure 3B). In terms of the stimulation strength, tDCS at current strengths of 0.7 mA or 1.2 mA significantly reduced spasticity, but the current strength of 2.0 mA showed no significant effect on post-stroke spasticity (Figure 3C). tDCS uses a low-intensity current to act on the target brain area to change the charge distribution of neuron membrane potential, resulting in depolarization or hyperpolarization, thereby changing the excitability of the cerebral cortex [38]. The anodal of tDCS is placed on the affected side to increase the excitability of the target brain area, and the cathodic is placed on the unaffected side to suppress the excitability of the target brain area. Studies have shown that anodal stimulation on the affected side can reduce limb spasticity symptoms in stroke survivors more than cathodal stimulation on the unaffected side [39]. The results of this meta-analysis are consistent with previous studies, which also showed a better effect of anodal tDCS on post-stroke spasticity. However, the mechanism of action of tDCS on post-stroke rehabilitation remains to be further investigated.

In the studies included in this meta-analysis, most of the brain regions stimulated by NIBS were the primary motor cortex [22,27,28,30], and a few studies were stimulated in the premotor cortex [23,30] and cerebellum [40]. The premotor cortex plays an important role in motor control and is another stimulation target besides the primary motor cortex [41,42]. The cerebellum works in concert with the cerebral cortex, is involved in motor control and has a role in the regulation of muscle tone [43]. The cerebellum may become a new target for NIBS in future studies. Although NIBS on different brain regions has rehabilitation effects on post-stroke spasticity, the interaction mechanism between different targets is still unclear. The mechanism of action between different targets needs to be further investigated in future studies.

There are several different scales for assessing spasticity in post-stroke patients in rehabilitation studies. Currently, the MAS is used in most studies, and its main purpose is to evaluate abnormal muscle tone, while a small number of studies use the Modified Tardieu Scale (MTS) as a spasticity assessment tool [44]. As the number of other scale studies (i.e., MTS) was too small, all studies included in this meta-analysis used MAS. However, both the MAS and MTS are subject to a certain degree of subjectivity, and more objective assessment methods need to be used in future research [45].

In patients after stroke, the balance between the two hemispheres of the brain is disrupted, resulting in hyperexcitability of the unaffected hemisphere and increased inhibition of the affected hemisphere [46]. Most of the reported findings showed that LF-rTMS had a positive effect on post-stroke spasticity [47–49]. Li et al. [50] showed that cTBS of the cerebellum reduced symptoms in patients with post-stroke spasticity. In addition, concomitant use of LF-rTMS and cTBS in post-stroke spastic patients resulted in better outcomes in rehabilitation. Different research results showed that different stimulation types of tDCS had certain therapeutic effects on patients with post-stroke spasticity [51–54]. The results of this meta-analysis are consistent with those of previous studies. Overall, NIBS for post-stroke spasticity is still mainly focused on the research of rTMS and tDCS, and the causal mechanisms underlying NIBS remain elusive. More comprehensive research is needed in the future.

Based on this meta-analysis, the results of non-randomized controlled trials of NIBS for post-stroke spasticity were also discussed. At this stage, no other NIBS have been found in RCTs of patients with post-stroke spasticity, and new techniques still need to be explored in future studies.

5. Conclusions

The results of the current meta-analysis are encouraging as they suggest that NIBS can promote rehabilitation in patients with post-stroke spasticity. At present, the NIBS applied to the field of post-stroke spasticity rehabilitation are mainly rTMS and tDCS. Other techniques, including transcranial alternating current stimulation (tACS) and transcranial ultrasound stimulation (TUS), still have limited evidence of significant variability in stimulation targets and stimulation parameters. Therefore, further in-depth study on the mechanism of action in the rehabilitation of post-stroke spastic patients is required. We hope that in the future, NIBS can be optimized and applied safely and efficiently to the rehabilitation of post-stroke spasticity.

Author Contributions: Conceptualization: X.W., L.G. and L.L. Data collection, analysis and interpretation: X.W., L.G., H.H., L.Y. and L.L. Drafting of manuscript: X.W., L.G. and L.L. Critical revision: X.W., L.G., L.Y. and L.L. Project Administration: L.L. All authors have read and agreed to the published version of the manuscript.

Funding: This work was supported by the National Natural Science Foundation of China (No.32071316, 32211530049), the Fundamental Research Funds for the Central Universities (Grant Nos. G2021KY05101, G2021KY05105, G2021KY05107,G2022WD01006), the Key Research and Development Project of Shaanxi province (2022SF-117), the Natural Science Foundation of Shaanxi province (2022-JM482), and the Education and Teaching Reform Funds for the Central Universities (No.22GZ230101).

Institutional Review Board Statement: Not applicable.

Informed Consent Statement: Not applicable.

Data Availability Statement: Not applicable.

Conflicts of Interest: The authors have declared that no competing interest exist.

References

1. Wissel, J.; Schelosky, L.D.; Scott, J.; Christe, W.; Faiss, J.H.; Mueller, J. Early development of spasticity following stroke: A prospective, observational trial. *J. Neurol.* **2010**, *257*, 1067–1072. [CrossRef] [PubMed]
2. Bavikatte, G.; Subramanian, G.; Ashford, S.; Allison, R.; Hicklin, D. Early Identification, Intervention and Management of Post-stroke Spasticity: Expert Consensus Recommendations. *J. Cent. Nerv. Syst. Dis.* **2021**, *13*, 11795735211036576. [CrossRef] [PubMed]
3. Bethoux, F. Spasticity Management after Stroke. *Phys. Med. Rehabil. Clin. N. Am.* **2015**, *26*, 625–639. [CrossRef] [PubMed]
4. Nam, H.S.; Koh, S.; Kim, Y.J.; Beom, J.; Lee, W.H.; Lee, S.U.; Kim, S. Biomechanical Reactions of Exoskeleton Neurorehabilitation Robots in Spastic Elbows and Wrists. *IEEE Trans. Neural. Syst. Rehabil. Eng.* **2017**, *25*, 2196–2203. [CrossRef]
5. Chen, Y.T.; Li, S.; DiTommaso, C.; Zhou, P.; Li, S. Possible Contributions of Ipsilateral Pathways From the Contralesional Motor Cortex to the Voluntary Contraction of the Spastic Elbow Flexors in Stroke Survivors: A TMS Study. *Am. J. Phys. Med. Rehabil.* **2019**, *98*, 558–565. [CrossRef] [PubMed]
6. Molero-Chamizo, A.; Salas Sánchez, Á.; Álvarez Batista, B.; Cordero García, C.; Andújar Barroso, R.; Rivera-Urbina, G.N.; Nitsche, M.A.; Alameda Bailén, J.R. Bilateral Motor Cortex tDCS Effects on Post-Stroke Pain and Spasticity: A Three Cases Study. *Front Pharmacol.* **2021**, *12*, 624582. [CrossRef]
7. Li, S. Spasticity, Motor Recovery, and Neural Plasticity after Stroke. *Front. Neurol.* **2017**, *8*, 120. [CrossRef]
8. Li, S.; Francisco, G.E.; Rymer, W.Z. A New Definition of Poststroke Spasticity and the Interference of Spasticity with Motor Recovery from Acute to Chronic Stages. *Neurorehabil. Neural. Repair.* **2021**, *35*, 601–610. [CrossRef]
9. Hara, T.; Shanmugalingam, A.; McIntyre, A.; Burhan, A.M. The Effect of Non-Invasive Brain Stimulation (NIBS) on Attention and Memory Function in Stroke Rehabilitation Patients: A Systematic Review and Meta-Analysis. *Diagnostics* **2021**, *11*, 227. [CrossRef]
10. Mori, F.; Koch, G.; Foti, C.; Bernardi, G.; Centonze, D. The use of repetitive transcranial magnetic stimulation (rTMS) for the treatment of spasticity. *Prog. Brain Res.* **2009**, *175*, 429–439.
11. Naghdi, S.; Ansari, N.N.; Rastgoo, M.; Forogh, B.; Jalaie, S.; Olyaei, G. A pilot study on the effects of low frequency repetitive transcranial magnetic stimulation on lower extremity spasticity and motor neuron excitability in patients after stroke. *J. Bodyw. Mov. Ther.* **2015**, *19*, 616–623. [CrossRef] [PubMed]

12. Theilig, S.; Podubecka, J.; Bösl, K.; Wiederer, R.; Nowak, D.A. Functional neuromuscular stimulation to improve severe hand dysfunction after stroke: Does inhibitory rTMS enhance therapeutic efficiency? *Exp. Neurol.* **2011**, *230*, 149–155. [CrossRef] [PubMed]
13. Wu, D.; Qian, L.; Zorowitz, R.D.; Zhang, L.; Qu, Y.; Yuan, Y. Effects on Decreasing Upper-Limb Poststroke Muscle Tone Using Transcranial Direct Current Stimulation: A Randomized Sham-Controlled Study. *Arch. Phys. Med. Rehabil.* **2013**, *94*, 1–8. [CrossRef] [PubMed]
14. Xu, P.; Huang, Y.; Wang, J.; An, X.; Zhang, T.; Li, Y.; Zhang, J.; Wang, B. Repetitive transcranial magnetic stimulation as an alternative therapy for stroke with spasticity: A systematic review and meta-analysis. *J. Neurol.* **2021**, *268*, 4013–4022. [CrossRef] [PubMed]
15. Alashram, A.R.; Padua, E.; Aburub, A.; Raju, M.; Annino, G. Transcranial direct current stimulation for upper extremity spasticity rehabilitation in stroke survivors: A systematic review of randomized controlled trials. *PM&R* **2022**, 14.
16. Huang, J.; Qu, Y.; Liu, L.; Zhao, K.; Zhao, Z. Efficacy and safety of transcranial direct current stimulation for post-stroke spasticity: A meta-analysis of randomised controlled trials. *Clin. Rehabil.* **2022**, *36*, 158–171. [CrossRef]
17. Page, M.J.; McKenzie, J.E.; Bossuyt, P.M.; Boutron, I.; Hoffmann, T.C.; Mulrow, C.D.; Shamseer, L.; Tetzlaff, J.M.; Moher, D. Updating guidance for reporting systematic reviews: Development of the PRISMA 2020 statement. *J. Clin. Epidemiol.* **2021**, *134*, 103–112. [CrossRef]
18. da Costa Santos, C.M.; de Mattos Pimenta, C.A.; Nobre, M.R. The PICO strategy for the research question construction and evidence search. *Rev. Lat. Am. Enfermagem.* **2007**, *15*, 508–511. [CrossRef]
19. Higgins, J.P.; Altman, D.G. Assessing risk of bias in included studies. In *Cochrane Handbook for Systematic Reviews of Interventions*; Higgins, J.P., Green, S., Eds.; Wiley: Hoboken, NJ, USA, 2008; pp. 187–241.
20. Higgins, J.P.; Altman, D.G.; Gøtzsche, P.C.; Jüni, P.; Moher, D.; Oxman, A.D.; Savovic, J.; Schulz, K.F.; Weeks, L.; Sterne, J.A.; et al. The Cochrane Collaboration's tool for assessing risk of bias in randomised trials. *BMJ* **2011**, *343*, d5928. [CrossRef]
21. Sterne, J.A.; Sutton, A.J.; Ioannidis, J.P.; Terrin, N.; Jones, D.R.; Lau, J.; Carpenter, J.; Rücker, G.; Harbord, R.M.; Schmid, C.H.; et al. Recommendations for examining and interpreting funnel plot asymmetry in meta-analyses of randomised controlled trials. *BMJ* **2011**, *343*, d4002. [CrossRef]
22. Askı, N.A.; Tosun, A.; Demirdal, U.S. Effects of low-frequency repetitive transcranial magnetic stimulation on upper extremity motor recovery and functional outcomes in chronic stroke patients: A randomized controlled trial. *Somatosens. Mot. Res.* **2017**, *34*, 102–107. [CrossRef]
23. Barros Galvão, S.C.; Borba Costa dos Santos, R.; Borba dos Santos, P.; Cabral, M.E.; Monte-Silva, K. Efficacy of Coupling Repetitive Transcranial Magnetic Stimulation and Physical Therapy to Reduce Upper-Limb Spasticity in Patients With Stroke: A Randomized Controlled Trial. *Arch. Phys. Med. Rehabil.* **2014**, *95*, 222–229. [CrossRef] [PubMed]
24. Chen, Y.J.; Huang, Y.Z.; Chen, C.Y.; Chen, C.L.; Chen, H.C.; Wu, C.Y.; Lin, K.C.; Chang, T.L. Intermittent theta burst stimulation enhances upper limb motor function in patients with chronic stroke: A pilot randomized controlled trial. *BMC Neurol.* **2019**, *19*, 69. [CrossRef] [PubMed]
25. Chen, Y.H.; Chen, C.L.; Huang, Y.Z.; Chen, H.C.; Chen, C.Y.; Wu, C.Y.; Lin, K.C. Augmented efficacy of intermittent theta burst stimulation on the virtual reality-based cycling training for upper limb function in patients with stroke: A double-blinded, randomized controlled trial. *J. Neuroeng. Rehabil.* **2021**, *18*, 91. [CrossRef] [PubMed]
26. Chervyakov, A.V.; Poydasheva, A.G.; Lyukmanov, R.H.; Suponeva, N.A.; Chernikova, L.A.; Piradov, M.A.; Ustinova, K.I. Effects of Navigated Repetitive Transcranial Magnetic Stimulation After Stroke. *J. Clin. Neurophysiol.* **2018**, *35*, 166–172. [CrossRef] [PubMed]
27. Gottlieb, A.; Boltzmann, M.; Schmidt, S.B.; Gutenbrunner, C.; Krauss, J.K.; Stangel, M.; Höglinger, G.U.; Wallesch, C.W.; Rollnik, J.D. Treatment of upper limb spasticity with inhibitory repetitive transcranial magnetic stimulation: A randomized placebo-controlled trial. *NeuroRehabilitation* **2021**, *49*, 425–434. [CrossRef]
28. Kuzu, Ö.; Adiguzel, E.; Kesikburun, S.; Yaşar, E.; Yılmaz, B. The Effect of Sham Controlled Continuous Theta Burst Stimulation and Low Frequency Repetitive Transcranial Magnetic Stimulation on Upper Extremity Spasticity and Functional Recovery in Chronic Ischemic Stroke Patients. *J. Stroke Cerebrovasc. Dis.* **2021**, *30*, 105795. [CrossRef]
29. Xu, D.; Cao, H.; Fan, Y.; Yan, D.; Su, M. Comparative Analysis of the Effect of Low-Frequency Repeated Transcranial Magnetic Stimulation and Extracorporeal Shock Wave on Improving the Spasm of Flexor after Stroke. *Evid.-Based Complementary Altern. Med.* **2021**, *2021*, 7769581. [CrossRef]
30. Andrade, S.M.; Batista, L.M.; Nogueira, L.L.; de Oliveira, E.A.; de Carvalho, A.G.; Lima, S.S.; Santana, J.R.; de Lima, E.C.; Fernández-Calvo, B. Constraint-induced movement therapy combined with transcranial direct current stimulation over premotor cortex improves motor function in severe stroke: A pilot randomized controlled trial. *Rehabil. Res. Pract.* **2017**, 6842549. [CrossRef]
31. Hesse, S.; Waldner, A.; Mehrholz, J.; Tomelleri, C.; Pohl, M.; Werner, C. Combined transcranial direct current stimulation and robot-assisted arm training in subacute stroke patients: An exploratory, randomized multicenter trial. *Neurorehabil. Neural. Repair.* **2011**, *25*, 838–846. [CrossRef]
32. Lee, S.J.; Chun, M.H. Combination transcranial direct current stimulation and virtual reality therapy for upper extremity training in patients with subacute stroke. *Arch. Phys. Med. Rehabil.* **2014**, *95*, 431–438. [CrossRef] [PubMed]

33. Mazzoleni, S.; Tran, V.D.; Dario, P.; Posteraro, F. Effects of Transcranial Direct Current Stimulation (tDCS) Combined with Wrist Robot-Assisted Rehabilitation on Motor Recovery in Subacute Stroke Patients: A Randomized Controlled Trial. *IEEE Trans. Neural. Syst. Rehabil. Eng.* **2019**, *27*, 1458–1466. [CrossRef] [PubMed]
34. Viana, R.T.; Laurentino, G.E.; Souza, R.J.; Fonseca, J.B.; Silva Filho, E.M.; Dias, S.N.; Teixeira-Salmela, L.F.; Monte-Silva, K.K. Effects of the addition of transcranial direct current stimulation to virtual reality therapy after stroke: A pilot randomized controlled trial. *NeuroRehabilitation* **2014**, *34*, 437–446. [CrossRef] [PubMed]
35. Lefaucheur, J.P.; Aleman, A.; Baeken, C.; Benninger, D.H.; Brunelin, J.; Di Lazzaro, V.; Filipović, S.R.; Grefkes, C.; Hasan, A.; Hummel, F.C.; et al. Evidence-based guidelines on the therapeutic use of repetitive transcranial magnetic stimulation (rTMS): An update (2014–2018). *Clin. Neurophysiol.* **2020**, *131*, 474–528. [CrossRef]
36. Iglesias, A.H. Transcranial Magnetic Stimulation as Treatment in Multiple Neurologic Conditions. *Curr. Neurol. Neurosci. Rep.* **2020**, *20*, 1. [CrossRef]
37. Dionísio, A.; Duarte, I.C.; Patrício, M.; Castelo-Branco, M. The Use of Repetitive Transcranial Magnetic Stimulation for Stroke Rehabilitation: A Systematic Review. *J. Stroke Cerebrovasc. Dis.* **2018**, *27*, 1–31. [CrossRef]
38. Brunoni, A.R.; Amadera, J.; Berbel, B.; Volz, M.S.; Rizzerio, B.G.; Fregni, F. A systematic review on reporting and assessment of adverse effects associated with transcranial direct current stimulation. *Int. J. Neuropsychopharmacol.* **2011**, *14*, 1133–1145. [CrossRef]
39. Leo, A.; Naro, A.; Molonia, F.; Tomasello, P.; Saccà, I.; Bramanti, A.; Russo, M.; Bramanti, P.; Quartarone, A.; Calabrò, R.S. Spasticity Management: The Current State of Transcranial Neuromodulation. *PM&R* **2017**, *9*, 1020–1029.
40. Harrington, A.; Hammond-Tooke, G.D. Theta Burst Stimulation of the Cerebellum Modifies the TMS-Evoked N100 Potential, a Marker of GABA Inhibition. *PLoS ONE* **2015**, *10*, e0141284. [CrossRef]
41. Traversa, R.; Cicinelli, P.; Pasqualetti, P.; Filippi, M.; Rossini, P.M. Follow-up of interhemispheric differences of motor evoked potentials from the 'affected' and 'unaffected' hemispheres in human stroke. *Brain Res.* **1998**, *803*, 1–8. [CrossRef]
42. Seitz, R.J.; Höflich, P.; Binkofski, F.; Tellmann, L.; Herzog, H.; Freund, H.J. Role of the premotor cortex in recovery from middle cerebral artery infarction. *Arch. Neurol.* **1998**, *55*, 1081–1088. [CrossRef] [PubMed]
43. Wang, C.C.; Wang, C.P.; Tsai, P.Y.; Hsieh, C.Y.; Chan, R.C.; Yeh, S.C. Inhibitory repetitive transcranial magnetic stimulation of the contralesional premotor and primary motor cortices facilitate poststroke motor recovery. *Restor. Neurol. Neurosci.* **2014**, *32*, 825–835. [CrossRef] [PubMed]
44. Sharma, N.; Cohen, L.G. Recovery of motor function after stroke. *Dev. Psychobiol.* **2012**, *54*, 254–262. [CrossRef]
45. Meseguer-Henarejos, A.B.; Sánchez-Meca, J.; López-Pina, J.A.; Carles-Hernández, R. Inter- and intra-rater reliability of the Modified Ashworth Scale: A systematic review and meta-analysis. *Eur. J. Phys. Rehabil. Med.* **2018**, *54*, 576–590. [CrossRef]
46. Chen, Y.; Wei, Q.C.; Zhang, M.Z.; Xie, Y.J.; Liao, L.Y.; Tan, H.X.; Guo, Q.F.; Gao, Q. Cerebellar Intermittent Theta-Burst Stimulation Reduces Upper Limb Spasticity After Subacute Stroke: A Randomized Controlled Trial. *Front Neural. Circuits.* **2021**, *15*, 655502. [CrossRef]
47. Kakuda, W.; Abo, M.; Kobayashi, K.; Momosaki, R.; Yokoi, A.; Fukuda, A.; Ito, H.; Tominaga, A.; Umemori, T.; Kameda, Y. Anti-spastic effect of low-frequency rTMS applied with occupational therapy in post-stroke patients with upper limb hemiparesis. *Brain INJ* **2011**, *25*, 496–502. [CrossRef] [PubMed]
48. Rastgoo, M.; Naghdi, S.; Nakhostin Ansari, N.; Olyaei, G.; Jalaei, S.; Forogh, B.; Najari, H. Effects of repetitive transcranial magnetic stimulation on lower extremity spasticity and motor function in stroke patients. *Disabil. Rehabil.* **2016**, *38*, 1918–1926. [CrossRef] [PubMed]
49. Málly, J.; Dinya, E. Recovery of motor disability and spasticity in post-stroke after repetitive transcranial magnetic stimulation (rTMS). *Brain Res. Bull.* **2008**, *76*, 388–395. [CrossRef]
50. Li, D.; Cheng, A.; Zhang, Z.; Sun, Y.; Liu, Y. Effects of low-frequency repetitive transcranial magnetic stimulation combined with cerebellar continuous theta burst stimulation on spasticity and limb dyskinesia in patients with stroke. *BMC Neurol.* **2021**, *21*, 369. [CrossRef]
51. Halakoo, S.; Ehsani, F.; Masoudian, N.; Zoghi, M.; Jaberzadeh, S. Does anodal trans-cranial direct current stimulation of the damaged primary motor cortex affects wrist flexor muscle spasticity and also activity of the wrist flexor and extensor muscles in patients with stroke?: A Randomized Clinical Trial. *Neurol. Sci.* **2021**, *42*, 2763–2773. [CrossRef]
52. Ochi, M.; Saeki, S.; Oda, T.; Matsushima, Y.; Hachisuka, K. Effects of anodal and cathodal transcranial direct current stimulation combined with robotic therapy on severely affected arms in chronic stroke patients. *J. Rehabil. Med.* **2013**, *45*, 137–140. [CrossRef] [PubMed]
53. Ehsani, F.; Mortezanejad, M.; Yosephi, M.H.; Daniali, S.; Jaberzadeh, S. The effects of concurrent M1 anodal tDCS and physical therapy interventions on function of ankle muscles in patients with stroke: A randomized, double-blinded sham-controlled trial study. *Neurol. Sci.* **2022**, *43*, 1893–1901. [CrossRef] [PubMed]
54. Del Felice, A.; Daloli, V.; Masiero, S.; Manganotti, P. Contralesional Cathodal versus Dual Transcranial Direct Current Stimulation for Decreasing Upper Limb Spasticity in Chronic Stroke Individuals: A Clinical and Neurophysiological Study. *J. Stroke Cerebrovasc. Dis.* **2016**, *25*, 2932–2941. [CrossRef] [PubMed]

MDPI
St. Alban-Anlage 66
4052 Basel
Switzerland
Tel. +41 61 683 77 34
Fax +41 61 302 89 18
www.mdpi.com

Brain Sciences Editorial Office
E-mail: brainsci@mdpi.com
www.mdpi.com/journal/brainsci

www.ingramcontent.com/pod-product-compliance
Lightning Source LLC
Chambersburg PA
CBHW061437210926
51850CB00008B/1540
9783036568393